OCCL BOX

STP 1173

Biomaterials' Mechanical Properties

Helen E. Kambic and A. Toshimitsu Yokobori, Jr., Editors

ASTM Publication Code Number (PCN):
04-011730-54

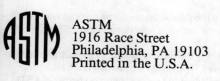

ASTM
1916 Race Street
Philadelphia, PA 19103
Printed in the U.S.A.

Library of Congress Cataloging-in-Publication Data

Biomaterials' mechanical properties / Helen E. Kambic and A.
Toshimitsu Yokobori, Jr., editors.
(STP ; 1173)
Includes bibliographical references and index.
ISBN 0-8031-1894-5
1. Biomedical materials—Mechanical properties. I. Kambic, Helen
E. II. Yokobori, A. Toshimitsu, 1951–   III. Series: ASTM
special technical publication ; 1173.
[DNLM: 1. Biocompatible Materials—congresses. QT 34 B61156
1994]
R857.M3B573   1994
610'.28--dc20   93-48490
                                                                       CIP

Photocopy Rights

Peer Review Policy

Each paper published in this volume was evaluated by three peer reviewers. The authors addressed
all of the reviewers' comments to the satisfaction of both the technical editor(s) and the ASTM
Committee on Publications.
The quality of the papers in this publication reflects not only the obvious efforts of the authors and the
technical editor(s), but also the work of these peer reviewers. The ASTM Committee on Publications
acknowledges with appreciation their dedication and contribution to time and effort on behalf of ASTM.

Printed in Fredericksburg, VA
February 1994

Foreword

Biomaterials science has attained great importance, particularly in the last two decades with the introduction of polyurethanes, metal components, novel plastics, coatings, and more recently with the advent of bioresorbable materials. Although there are hundreds of potential choices of materials and synthetic materials, each remains distinct with regard to their synthesis, additives, bulk and surface properties. As soon as the methods for production were formalized, engineers began testing them and clinicians were eager to implant them—but not necessarily in that order. Processing into prosthetic devices profoundly changed the mechanical properties and their implant behavior. Therefore, the search for the right combination of these properties continues.

ASTM

This publication, *Biomaterials' Mechanical Properties,* contains papers presented at the symposium of the same name, held in Pittsburgh, PA on 5–6 May 1992. The symposium was sponsored by ASTM Committee F–4 on Medical and Surgical Materials and Devices and its Subcommittee F4.04 on Cardiovascular Implants and Materials. Helen E. Kambic, from The Cleveland Clinic Foundation, and A. Toshimitsu Yokobori, Jr., from Tohoku University, Japan, presided as symposium co-chairs and are co-editors of the resulting publication.

The specific aims of the symposium were (1) to review our current test methods, (2) to identify new testing techniques, and (3) to promote an interchange between manufacturers, basic scientists and clinicians. To promote these aims, several prominent scientists from industry and academia were invited to present papers in each of the sessions. The international flavor of the meeting was spearheaded by Dr. T. Yokobori, Professor and Dean, School of Science and Engineering at Teikyo University, Utsonomiya, Japan.

The technical sessions focused on testing methods that emphasized an understanding of material properties and exploiting this knowledge to serve as an experimental database for future analysis and design.

The Session Chairs were M. Saitoh (Sendai, Japan), P. Marlowe (FDA, USA), J. Lee (Toronto, Canada), R. Benson (Knoxville, TN), Y. Miyasaha (Sendai, Japan), S. Teoh (Singapore), S. Niwa (Aichi, Japan), S. Brown (Cleveland, OH), K. Hayashi (Sapporo, Japan), Y. Tanabe (Nigata, Japan), H. Watanabe (Kyoto, Japan), M. Nakamura (Osaha, Japan), S. Niwa (Aichi, Japan), H. Kambic (Cleveland, OH), A.T. Yokobori (Sendai, Japan), and T. Yokobori (Utsonomiya, Japan).

The first Student Prize Competition was introduced at this meeting. A stipend and plaque were presented to the winning student paper based on the theme of the symposium. The student presentation was given in the technical session. The concept of the competition was inaugurated by D. Marlowe (FDA–Rockville, MD), J. Black (Clemson, SC), R. Hori (Zimmer, Inc.–Warsaw, IN), M. Mayor (Darmouth, NH), and K. St. John (Jackson, MS).

A workshop was held at the end of the formal presentations, and mathematical modeling, government and academic sponsorship of research, testing protocols, biostatistics, product-oriented research, and quality assurance issues were debated.

We would like to express our thanks to several people: D. Savini (ASTM) for her suggestions throughout the symposium planning process; T. Pravitz and K. Dernoga (ASTM) for manuscript submissions and publications; and our numerous reviewers, to whom we are enormously indebted.

The Editors

Contents

FUTURE DIRECTIONS

Overview

Biomaterials perform diverse biological functions. Understanding the process controlling the mechanical properties is important for materials in medical device use. The mechanical properties of coatings and composites depend on their deformation and fracture mechanisms. When stresses are applied that exceed the yield strength, plastic deformation can occur resulting in mechanical damage. As a majority of structural metallic materials reside in aqueous environments, the corrosion and degradation of metallic systems can result in device failure oftentimes coupled with the migration of particulate debris. The impact of device failure on the well-being of an implant recipient can be traumatic. Such findings have demanded more stringent acceptance criteria for mechanical and chemical properties of both surface and bulk materials.

In planning this book, the editors chose to attract contributors not only from the cardio-vascular areas, but to include scientific and clinical interests and common goals in the areas of urological, orthopedic, and polymeric research. The choice of test methods, experimental design data analyses, and selection of test models presented a range from cellular to implant devices. In order to define the proper test configurations, judgments were made as to which test criteria and test methods were identified. The criteria and the application of engineering principles would become clear and comprehensible to potential regulators and users in the medical community.

Therefore, this Special Technical Publication was compiled as a review of the 1992 Symposium on Biomaterials' Mechanical Properties held in Pittsburgh, Pennsylvania.

The Table of Contents is composed of a collection of 24 papers which have been grouped into 6 major categories. These include: (1) methodologies for testing cardiovascular materials, (2) adhesives, films, and plastics, (3) the evaluation of metallic materials and bone, (4) composite materials, (5) urologic materials, and (6) future directions.

Cardiovascular Materials

One fundamental assumption underlying the mechanical approach to the analysis of cardiovascular materials is that they undergo cyclic deformation and require a blood-compatible surface. Hayashi begins with a look at fatigue properties that are crucial to the endurance, reliability, and safety of implants. Using the segmented polyether urethanes as a model, he has outlined the evaluation of materials by application of different test environments, temperature, and cyclic rate on the tensile and fatigue properties. Computer data acquisition and processing have established a relevant database for comparison with future accelerated endurance test methods.

Two papers in this group have focused on the durability of materials in heart valves. Lee et al. have combined structural analyses (biochemical and histological) with mechanical testing for the examination of the viscoelastic behavior of collagenous bioprosthetic tissues. Implementing a high strain rate uniaxial test apparatus, large deformation cyclic loading and small deformation forced vibration studies at frequencies of up to 10 Hz were applied. Stress relation studies with loading times of 0.1 s or less are used to characterize various treatments of collagenous tissues used for heart valves. They have correlated changes in extensibility and stress relaxation behavior with mechanical properties. Based on these results, they suggest a high strain rate by biaxial testing for future studies.

Teoh et al. have designed a test rig to simulate the impact-sliding action mechanism of wear between the struts and disc occluder of a mechanical heart valve. Performed at body temperatures and 3 Hz, the design accelerates wear. The areas of contact are held constant and wear profiles are monitored using a surface profilometer and visualized by SEM. This method has the advantage of early wear detection.

Microstructural defects introduced into vascular grafts made from expanded PTFE by the use of running sutures or forcep compression reduce the internodal distance adjacent to the anastomosis. Holubec et al. have reported that impaired healing results when the internodal distance is reduced to 10 μm or less. Analysis of the optimum PTFE ultrastructure and cellular ingrowth on healing was evaluated in dog and rat models. Such studies are pertinent to the development of a small vascular prosthesis of 4 mm or less in internal diameter.

Yokobori et al. evaluated the effects of encapsulation of the vascular substitute and of sutures on the anastomotic strength. Using a pulsatile pressure flow test system, the *in vitro* tensile anastomotic strength and the *in vitro* pulsatile flow through pressure tests (Δ p 110–294 mmHg) were performed on polyester vascular grafts. Identical suture techniques were used, and grafts were implanted in dogs and tested after three months. Although the *in vitro* tests confirmed the strength of the vascular graft, *in vivo* tests were necessary to describe the enhanced effect on strength due to tissue adhesion and encapsulation.

Adhesive Films and Plastics

A prediction of material failure and the optimal stresses used in the design of components to prevent premature failure are concerns expressed by Teoh in his paper concerning the design stresses of medical plastics. The modeling of the creep rupture behavior of plastics has identified upper stress values prior to fracture and lower stress limits maintained without failure. Based on these data, Delrin® was given as an example with stress limits corresponding to its applicability in mechanical heart valves but not in joint prostheses.

The formation of bonded interfaces may produce microscopic flaws which could promote interfacial failures. Moon et al. investigated the mechanical properties of tooth adhesive resins to determine if bond strengths approach the cohesive strength of the materials and for finite element evaluation of polymerization shrinkage bond stress. Data were obtained for the elastic moduli, breaking strength, and deformation. They conclude that strength values could limit the bond strength.

Peterson presented a technical report on problems correlating porous coating pull-off strength results with the use of test coupons. The use of Taguchi methods was described to isolate the variables causing test result differences.

Evaluation of Metallic Materials

Joint prostheses must fulfill demands regarding tissue compatibility and particular mechanical properties. Bone tissue is a dynamic material having the potential to adapt to its environment. Bone research has contributed greatly to our understanding of bone mechanics. The papers in this section address the challenges in joint replacement, namely, adverse bone remodeling and the generation of particulate debris that arise from metal/bone fretting or abrasion.

Bhambri and Gilbertson have evaluated the fretting fatigue behavior of head/taper combinations used for total hip replacements. Fatigue tests were performed with simulated body fluids within a cell designed to retain particles greater than 0.25 μm. SEM and EDAX were used to characterize the particles. The advantages of a surface nitriding treatment were discussed to reduce fretting.

In order to study the viscoelastic properties of bone, Tanabe et al. assumed that the behavior of bone could be represented by a three-element standard linear model. Experimental data obtained by analysis of the split-Hopkinson pressure bar (SHPB) tests were confirmed by results from experiments and ultrasonic measurements done on bovine femoral bone. These methods may reduce the time required to characterize mechanical properties of bone.

The strength of regenerate bone was evaluated by Miyasaka et al. Experimental callotasis was developed in a rabbit femoral model. The developed callus showed hysteresis in uniaxial tests and stress relaxation. The technique of external fixation, the rate of destruction, and the quality of the callus are important parameters in the use of the callotasis method and in the evaluation of the viscoelastic model for the developing elongated callus.

Higo and Tomita described a fatigue test employing a four-point side notch bend specimen for evaluating the components of artificial joints. Corrosion was measured by comparing fatigue in an air environment to that of physiological saline. Galvanic pico-corrosion tests and crevice corrosion were examined.

Flemming et al. identified a fretting component at the cone-taper interface of modular total hips that may be a factor in the corrosion observed in this area. Interface fretting was studied by measuring current during the cyclical loading of hips in a universal testing machine. The taper fretting current was measured and compared for two different hip designs. The current mechanical test method was the most appropriate method to study corrosion of the hip cone and taper. This method was applied to study the variability of neck extensions and its contribution to the resulting corrosion. This paper was chosen as the first winner in the newly inaugurated Student Paper Competition sponsored by the ASTM Committee F–4 on Medical and Surgical Devices and Materials. The competition is open to all students of members of the ASTM Committee F–4. This award includes a $500 stipend and award certificate. Mr. Flemming is a graduate student of Dr. S. Brown, Department of Biomedical Engineering, Case Western Reserve University, Cleveland, OH.

Nakamura et al. introduced the importance of using *in vitro* cytotoxic studies in the evaluation of materials in the oral environment. Dental amalgams were subject to dynamic extraction with suspended, freely moving, and static specimens using various media and temperature conditions. Extracts from all materials were evaluated by cell culture and atomic absorption spectroscopy. The *in vitro* method is suggested as a candidate simulation test that may be effective in evaluating the adhesive strength of cells on biomaterials.

Ligaments support the joints, and injury to the anterior cruciate ligament (ACL), for example, destabilizes the knee, often leading to osteoarthritis. Stewart et al. examined ligament implant fixation devices. A quantification of loads placed on these tissues relative to normal tissue function and the method of device fixation are topics related to rehabilitation and healing.

Composite Materials

The use of soft or hard tissue composite materials imposes specific mechanical and biocompatibility demands. They permit a greater manipulation of their stiffness to accommodate implant design. Latour and Black have outlined a collaborative effort for determining the bond strength and environmental resistance between fiber-reinforced polymer composite materials for medical applications. Test fiber microdroplet samples under both static and dynamic loading and conditions for diffusional equilibrium reduce the time required for testing. This method should be useful for the development of composite biomaterials resistant to *in vivo* mechanical degradation.

The accelerated degradation of polymer composites was also reported by Jockisch et al. Carbon fiber reinforced PEEK injection molded bendbars, cut in four sections of the bendbar, were used to evaluate local microstructural variations in composites. Fracture surfaces and flexure testing of the miniflexbars were sensitive to local variations in microstructure. Small-scale specimens may be valuable in the analysis of mechanical properties of composites.

Gilbert and Dong have introduced a novel method that uses stress relaxation experiments whereby strain is applied to a sample, and the stress decay response is measured over time with analog-to-digital data acquisition. Laplace transformation techniques are employed. A three-dimensional relationship between complex modulus, frequency, and temperature can be constructed. The changes in stiffness of a material can be monitored under a variety of experimental conditions.

The problem of calcium salt deposits and the failure of biomedical polyurethanes was addressed by Wong and Benson. The fracture behavior of Biomer® and Pellethane® indicate that with a high concentration of salt, the salt disrupts the intermolecular faces leading to structural changes manifested in the strain energy to failure.

Leadbetter et al. introduce the use of absorbable microcomposites and fiber-reinforced composites with hybridized interfaces. The strength of interfacial bonding is crucial for these composites. Absorbable materials may offer the advantage of eliminating second surgeries and may replace metallic components with their apparent corrosive problems.

Urologic Materials

The three papers in this section on the biomechanics of the ureters and urinary calculi seem to be a point of departure for the entire book because the topic deals with *in vivo* tissue testing. The papers of Uchida et al. and Watanabe et al. in this section deal with the problem of the generation of urinary calculi in the kidney and ureter. Conventional therapy suggests open surgery, but attempts for extracting the calculi require data on the calculi themselves and on the properties of the ureter.

Uchida et al. identified a program for the intracorporeal destruction of urinary calculi with a technique they called "microexplosion lithotripsy." The chemical analysis and compressive tensile strengths of calculi were determined under wet and dry conditions. Based on these data, a transmitted shock wave exceeding the compressive strength of the calculus causes the destruction of urinary calculi and release of gas bubbles. These techniques may be applicable for the removal of calculi measuring 7 mm in diameter and below.

Tension and pressure testing of cadaver ureters was performed by Watanabe et al. to examine the transverse and longitudinal properties of the ureter and maximum increase in diameter prior to leaking. Samples from the longitudinal direction were four times stronger than those in the transverse direction. Damage to the ureter may go undetected under certain conditions.

The third paper in this group from Saitoh et al. analyzed the *in vivo* mechanical properties of the canine, the normal bladder, the denervated bladder, and denervated bladder two weeks after denervation. Mechanical data were obtained using suture markers placed on the bladder. A computer analysis based on Glantz's mathematical model for smooth muscle was used to evaluate changes in the stress strain curves. The mechanical properties of the bladder are essentially viscoelastic.

Future Directions

The last section of this book poses a question as to how the biomaterials community will address the issues of quality, safety, and efficacy in the experimental testing of materials. This area of increasing interest to clinicians, device manufacturers, and basic scientists. The aforementioned papers in this STP attest to illustrate the challenges and complexities of biomaterials testing. The listing here is far from complete. While the transition from experimental research to clinical or market acceptance depends on good design, adequate testing, and quality control assurance, of utmost importance are good manufacturing and laboratory procedures. Unless we outline these priorities, how and what we test may be meaningless. This section also highlights research opportunities in areas involving biomaterials-based technologies, tissue engineering, and cutting-edge methodologies.

Helen E. Kambic, M.S.

The Cleveland Clinic Foundation
Cleveland, OH
symposium co-chair and co-editor

A. T. Yokobori, Jr., Ph.D.

Tohoku University
Sendai, Japan
symposium co-chair and co-editor

Cardiovascular Materials

Kozaburo Hayashi[1]

Fatigue Properties of Segmented Polyether Polyurethanes for Cardiovascular Applications

REFERENCE: Hayashi, K., **"Fatigue Properties of Segmented Polyether Polyurethanes for Cardiovascular Applications,"** *Biomaterials' Mechanical Properties, ASTM STP 1173,* H. E. Kambic and A. T. Yokobori, Jr., Eds., American Society for Testing and Materials, Philadelphia, 1994, pp. 9–18.

ABSTRACT: Effects of temperature (24°, 37°, and 50°C) and cyclic rate (0.8, 2, and 5 Hz) on fatigue behavior were studied on two different segmented polyether polyurethanes immersed in a plasma-analogous cholesterol-lipid solution. Dynamic fatigue tests were carried out under conditions of 50% mean strain and 10% strain amplitude. Changes in the mean stress and the ratio of stress amplitude to strain amplitude were significantly larger at 50°C than at 24° and 37°C. In the initial stage of fatigue testing, changes in these variables appeared earlier at higher cyclic rates. However, the long-term dynamic fatigue behavior was dependent on the duration of testing rather than on the repetition number or the cyclic rate. These results imply that the fatigue testing in the cholesterol-lipid solution of 50°C at the cyclic rate of 5 Hz might be useful for the prediction of long-term behavior of these materials under actual service inside the body.

KEYWORDS: segmented polyether polyurethane, elastomer, cholesterol-lipid solution, servo-hydraulic tester, stress relaxation, fatigue test, accelerated testing, durability

Segmented polyether polyurethanes are believed to be some of the most promising materials for cardiovascular implants because they possess two basic properties required of candidate materials: excellent mechanical properties and blood compatibility [1]. Since materials used in cardiovascular devices and their components undergo cyclic deformation while in contact with blood, their fatigue properties are extremely important for the guarantee of long-term reliability and safety. Although there are many reports on the blood- and bio-compatibilities of polyurethanes, their mechanical properties, particularly their fatigue properties, have not been well documented.

The author and his coworkers have been doing a series of studies on the basic tensile and fatigue properties of several elastomeric polymers including segmented polyether polyure-thanes [2–7]. For the guarantee of long-term performance of implants, significant time and cost must be expended to obtain those reliable durability data if fatigue tests are performed at the cyclic rate experienced inside the body. To solve this problem, we need to develop accel-erated-time test methods and to establish criteria for the prediction of material life. Aiming to obtain basic data for the design of cardiovascular prostheses as well as for the development of accelerated durability test and evaluation methods, effects of test temperature and cyclic rate on fatigue behavior were studied on two kinds of segmented polyether polyurethanes that are being used clinically in cardiac prostheses. This paper deals with the results obtained from the static and dynamic fatigue tests of these materials.

[1] Professor, Department of Mechanical Engineering, Faculty of Engineering Science, Osaka University, Toyonaka, Osaka 560, Japan.

Method

Materials

The materials studied are Toyobo TM5[2] and Biomer®[3] which are being used clinically in left ventricular assist devices and artificial hearts based on the favorable experiences with these materials in animal experiments [8,9].

Toyobo TM5 is a segmented polyether polyurethane that is usually prepared as a 15% by weight solution in dimethyl formamide. The soft segment of this material is composed of polytetramethylene glycol and 4,4'-diphenylmethane diisocyanate (MDI); the hard segment contains propylene diamine and MDI. The molecular weight of the soft segment is 2000.

Biomer is a similar segmented polyether polyurethane to Toyobo TM5, and it is prepared as a 30% by weight solution in dimethyl acetamide. The soft segment consists of polytetramethylene oxide and MDI, while the hard segment contains ethylene diamine and MDI. The molecular weight of the soft segment is estimated to be around 1800.

The procedures for fabricating sample sheets of 0.5 to 1.0 mm in thickness have been reported elsewhere [2,3]. These sample sheets were cut with a special punch to a dumbbell shape (gage length: 16.0 mm, width: 5.0 mm) which has almost the same dimensions as those of the specimen standardized by ASTM Test Method for Tensile Properties of Plastics by Use of Microtensile Specimens (D 1708).

Material Test System

A servohydraulic testing machine was used for static and dynamic fatigue tests in combination with a video dimension analyzer. Details of the test system have been reported elsewhere [10]. Although the test machine has a capability of testing materials under the maximum dynamic load of ±800 kg, the force transducer conditioner allows dynamic testing to be carried out under the maximum load of ±2 kg with less than ±0.25% total error when a low capacity load cell (±20 kg) is used. Smooth application of force and deformation is possible with this test machine because hydrostatic bearings are used on the piston rod inside the actuator. Therefore, a large piston stroke (±125 mm) or small force, or both, can be applied to a test specimen in a very smooth fashion.

In this test machine, a differential transformer is installed inside the piston cylinder to monitor the piston stroke. In the present study, however, a TV camera and a video dimension analyzer were used for the accurate measurement of true deformation developed in the parallel part of a specimen without contacting the specimen.

Test Condition

Dynamic fatigue tests were carried out under conditions of 50% of mean strain (ε_m) and 10% of strain amplitude (ε_a) in a strain-control, sine-waveform mode. For the study of temperature effects, specimens were immersed in a plasma-analogous cholesterol-lipid solution [2] of 24°, 37°, or 50°C; the cyclic rate of 2 Hz was selected for this series of dynamic tests. To study the effects of cyclic rate, additional fatigue tests were carried out at the cyclic rates of 0.8 and 5 Hz on the specimens immersed in the same solution kept at 37°C. All fatigue tests were continued until 5×10^6 cycles. The mean stress (σ_m) and the ratio of stress amplitude (σ_a) to strain amplitude (ε_a) were measured during the dynamic fatigue testing.

[2] Toyobo Co., Osaka, Japan.
[3] Ethicon, Somerville, NJ.

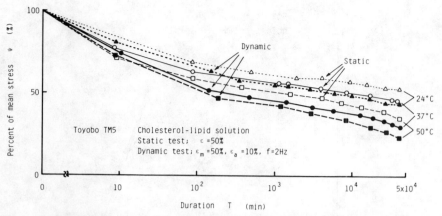

FIG. 1—*Static and dynamic stress relaxation behavior of Toyobo TM5 polyurethane at three different temperatures.*

Static fatigue tests, that is, static stress relaxation tests, were performed for about a month applying a constant 50% strain to the specimens immersed in the cholesterol-lipid solution kept at 24°, 37°, or 50°C. The stress developed by this strain was measured periodically.

Results

Effects of Environmental Temperature

Figure 1 shows temporal changes of the mean stress measured during the dynamic fatigue testing and those of the stress during the static relaxation testing which were carried out on Toyobo TM5 polyurethane at different temperatures. The stress decreased markedly within 3 h and then continued to decreased gradually for one month. The higher the ambient temperature was, the greater the stress decrease was; the dynamic stress relaxation was greater than the static one regardless of the test temperature.

Effects of temperature on the dynamic relaxation of Biomer are shown in Fig. 2. The stress

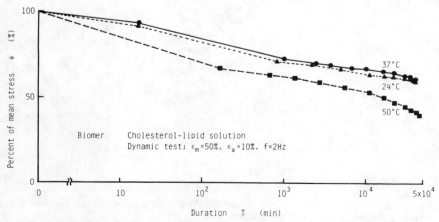

FIG. 2—*Dynamic stress relaxation behavior of Biomer at three different temperatures.*

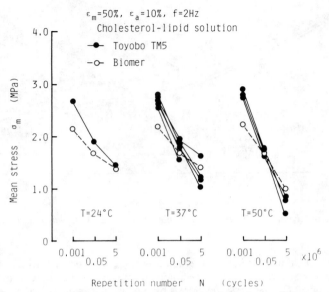

FIG. 3—*Mean stress measured at three repetition numbers during fatigue testing at different temperatures.*

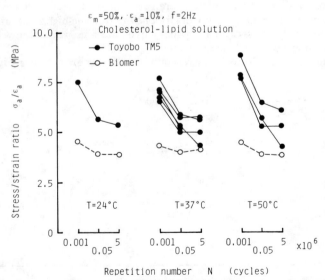

FIG. 4—*Ratio of stress amplitude to strain amplitude (stress/strain ratio) measured at three repetition numbers during fatigue testing at different temperatures.*

TABLE 1—*Percent ratios of mean stress and stress/strain ratio at 5 × 10⁶ cycles to their initial values. Testing was carried out in the cholesterol-lipid solution under conditions of 50% mean strain, 10% strain amplitude, and 2 Hz cyclic rate.*

	Mean Stress, %		Stress/Strain Ratio, %	
	Toyobo TM5	Biomer	Toyobo TM5	Biomer
24°C	54.0	64.5	71.3	86.6
37°C	46.3 ± 9.1[a]	64.9	73.8 ± 7.4[a]	95.9
50°C	24.5 ± 5.5[b]	44.5	64.0 ± 8.1[b]	87.2

Mean ± standard deviation.
[a] n(specimen number) = 4.
[b] n = 3.

decreased gradually at every temperature in this material, too, although almost no difference was observed in the relaxation behavior between 24° and 37°C. The stress reduction was much greater at 50°C than at 24° and 37°C. The reduction of stress in this material was significantly smaller than that in TM5 polyurethane at each temperature.

The mean stress measured during the dynamic fatigue testing is plotted against the repetition number in Fig. 3. As was shown in Figs. 1 and 2, both the materials demonstrated a large reduction of the mean stress, which was greater at higher ambient temperature. The degree of the stress relaxation was less in Biomer than in Toyobo TM5.

Figure 4 shows changes in the ratio of stress amplitude to strain amplitude, the stress/strain ratio for short, which is a kind of dynamic elastic modulus. The stress/strain ratio decreased markedly in Toyobo TM5 and somewhat slightly in Biomer in the early period of fatigue testing, that is until 5 × 10⁴ cycles. However, the decrease became much less between 5 × 10⁴ and 5 × 10⁶ cycles with the exception of two specimens of TM5 polyurethane. As a whole, changes in the stress/strain ratio were again much smaller in Biomer than in Toyobo TM5 polyurethane. There seemed to be no significant differences in the change of the dynamic elasticity between 24° and 37°C in the two materials.

Changes in the mean stress and the stress/strain ratio caused by 5 × 10⁶ cycles of deformation at different temperatures are summarized in Table 1. Difference of temperature between 24° and 37°C had no significant influence on the dynamic material behavior. However, the elevation of test temperature to 50°C enhanced the stress relaxation greatly in both the materials. It is obvious that the material behavior is much more stable in Biomer than in Toyobo TM5.

Effects of Cyclic Rate

Figures 5 and 6 show effects of the cyclic rate on the temporal changes of the mean stress in Toyobo TM5 and Biomer polyurethanes, respectively. With increase in the cyclic rate, the reduction of stress increased if compared at the same period of time: the stress relaxation appeared earlier at higher cyclic rates. Difference of the stress relaxation was smaller between 0.8 and 2 Hz rather than between 2 and 5 Hz; in Biomer, there was almost no difference between 0.8 and 2 Hz. Again, the stress reduction was much smaller in Biomer than in Toyobo TM5 polyurethane at each cyclic rate.

In Figs. 7 and 8, the mean stress and the ratio of stress amplitude to strain amplitude are plotted against the repetition number, respectively. The repetition number of 5 × 10⁶ is equivalent to around 1740, 700, and 280 h for the cyclic rates of 0.8, 2, and 5 Hz, respectively. At

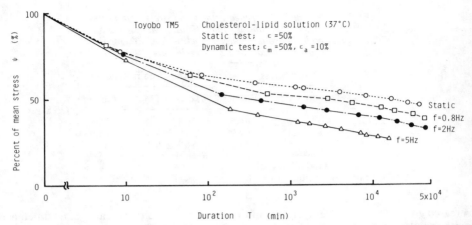

FIG. 5—*Stress relaxation behavior of Toyobo TM5 polyurethane observed under static load condition and during cyclic deformation at different frequencies.*

this repetition number, the testing at 0.8 Hz gave lower mean stresses than those at 2 and 5 Hz in both the materials; however, almost no differences were observed between 2 and 5 Hz testing. The stress/strain ratio decreased greatly until 5×10^4 cycles in all cases except for the Biomer specimen tested at 2 Hz, although there were much less changes between 5×10^4 and 5×10^6 cycles. The stress/strain ratio at 5×10^6 cycles was somewhat larger in the specimens tested at 5 Hz than those tested at the other cyclic rates.

Table 2 shows changes in the mean stress and the stress/strain ratio caused by 5×10^6 cycles of deformation given at different cyclic rates. As a whole, changes in these parameters were much larger in the specimens cyclically deformed at 0.8 Hz than in those tested at 2 and 5 Hz; there were almost no differences between 2 and 5 Hz except for the stress/strain ratio in Biomer.

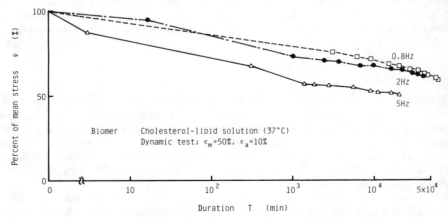

FIG. 6—*Dynamic stress relaxation behavior of Biomer at three different cyclic rates.*

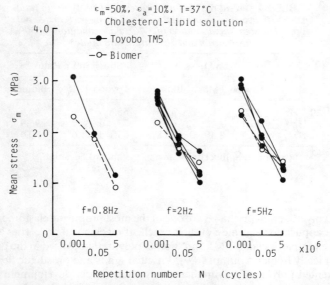

FIG. 7—*Mean stress measured at three repetition numbers during fatigue testing at different cyclic rates.*

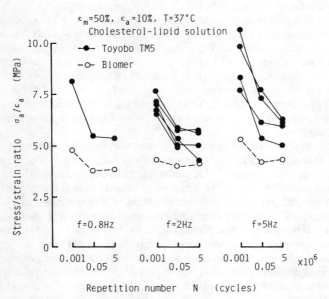

FIG. 8—*Stress/strain ratio measured at three repetition numbers during fatigue testing at different cyclic rates.*

TABLE 2—*Percent ratios of mean stress and stress/strain ratio at 5 × 10⁶ cycles to their initial values. Testing was carried out in the cholesterol-lipid solution of 37°C under conditions of 50% mean strain and 10% strain amplitude.*

	Mean Stress, %		Stress/Strain Ratio, %	
	Toyobo TM5	Biomer	Toyobo TM5	Biomer
0.8 Hz	37.9	42.5	65.8	82.9
2 Hz	46.3 ± 9.1[a]	64.9	73.8 ± 7.4[a]	95.9
5 Hz	46.9 ± 8.4[a]	58.8	63.1 ± 11.0[a]	80.4

[a] n(specimen number) = 4, mean ± standard deviation.

Discussion

Segmented polyether polyurethanes are one of the most promising elastomeric polymers for cardiovascular applications because of their excellent mechanical properties and blood compatibility. For example, Toyobo TM5 and Biomer polyurethanes used in the present study are being used clinically in blood pumps [8,9]. Vascular grafts and prosthetic heart valves fabricated of segmented polyether polyurethanes have been under development in recent years [1,11,12]. These components undergo cyclic deformation of fairly large strains while in contact with blood. Since the materials used in these components have to maintain their performance for prolonged periods of time, stability of the mechanical properties during service is extremely important. However, there is a paucity of information related to the fatigue properties of segmented polyether polyurethanes, particularly those under the condition that the materials are in contact with blood at body temperature, because it is very difficult to carry out long-term *in vitro* fatigue testing in blood.

To overcome this problem, the author and his collaborators have been using a synthetic cholesterol-lipid solution as a substitute for blood [2]. The composition of this solution is analogous to that of plasma except that the former solution contains no protein nor enzyme. We compared the tensile properties of Toyobo TM5 polyurethane specimens retrieved from the blood pumps that were implanted in goats for 6 to 72 days with those cyclically deformed by an *in vitro* fatigue testing in the same cholesterol-lipid solution of 37°C as that used in the present study [4]. The results obtained were substantially similar in both cases. This plasma-analogous solution is useful for the *in vitro* mechanical testing of materials that are used in contact with blood.

It is not difficult to perform fatigue testing of materials for a few months at the frequency of the heart rate, that is 1 to 2 Hz. For the prediction of fatigue life of a material, however, we need to accumulate a huge amount of reproducible and reliable data by doing fatigue tests for much longer periods of time. Also, it is necessary to determine the relationship between the stress or strain applied and the cyclic number to failure. For the guarantee of long-term performance of implants, significant time and cost must be expended to obtain those reliable durability data if fatigue tests are performed at the cyclic rate of 1 to 2 Hz. To solve this problem, we need to develop accelerated-time test methods and to establish criteria for the prediction of material life. Because the mechanical properties of elastomeric polymers are quite sensitive to temperature and strain rate, we should accumulate basic data on the effects of environmental temperature and cyclic rate for the development of accelerated test and evaluation methods.

In the initial stage of fatigue testing of Toyobo TM5 polyurethane, changes in the mean stress were different between 24° and 37°C (Fig. 1); stress relaxation was greater at 37°C than at 24°C if compared at the same period of time. After fatigue testing of 5×10^6 cycles, however, there was no significant difference in the mean stress between these two temperatures, as shown in Fig. 3 and Table 1. Similar results were observed of Biomer as well, although there was no difference in the stress relaxation curves between 24° and 37°C in this material, even in the early stage of fatigue testing. Elevation of temperature to 50°C accelerated the stress relaxation significantly in both the materials throughout the test period; at 5×10^6 cycles, the mean stress was much lower at 50°C than at 24° and 37°C. The stress/strain ratio, that is, the dynamic elastic modulus, also decreased in the early stage of fatigue testing regardless of temperature, as shown in Fig. 4; again, the decrease was larger at 50°C than at 24° and 37°C. However, no essential change was observed in the stress/strain ratio between 5×10^4 and 5×10^6 cycles at every temperature. Table 1 indicates that the changes of the stress/strain ratio caused by the cyclic deformation were much smaller than those of the mean stress. As a whole, the influences of temperature on the stress relaxation and dynamic elastic modulus were greater in Toyobo TM5 than in Biomer.

If the mechanical properties of a material are independent of cyclic rate for a prolonged period of time, durability of the material can be evaluated from the accelerated tests at increased cyclic rates. If compared at the same cyclic number, for example, at 5×10^6 cycles, the mean stress and the stress/strain ratio seemed to be larger at higher cyclic rates, as shown in Figs. 7 and 8. Table 2 indicates that the decreases in the mean stress and the stress/strain ratio caused by the cyclic deformation of 5×10^6 times were greater at 0.8 Hz than at 2 and 5 Hz; no significant differences were observed between the results obtained at 2 and 5 Hz with only one exception in the stress/strain ratio of Biomer. These results imply that the fatigue behavior of these materials is dependent on time, and it is true in the early period of fatigue testing, as shown in Figs. 5 and 6. After being deformed cyclically for prolonged periods of time, however, the mean stress and the stress/strain ratio seemed to settle down at certain values regardless of cyclic rates (see Fig. 12 in Ref 6).

Conclusion

Changes in the mean stress and the ratio of stress amplitude to strain amplitude were significantly lower at 50°C than at 24° and 37°C, and were greater under dynamic load condition than under static condition at every temperature. In the initial stage of cyclic deformation, changes in these variables appeared earlier at higher cyclic rates. However, the long-term dynamic fatigue behavior was dependent on the duration of testing rather than on the repetition number or the cyclic rate. These results imply that the fatigue testing in the cholesterol-lipid solution of 50°C at the cyclic rate of 5 Hz might be useful for the prediction of long-term behavior of these materials under actual service inside the body. Additional long-term fatigue tests under these conditions are suggested for the development of accelerated material test and evaluation methods.

References

[1] Lelah, M. D. and Cooper, S. L., *Polyurethanes in Medicine,* CRC Press, Boca Raton, FL, 1986.
[2] Hayashi, K., Matsuda, T., Takano, H., and Umezu, M., "Effects of Immersion in Cholesterol-Lipid Solution on the Tensile and Fatigue Properties of Elastomeric Polymers for Blood Pump Applications," *Journal of Biomedical Materials Research,* Vol. 18, No. 8, 1984, pp. 939–951.
[3] Hayashi, K., Takano, H., Matsuda, T., and Umezu, M., "Mechanical Stability of Elastomeric Polymers for Blood Pump Applications," *Journal of Biomedical Materials Research,* Vol. 19, No. 2, 1985, pp. 179–193.
[4] Hayashi, K., Matsuda, T., Takano, H., et al., "Effects of Implantation on the Mechanical Properties of the Polyurethane Diaphragm of Left Ventricular Assist Devices," *Biomaterials,* Vol. 6, No. 2, 1985, pp. 82–88.

[5] Hayashi, K., Matsuda, T., Nakamura, T., et al., "Mechanical and ESCA Studies of Segmented Poly-ether Polyurethanes with Various Molecular Weights for Blood Pump Application," *Progress in Artificial Organs—1985,* Y. Nose, C. Kjellstrand, and P. Ivanovich, Eds., ISAO Press, Cleveland, OH, 1986, pp. 989–993.

[6] Hayashi, K., "Tensile and Fatigue Properties of Segmented Polyether Polyurethanes," *Polyure-thanes in Biomedical Engineering II,* H. Planck, I. Syre, M. Dauner, and G. Egbers, Eds., Elsevier, Amsterdam, 1987, pp. 129–149.

[7] Hayashi, K., "Mechanical Properties of Segmented Polyether Polyurethanes for Blood Pump Appli-cations," *Artificial Heart 2,* T. Akutsu, Ed., Springer-Verlag, Tokyo, 1988, pp. 13–17.

[8] Takano, H., Nakatani, T., Taenaka, Y., and Umezu, M., "Development of the Ventricular Assist Pump System: Experimental and Clinical Studies,"*Artificial Heart 1,* T. Akutsu, Ed., Springer-Ver-lag, Tokyo, 1986, pp. 141–151.

[9] DeVries, W. C., Anderson, J. L., Joyce, L. D., et al., "Clinical Use of the Total Artificial Heart," *New England Journal of Medicine,* Vol. 310, 1984, pp. 273–278.

[10] Hayashi, K. and Nakamura, T., "Material Test System for the Evaluation of Mechanical Properties of Biomaterials," *Journal of Biomedical Materials Research,* Vol. 19, No. 2, 1985, pp. 133–144.

[11] Reul, H. M. and Ghista, D. N., "The Design Development, In Vitro Testing, and Performance of an Optimal Aortic Valve Prosthesis," *Biomechanics of Medical Devices,* D. N. Ghista, Ed., Marcel Dekker, New York, 1981, pp. 257–300.

[12] Hayashi, K., Takamizawa, K., Saito, T., et al., "Elastic Properties and Strength of a Novel Small-Diameter, Compliant Polyurethane Vascular Graft," *Journal of Biomedical Materials Research: Applied Biomaterials,* Vol. 23, No. A2, 1989, pp. 229–244.

J. Michael Lee,[1] *Sean A. Haberer,*[2] *Christopher A. Pereira,*[1]
Wendy A. Naimark,[1] *David W. Courtman,*[3] *and Gregory J. Wilson*[4]

High Strain Rate Testing and Structural Analysis of Pericardial Bioprosthetic Materials

REFERENCE: Lee, J. M., Haberer, S. A., Pereira, C. A., Naimark, W. A., Courtman, D. W., and Wilson, G. J., **"High Strain Rate Testing and Structural Analysis of Pericardial Bioprosthetic Materials,"** *Biomaterials' Mechanical Properties, ASTM STP 1173,* H. E. Kambic and A. T. Yokobori, Jr., Eds., American Society for Testing and Materials, Philadelphia, 1994, pp. 19–42.

ABSTRACT: Characterization of the viscoelastic behavior of pericardial biomaterials for heart valve or patching applications demands testing under loading times or frequencies typical of those that occur in physiological function or in a bioprosthetic device. We have used a servo-hydraulic testing system to evaluate the behavior of these materials under loading times as low as 0.05 s, frequencies up to 10 Hz and strain rates exceeding 24 000 %/min. Mechanical tests included large deformation cyclic loading, stress relaxation experiments, and small deformation forced vibration. This paper reviews our experience with these tests, interpreted using results from collagen denaturation temperature testing and biochemical analysis, in three distinct studies:

(1) examination of the effects of glutaraldehyde, poly (glycidyl ether) (a diepoxide compound), and cyanamide on bovine pericardium,

(2) comparison of bovine and porcine pericardia, and

(3) evaluation of the effects of extraction of cellular components from bovine pericardium.

These tools provide better means toward understanding the viscoelastic properties of these materials and the structural/functional relationships that determine those properties.

KEYWORDS: viscoelasticity, mechanical testing, heart valves, crosslinking, glutaraldehyde, servohydraulic testing, collagen, pericardium, bioprostheses, soft tissues

The pericardium is the sac that surrounds the heart in the thorax. As its older German name "hertzbeutel" or "heart bag" implies, it fits snugly about the heart and is attached to the great vessels and other attachment ligaments. Twenty-five years ago, the viscoelastic behavior of the pericardium was a subject that engendered little interest. However, this view has changed for three reasons. First, while the pericardium was long thought to have no physiological function beyond keeping the heart in place in the thorax, this view has changed markedly. The pericardium is now understood to be important in normal and pathological cardiac function, its principal physiological roles involving limitation of the expansion of the cardiac chambers in diastole and coupling of left and right diastolic filling volumes [1]. Second, since 1975, glutar-

---

[1] Associate professor, tissue mechanics technician, and Ph.D candidate, respectively, Centre for Biomaterials, University of Toronto, Toronto, Ontario, Canada M5S 1A1.

[2] Applications engineer, Instron Canada, Burlington, Ontario, Canada L7L 4X8.

[3] Ph.D candidate, Department of Pathology, University of Toronto, Conacher Research Wing, Toronto General Hospital, Toronto, Ontario, Canada M5G 2C4.

[4] Professor and senior staff pathologist, The Hospital for Sick Children, Toronto, Ontario, Canada M5G 1X8.

aldehyde treated bovine pericardium has been used in the construction of bioprosthetic heart valves. Pericardial xenograft valves give hemodynamic performance satisfactory for use as mitral replacements, and—despite problems with mechanical design in the first generation— second generation pericardial valves have remained as rivals to the porcine aortic valve xeno- grafts [2,3]. Third, both autogenous pericardium and glutaraldehyde treated pericardium (from cattle, pigs, horses, and even yaks) have found wide use as patching materials [4–7]. These materials have been used creatively for repair of congenital heart defects, for pericardial closure, for replacement of chordae tendineae, and formation of conduits for vascular repair.

In any cardiovascular application, pericardial materials must sustain dynamic loads for the lifetime of the structure. The mechanical properties of the material are therefore of paramount importance for success. The mechanical properties of fresh pericardial tissues and of pericar- dial bioprosthetic materials have been explored by several authors. Uniaxial tensile testing has been performed on both fresh and treated tissues [8–12], and biaxial testing has been per- formed on fresh tissues only [13,14]. Pericardial materials have been shown to possess non- linear stress-strain behavior, to be anisotropic, and to display viscoelastic behavior including stress relaxation, creep, and cyclic hysteresis. Nonetheless, the degree of viscoelasticity of these materials has likely been underestimated in experiments to date due to the long loading times employed. The studies described were conducted with loading times in the range of seconds to minutes—therefore under relatively low strain rates, typically reaching an upper limit of a few hundred percent per minute. In most cases, the minimum loading times reflected the lim- itations of the testing apparatus; for instance, a screw-driven tensile testing machine. There is little published evidence of the period over which heart valve leaflet material is loaded during valve closure. However, the strain rate in trileaflet valves has been estimated to be approxi- mately 15 000 %/min [15]. The overall objective of the present studies was to use mechanical testing under physiologically relevant time frames to better characterize the viscoelastic behav- ior of pericardial materials. In the experiments described below, strains of 10 to 20% were achieved in a minimum time of 0.05 s for a maximum strain rate of 24 000 %/min—exceeding that expected *in vivo*.

Since their first use, pericardial bioprosthetic materials have relied on glutaraldehyde cross- linking to improve *in vivo* stability and resistance to degradation. The glutaraldehyde treat- ment is nominally intended to: (1) reduce immunogenicity of the materials, (2) increase resist- ance to degradation by host and bacterial enzymes, and (3) sterilize the materials. Each of these goals is incompletely achieved. Ultimately, structural degeneration of the material by tearing, delamination, and calcification (especially in young patients) remains the primary limitation to the implantation lifetime of these materials. It is unfortunately now clear that glutaralde- hyde treatment itself contributes to calcification of these materials [16,17]. However, in func- tional implants, it is unclear to what extent the changes in mechanical properties produced by crosslinking influences the degradation of these materials. One may speculate that changes in flexural behavior could lead to local buckling and fatigue damage to collagen fibers [18]. Alter- natively, delamination could result, leading to increased infiltration of blood components and calcification at sites of cellular debris. While neither of these latter mechanisms has been con- vincingly demonstrated, the linkage of glutaraldehyde treatment and degeneration has accel- erated the search for alternative tissue stabilization techniques. Several alternative crosslinking reagents have been explored in different applications, including: (1) diepoxides [19,20], (2) diisocyanates [21], (3) carbodiimides [22], and (4) diisothiocyanates [23]. The first study pre- sented examines the effects of both glutaraldehyde and alternative crosslinking agents on the high strain rate viscoelastic behavior of bovine pericardial materials.

It has long been known that significant anatomical differences exist beween the pericardia of different species—even among mammals. These include gross differences in thickness, appearance, folds, and attachments. While these anatomical differences undoubtedly have functional importance, their purposes are not clear. Further, it remains a matter of dispute whether significant mechanical differences exist between the pericardial tissues of domestic mammals [11–13]. In the second study, we have used high strain rate methods and biochemical analysis to explore the structural/mechanical differences between bovine and porcine pericardia, both of which have been used for preparation of bioprosthetic materials.

Finally, if we wish to reduce immunological recognition and calcification of pericardial biomaterials—yet preserve mechanical function—extraction of cellular components may be a potential alternative to glutaraldehyde crosslinking. This approach was first explored for "acellular matrix" vascular graft construction by Brendel and colleagues [24], and later by Wilson et al. [25]. A modification of this technique has recently been described by Courtman et al. [26] for preparation of an acellular pericardial material which may be used with or without crosslinking. The third study explores the effects of this extraction protocol on the biochemical makeup of the material and its high strain rate viscoelastic behavior.

The work presented represents a synopsis and review of three studies in our laboratory that have employed high strain rate testing of pericardial biomaterials. Our objectives in each case have been to: (1) more accurately assess the viscoelastic behavior of pericardial materials before and after processing for bioprosthetic function, and (2) to link structural (and predominantly biochemical) information on the materials to their mechanical function.

Mechanical and Structural Testing Methods

Each of three studies presented employed the high strain rate testing methodology developed originally by Haberer et al. [27]. As well, each class of material examined was tested for collagen denaturation temperature using a customized six sample tester developed in our laboratory. These common experimental methods and the applied statistical analysis are described in this section. The specific materials examined in each of the three studies are presented in the respective sections which follow.

Instrumentation and Methods for High Strain Rate Testing

Test strips 20 by 4 mm were cut from each ventral pericardial sample in the base-to-apex direction and mounted for a nominal gage length of 10 mm between screw-tightened, sandpaper-lined brass grips. For later determination of the actual gage length and width, each tissue strip was loaded to 0.5 g and photographed using a 55-mm Micro lens (Nikkor). The length at 0.5-g load was defined as the gage length in order to improve reproducibility of the data and to allow better understanding of the effects of crosslinking [28]. The thickness of the tissue was measured on an adjacent region of the tissue using a Mitutoyo nonrotating thickness gage (precision 0.01 mm) [10,11]. During testing, the test strips were held in a tissue bath filled with Hanks solution and maintained at a temperature of 37.0 ± 0.2°C using a RTD temperature sensing probe and temperature controller (Cole-Parmer).

The mechanical experiments were performed on a uniaxial servohydraulic testing machine (Instron Model 1331 load frame with Series 2150 controller). The tissue tank and instrumentation which were mounted on the testing machine are shown in Fig. 1. A 250-g load cell (Sensotec, Model 31/4680) and the top sandpaper-lined brass grip for the tissue were attached to a steel rod held in the top hydraulic grip of the Instron. The bottom tissue grip was connected to the tissue bath which was in turn attached by C-clamps to an aluminum platform held by the bottom hydraulic grip. Since the tissue bath was moved very rapidly by the actuator during testing, we initially expected that fluid motion would be a problem. This was not the case, perhaps because the tank moved only vertically and side-to-side waves were not produced.

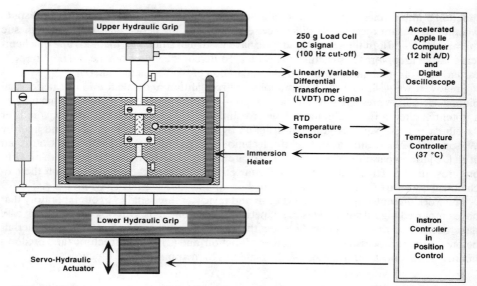

FIG. 1—*High strain rate testing apparatus. The apparatus is mounted onto an Instron servohydraulic testing machine, held by the upper and lower hydraulic grips.*

Ultimately, no baffles were required, and control studies confirmed that testing with or without fluid produced identical results.

The deflection of the actuator (and hence the extension of the specimen) was measured by a DC linearly variable differential transformer (LVDT, Intertechnology Model SE 374). The body of the LVDT was supported by a frame attached to the unmoving top grip of the Instron while the core was screwed into the platform beneath the bath. The LVDT therefore measured the relative movement between the upper and lower grips and thereby the change in length of the specimen. While it should have been possible to use the feedback signal from the internal LVDT in the actuator, the signal from this particular machine was unacceptably noisy. Supplied with a DC excitation voltage, the LVDT produced a DC output of 0 to 5 V. The load cell was connected to an excitation amplifier (Sensotec, Model 4500) which similarly produced a DC voltage output of 0 to 5 V.

The load signal initially contained a high noise level that overwhelmed the recorded data. This noise, identified by spectral analysis as being centered at 220 to 250 Hz, was identified as being due to load frame resonance and was successfully corrected using a fifth order low-pass Butterworth filter. This filter produced a very sharp cutoff at 100 Hz, ten times our maximum vibrational frequency.

Signals from the load cell and the LVDT were displayed during testing on a digital storage oscilloscope (Gould, Model 1425). The signals were also input into a 16-channel, 12-bit analog-to-digital (A/D) converter (Applied Engineering) in an accelerated Apple IIe computer (Applied Engineering, Transwarp, 3.6 times acceleration). The rate of data acquisition for these experiments was 430 pairs of data points per second (deflection/load). The deflection and load signals were sampled sequentially. This feature was problematic since, when higher frequency (1 or 10 Hz) signals were sampled, an apparent hysteresis was introduced. This effect was corrected using the results of an experiment in which the voltage from a waveform generator was delivered to both A/D channels, and the time lag introduced during sampling measured. A numerical correction was then developed that corrected both for this effect and for the small but constant phase shift introduced by the Butterworth filter on the load signal.

The Instron controller was operated solely in stroke mode (displacement control using feedback from the LVDT in the servohydraulic actuator). Load control was not employed since it was felt to be unwise to control a large servohydraulic system with feedback from a very sensitive load cell. This cautious approach ruled out creep testing for these studies.

Mechanical Testing Protocol

Three types of tests were performed on each tissue sample: (1) large deflection cyclic loading (stress-strain curve measurement), (2) stress relaxation, and (3) small deflection forced vibration (Fig. 2). The order of application of these tests was not randomized. The rationale and potential consequences of this choice are discussed (see Discussion). Prior to each test, the test strip was preconditioned by 25 ramp loading cycles between 0 and 80 g at a frequency of 1 Hz. The cyclic load-elongation response under a ramp deflection was then measured at 0.01, 0.1, 1 and 10 Hz between 0 and 80 g: a total of four tests. It is important to note that the loading time in each case was one half of the period of the waveform; for instance, in a 1-Hz test, the loading time was 0.5 s. One hundred data pairs (deflection/load) encompassing one complete cycle were recorded at each frequency.

After completion of the cyclic loading tests, stress relaxation tests were performed. The preconditioned strip was loaded using a ramp with loading time of 100, 10, 1, or 0.1 s to a load

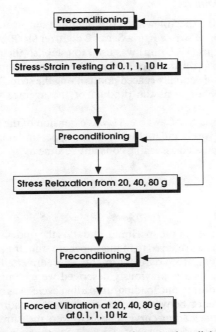

FIG. 2—*High strain rate testing protocol. This protocol was used in all the tests described in this paper. However, the initial experiments described in Study 1 also included stress-strain and forced vibration experiments at 0.01 Hz.*

of 20, 40, and 80 g—a total of twelve tests for each specimen. Before each test, the extension required to produce the desired initial load (say, 80 g) was established. The extension was then ramped to that value in the chosen time interval (say, 1 s). Once the desired load was achieved, the strip was held at the corresponding extension for 100 s. It is important to note that, using these methods, the loading time was constant irrespective of the initial load; for example, in 1-s loading time tests, the specimen was loaded to 20 g in 1 s and to 80 g in 1 s. Data collection consisted of two sets of 100 pairs of data points. The first 100 points were collected during loading and the subsequent 100 during load decay.

Forced vibration testing was next performed at 0.01, 0.1, 1, and 10 Hz about extensions corresponding to mean loads of 20, 40, and 80 g—a total of twelve tests. The tissue was extended from zero load to one of the aforementioned mean loads and the required extension measured. The tissue was then vibrated sinusoidally with a small defection (~ 0.05 mm) about the extension corresponding to the chosen mean load. The mean load relaxed during each forced vibration experiment. For the 10-Hz and 1-Hz experiments, the relaxation was negligible; for the 0.1-Hz tests, the relaxation required that the first two cycles or so be used for analysis since they best corresponded to the chosen mean load. Two hundred pairs of data points (approximately six cycles) were measured for each test. In total, then, 28 tests were performed on each tissue strip. For completeness, this regimen was used as stated in Study 1; however, in the other two studies, the 0.01-Hz stress-strain and forced vibration studies were omitted, since the 100-s loading time was nonphysiological and to streamline the experiments.

Analysis of Mechanical Data

Photographic prints of the specimen and grips obtained during testing were digitized on an Apple IIe computer equipped with a Kurta Series 2 digitizer (1000 points/in. resolution). The width of the machined grips (19.1 mm) was used to establish the photo magnification. The gage length was calculated as the distance between the top and bottom grips. The width of the tissue was averaged across six equally spaced points along the strip. The cross-sectional area of the specimen, A_0, was obtained as the product of the average width and the measured thickness.

Strain, ε, was calculated as $\Delta L / L_0$ where ΔL was extension of the specimen and L_0 the gage length. Nominal stress, σ_n, was calculated as the force (F) per unit nominal cross-sectional area (A_0). True stress σ was calculated assuming constant volume as

$$\sigma = \frac{FL}{A_0 L_0}$$

where L is the deformed length of the specimen, and A_0 is the undeformed cross-sectional area as calculated above. All stresses referred to in this paper are true stresses calculated in this manner. Load/extension/time data from the experiments were converted to stress/strain/time data on computer and the phase shifts previously described were eliminated. Percent hysteresis (percent strain energy lost during one loading/unloading cycle) was calculated from the stress-strain curves as the difference between the areas under the loading and unloading curves divided by the area under the loading curve. The areas were measured from plots of the stress-strain curve using a planimeter (Eugene Dietzgen Co.). Stress-strain curves to a maximum load of 80 g and percent hysteresis were obtained for each specimen under each test frequency.

For stress relaxation experiments, the percent stress remaining at a time t was calculated from load/time data as the ratio of the stress at time t, $\sigma(t)$, to the stress at the time of maximum stress (defined as $t = 0$), $\sigma(0)$. Approximately 100 data points were calculated and plotted against $\log_{10}(t)$ from 0.01 to 100 s. Plotting on a log time axis allowed better assessment of the presence of any relaxation asymptote and conclusions to be drawn regarding the relaxation spectrum of the material (see Discussion). The data for each treatment group were averaged at loads of 20, 40, and 80 g and loading times of 100, 10, 1, and 0.1 s.

The forced vibration data were analyzed using the equations for sinusoidal loading. The applied stress was taken to vary with time according to

$$\sigma(t) = \sigma_m + \sigma_0 \sin (2\pi ft + \alpha)$$

where $\sigma(t)$ is the stress at time t, σ_m is the mean stress, σ_0 is the amplitude of the stress sinusoid, f is the frequency (in Hz), and α is the phase angle of the stress. The corresponding strain could then be described by

$$\varepsilon(t) = \varepsilon_m + \varepsilon_0 \sin (2\pi ft + \beta)$$

where $\varepsilon(t)$ is the strain at time t, ε_m is the mean strain, ε_0 is the amplitude of the strain sinusoid, and β is the phase angle of the strain. From these two equations the phase lag ϕ of the strain behind the stress could be calculated as $\phi = \alpha - \beta$, and the magnitude of the complex dynamic modulus, $|E^*|$ calculated as the ratio σ_0/ε_0. Furthermore, the storage modulus E_S and the loss modulus E_L could be calculated from the following equations

$$E_S = \frac{\sigma_0}{\varepsilon_0} \cos (\phi) \qquad E_L = \frac{\sigma_0}{\varepsilon_0} \sin (\phi)$$

The storage modulus, E_S, can be identified as the in-phase, elastic, or real component of the complex dynamic modulus, while the loss modulus, E_L, can be identified with the out-of-phase, viscous, or imaginary component of the dynamic modulus. Their ratio, tan (ϕ), therefore gives an estimate of the viscoelastic character of the material: tan $(\phi) = 0$ for an elastic solid and goes to one for a viscous fluid.

A computer program was used to visually display the stress-time data and an initial estimated sinusoidal fit. The stress parameters σ_0 and σ_m were first calculated as

$$\sigma_0 = \frac{\sigma_{max} - \sigma_{min}}{2} \qquad \sigma_m = \frac{\sigma_{max} + \sigma_{min}}{2}$$

where σ_{max} and σ_{min} were the maximum and minimum values of the stress data. The values of σ_0 and α were then adjusted individually while the experimental data points and fitted stress-time curve were superimposed on screen. When a close match was obtained, the values of σ_0 and α were saved. After the stress parameters were calculated, ε_0 and ε_m were calculated from the maximum and minimum values of the strain-time data as

$$\varepsilon_0 = \frac{\varepsilon_{max} - \varepsilon_{min}}{2} \qquad \varepsilon_m = \frac{\varepsilon_{max} + \varepsilon_{min}}{2}$$

The strain sinusoids were similarly fitted and the values of ε_0 and β saved. The saved stress and strain parameters σ_0, ε_0, α, and β were then used to calculate the dynamic modulus, phase angle, and loss and storage moduli as above.

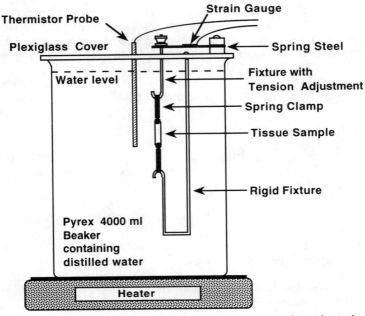

FIG. 3—*Denaturation temperature tester. The diagram shows one of six identical sample holders located around the central thermistor probe. Data acquisition from the thermistor and the six force transducers was accomplished by computer.*

Denaturation Temperature Testing

Collagen denaturation temperature T_d was measured as an indicator of the stability of the collagen triple helix in each material. Strip specimens from each treatment group were examined using a custom-built device which permitted testing of six specimens at once (Fig. 3). Each test strip was clamped between two spring clamps and mounted in the device. The lower clamp was fixed, while the upper clamp could be screw-adjusted to extend the specimen, the required force being measured by a strain gaged cantilever load cell. The upper assembly with its six mounted specimens was then lowered into a beaker containing distilled water at room temperature. Each strip was extended to a nominal load of 200 g and held at this extension. As the force relaxed, the water was heated at 1°C/min until the collagen in the specimen denatured; i.e., changed from its triple helical structure to a random coil. Since the specimen was constrained to length, the force rose rapidly at this temperature. Force/temperature pairs were recorded using an Apple IIe computer with an 8-bit A/D card (Applied Engineering) as per the aforementioned mechanical tests. These curves were plotted and the inflection point in the curve was taken to be T_d.

Statistical Analysis

Analysis of variance (ANOVA) with multiple comparisons was performed on all the data to obtain differences with treatment or species (Statview SE + Graphics or Statview II, Abacus Concepts). A two-way analysis of variance was used for stress-strain and hysteresis results where the variables were treatment or species and frequency only. The other results, obtained from stress relaxation and forced vibration tests, were analyzed using a three-way analysis of variance where the variables were treatment or species, frequency or loading time, and initial or mean load. An F-test was then used to determine if any of the variables showed a significant difference. If the F-test was positive, Fisher's least significant difference test for multiple comparisons was used to determine individual differences with each significant variable. Its approach to correction for multiple comparisons is identical to that used in Bonferroni corrected t-tests. A critical confidence level of $p = 0.05$ was used throughout this paper. Data are presented as the mean $\pm$ the standard error of the mean (SE).

Study 1: Testing of Pericardial Bioprosthetic Materials

Objective

The objective of our first study was to determine the degree of viscoelastic behavior of pericardial biomaterials when examined under physiologically relevant loading times; i.e., under higher strain rates than were typical in previous experiments. It was important in these studies to be able to accurately determine both the loading times in stress relaxation experiments and the applied frequencies in stress-strain and vibrational studies. Further, we sought to compare the viscoelastic behavior observed in these experiments with that observed in earlier low strain rate studies of fresh and glutaraldehyde-treated pericardium. Therefore, these experiments included the extra loading time of 100 s and vibrational frequency of 0.01 Hz—a wide enough range of times/frequencies for conclusions to be drawn regarding the importance of high strain rate testing in describing viscoelastic behavior.

Materials

Twenty hearts and intact pericardia were obtained fresh from slaughter of calves aged 6 to 8 months and transported in buckets filled with Hanks solution (pH 7.4, 310 mOs). The ventral surface of the pericardium was stripped of adherent fat and a rectangle of pericardium approximately 8 cm by 8 cm was harvested. To minimize the effects of tissue anisotropy [10,13] and inhomogeneity, the same anatomic region was used for each specimen. Furthermore, before excision, the base-to-apex direction was marked for reference using two sutures along the line defined by the aortic root and the apex of the heart. The twenty specimens were divided into four treatment groups of five specimens each. The treatments included: (1) no fixation (fresh); (2) 48 h in 0.5% glutaraldehyde at pH 7.5; (3) 48 h in 1% Denacol EX-512 poly (glycidyl ether), a diepoxide reagent, at pH 11; and (4) 48 h in 1% cyanamide, a carbodiimide reagent, at pH 5.4. These procedures have been previously described in detail by Pereira et al. [20]. The carbodiimide and diepoxide reagents have each previously been suggested as alternative chemical crosslinking reagents to replace glutaraldehyde [20,22].

Results

The large deformation stress-strain response for all treatments was nearly unaffected by loading frequency. While there were no significant differences with frequency, the stress-strain curve at 10 Hz was shifted to the left for all treatments (compare Figs. 4 and 5). For example, decreasing loading time to 0.05 s from 0.5 s (and hence increasing strain rate by ten times) resulted in a reduction of approximately 15% in extensibility for fresh tissue and glutaraldehyde treated tissues. While there was no significant effect of treatment on calculated hysteresis, there was a large and significant increase in hysteresis for all treatments at 10 Hz—percentage losses rose from an average of 15% to nearly 30%, representing substantially viscoelastic behav-

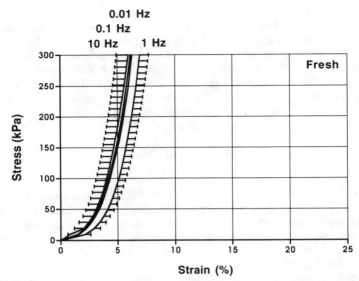

FIG. 4—*The stress-strain curves for fresh bovine pericardium were independent of loading frequency (and therefore of strain rate) for frequencies between 0.01 and 10 Hz. The loading times were 0.05, 0.5, 5, and 50 s for frequencies of 10, 1, 0.1, and 0.01 Hz. n = 5 for each group. Mean strain ± SE.*

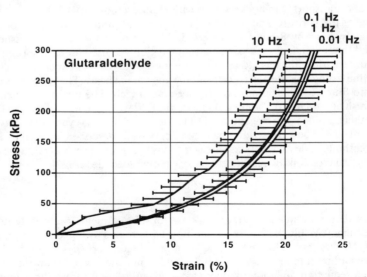

FIG. 5—*The stress-strain curves for the chemically treated pericardium were also independent of loading frequency. Curves for glutaraldehyde treated bovine tissue are shown. The loading times were 0.05, 0.5, 5, and 50 s for frequencies of 10, 1, 0.1, and 0.01 Hz. n = 5 for each group. Mean strain ± SE.*

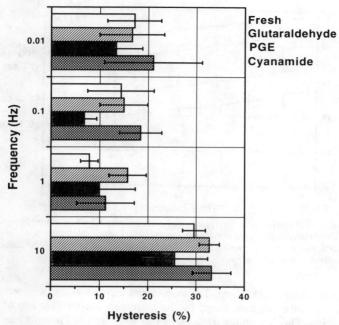

FIG. 6—*Hysteresis was significantly increased for loading times of 0.05 s (10 Hz) compared to loading times of 0.5 s (1 Hz), 5 s (0.1 Hz), or 50 s (0.01 Hz).* n = 5 *for each group. Mean ± SE.*

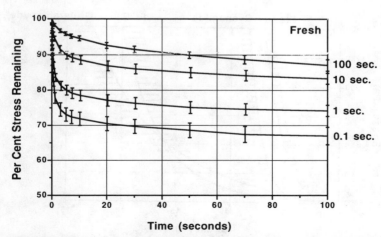

FIG. 7—*The degree of stress relaxation observed increased significantly as loading time decreased (*p *< 0.01). Curves for fresh bovine pericardium are plotted against time on a linear scale, zero time taken to be the time that the initial load of 80 g was achieved.* n = 5 *for each loading time. Mean ± SE.*

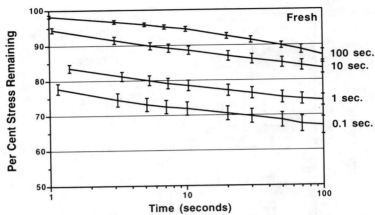

FIG. 8—*The stress relaxation data for fresh bovine pericardium from Fig. 7 are plotted against* $\log_{10}$ *of time. The linearity of the relaxation curves demonstrates that no single relaxation time (as in, for instance, a Maxwell or standard linear solid model) is sufficient to describe the relaxation behavior of these materials.* n = 5 *for each loading time. Mean* ± *SE.*

ior under large deformations (Fig. 6). The viscoelastic character of the material under large deformations was further demonstrated by the increased stress relaxation observed under more rapid loading. This is seen for fresh tissue in Figs. 7 and 8. These figures show that, as the loading time decreased, the percent stress remaining at a given time also decreased; i.e., greater relaxation was observed. Decreasing the loading time from 10 s to 0.1 s significantly increased the observed relaxation by approximately 25% for fresh tissue and by 20% for glutaraldehyde treated tissue.

Both glutaraldehyde and epoxide treated materials were significantly more extensible than those from the other groups (Fig. 9). At a stress of 300 kPa, fresh tissue showed a mean strain

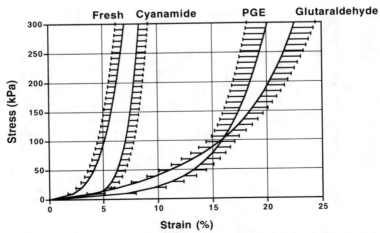

FIG. 9—*Stress-strain data at 1 Hz showed that both glutaraldehyde and poly (glycidyl ether) produced significant crosslinking of bovine pericardium while cyanamide did not* ($p < 0.001$). *The long, ramping shape of the curves for the crosslinked material reflects recovery of fixation shrinkage during loading.* n = 5 *for each group. Mean strain* ± *SE.*

of 7.0 ± 0.8% compared to a mean strain of 22.5 ± 1.9% for glutaraldehyde treated tissue and 20.1 ± 1.4% for epoxide treated tissue. The shapes of the curves were also affected by the aldehyde and epoxide treatments. Fresh tissue and cyanamide treated materials exhibited a rapid rise in stress with increasing strain after an initial low slope region; however, both the glutaraldehyde and epoxide treated tissues showed a long, ramping low stress response with a more gradual rise in stress with increasing strain. The tissue treatment also significantly affected the observed stress relaxation (Fig. 10). Epoxide treated and glutaraldehyde treated tissues showed significantly decreased relaxation compared to fresh tissue. At 100 s, the epoxide treated tissue showed the least relaxation with 80.6 ± 0.6% stress remaining (versus 66.4 ± 5.0% for fresh tissue). The cyanamide fixed tissue exhibited the greatest relaxation with 57.7 ± 6.0% stress remaining at 100 s—a value significantly different from those of all the other treatment groups.

In contrast to the marked viscoelastic behavior observed in stress relaxation and hysteresis experiments, the materials were surprisingly elastic in forced vibration, with the phase angle ϕ falling between 2 and 12° (Fig. 11). The small phase angles and the independence of phase angle on vibrational frequency were both in direct contrast with the increasing hysteresis observed with increasing frequency in the large deformations imposed in stress-strain testing. Comparison of calculated storage and loss moduli strongly illustrated the dominance of the elastic component under forced vibration: for all treatment groups, the loss modulus was less than 15% of the storage modulus. While the dynamic modulus increased with increasing mean load, reflecting the concave upward shape of the stress-strain curve, frequency of vibration had no effect on this parameter. Glutaraldehyde was the sole treatment to produce a significantly different (i.e., lower) dynamic modulus from those of the other treatment groups (Fig. 12).

Study 2: Comparison of Bovine and Porcine Pericardia

Objective

Bovine and porcine pericardium both have been used in the preparation of bioprosthetic materials [29,30]. However, since species-related differences in mechanical behavior have been suggested in the literature, we sought to determine whether such differences exist in the

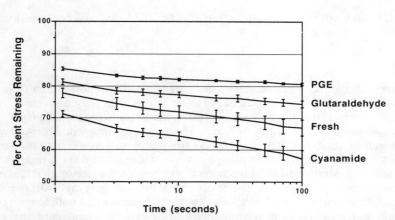

FIG. 10—*Crosslinking by glutaraldehyde and poly (glycidyl ether) both significantly reduced the observed stress relaxation under an initial load of 80 g, but did not alter the curve shape. Cyanamide treatment increased relaxation, perhaps indicating some destabilization of the collagen in the acid buffer. n = 5 for each group. Mean ± SE.*

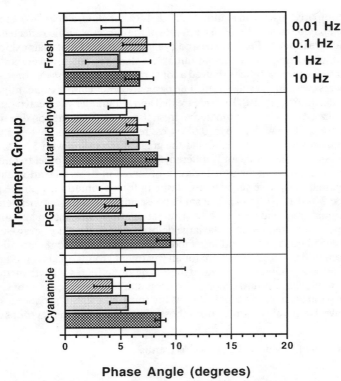

Phase Angle (degrees)

FIG. 11—*The phase angle ϕ measured at 80 g mean load was very small, indicating nearly elastic behavior in small deformations. The phase shift was independent of the applied frequency indicating that relaxation behavior extends to characteristic times at least as low as 0.1 s. n = 5 for each group. Mean ± SE.*

viscoelastic behavior of these two species in particular, and to examine the structural differences that underpin these properties.

Materials

Intact pericardia with enclosed hearts were harvested immediately post-mortem from calves and pigs (approximately 6 months old and 140 to 150 kg and 65 to 74 kg, respectively) at local abbatoirs. Pericardia and hearts were transported in Hanks physiological saline (pH 7.4, 310 mOs) and prepared for use promptly on return. The maximum time period between retrieval and completion of mechanical testing was 6 h. Ventral samples of tissue were cleaned, marked, and harvested as above: approximately 8 by 8 cm in calves, and 5 by 5 cm in pigs. Each specimen was subdivided into sections for mechanical, biochemical, and histological analysis. For mechanical testing, two 20 by 4 mm base-to-apex strips were cut from the center of each pericardial sheet. One strip from each heart was tested mechanically and both strips were then fixed in buffered formalin prior to preparation for histological analysis. A third strip was subjected to denaturation temperature testing. For collagen analysis, five specimens were taken with an 8-mm cork bore punch from the right and left upper and lower corners and the center of each sheet of pericardium. These specimens were then freeze-dried. The remaining tissue was sectioned into four pieces and used for determining the water content of the tissue and for subsequent collagen extractions and typing. The biochemical analysis and results have been described by Naimark et al. [*31*].

Results

Bovine pericardial tissue was both grossly more opaque than porcine tissue and significantly thicker (0.42 ± 0.01 mm versus 0.20 ± 0.01 mm, $p < 0.0005$). The thinner porcine tissues were also significantly less extensible than the bovine tissues ($p < 0.01$, Fig.13). At 1 Hz, porcine tissue (4.4 ± 0.5% strain at 300 kPa) was significantly less extensible than bovine tissue (8.9 ± 0.9% strain). This statistical trend was observed from 100 to 400 kPa and 0.1 to 10 Hz.

The frequency of cyclic loading had no significant effect on the stress-strain curves for either species, although there was again an overall shift to the left with increased frequency. For example, the mean strain for bovine tissue at 1.0 Hz was 8.9 ± 0.9%, decreasing to 7.9 ± 0.7% at 10 Hz.

In forced vibration, the magnitude of the dynamic modulus (E^*) also varied significantly with species ($p = 0.0001$, Fig. 14) regardless of initial load or frequency of vibration. Since a

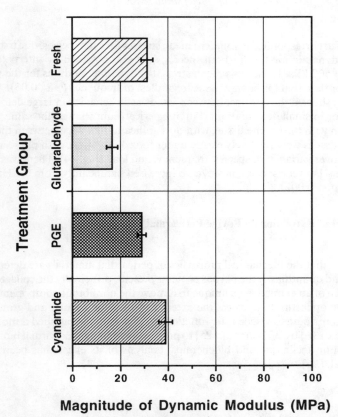

FIG. 12—*The magnitude of the dynamic modulus |E*| under 80 g mean load was only altered significantly by glutaraldehyde treatment (*p < 0.05*). n = 5 for each group. Mean ± SE.*

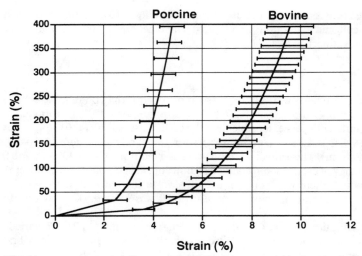

FIG. 13—*The thinner porcine pericardium was significantly less extensible than the thicker bovine pericardium (p < 0.01). n = 8 for each group. Mean strain ± SE.*

given mean load corresponded to different mean stresses for each species, due to the differences in thickness, dynamic moduli for both species were also obtained by interpolation under a mean stress of 500 kPa. Under this mean stress, the dynamic modulus for the porcine tissue was 40% larger than that for bovine tissue, regardless of frequency ($p < 0.05$).

Both tissues showed the contrast between viscoelastic behavior in large deformations and elastic behavior in small deformations. Porcine pericardium showed the same marked stress relaxation seen with the bovine tissue, with no significant difference between the two species. As well, both tissues were relatively elastic under forced vibration, with phase angles ranging from 4 to 20° over variables of species, frequency, and load (Fig. 14). There was no difference in phase angle ϕ between species; however, ϕ increased significantly from 0.1 Hz to 10 Hz for both species ($p < 0.002$).

Study 3: Effect of Extraction on Bovine Pericardial Materials

Objective

It is assumed that the mechanical properties of pericardial materials are determined by the architecture and quantities of the fibrous proteins present, principally the collagen and elastin. The application of an extractive technique to remove the nonfibrous components of the tissue offers a unique opportunity to assess the extent to which the cellular and ground substance components contribute to viscoelastic function. In this study, we applied a modified version of the technique used by Wilson et al. [25] to prepare an acellular pericardial biomaterial. This gentler extraction technique and biochemical analysis of its effects has been described by Courtman et al. [26].

Materials

Seventeen hearts with intact pericardia were obtained fresh from slaughter of 6 to 9 month old calves. The hearts were transported to the laboratory in phosphate buffered saline at room temperature. Ventral rectangular samples approximately 5 cm by 5 cm were harvested from each heart as previously described. Each pericardial specimen was divided into two sections: the first analyzed fresh and the second analyzed after cell extraction. Samples from nine hearts went through mechanical analysis and denaturation temperature testing, while samples from eight hearts went through biochemical analysis.

Results

After extraction, the pericardial materials were 25% thicker; however, there was no significant change in the collagen denaturation temperature from the fresh tissue. The stress-strain results for the fresh and extracted tissues were also not statistically separable. While the stress-strain behavior of the acellular pericardial material remained strain rate independent, the slight decrease in extensibility with increasing strain rate became more consistent. Forced vibration tests also showed no significant differences between fresh and extracted materials (Fig. 15). In both materials, dynamic moduli increased with increasing mean load (reflecting

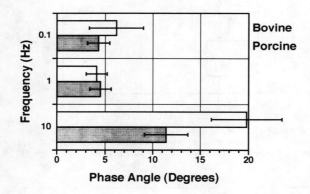

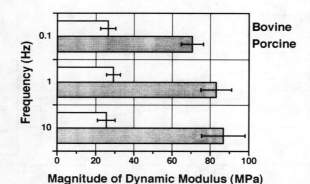

FIG. 14—(a) *Forced vibration testing showed no differences in the phase angle* φ *between bovine and porcine pericardium. While* φ *increased significantly at 10 Hz, the large value for bovine tissue at 10 Hz appears to be an anomaly not seen in the other studies presented here.* (b) *A difference between the two species was seen in the magnitude of the dynamic modulus* |E*|, *shown here for 80 g mean load. Porcine tissue was significantly stiffer in vibration (*p < 0.0005). n = 8 *for each group.*

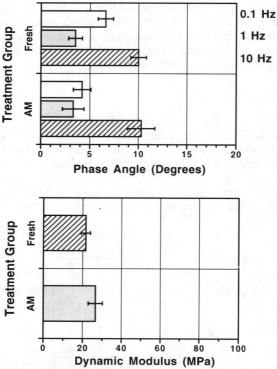

FIG. 15—*Neither the magnitude of the dynamic modulus* |E*| *(shown for 80 g mean load, 1 Hz) nor the phase angle* φ *(shown for 80 g mean load) for bovine pericardium were altered by the extraction process. ACM = acellular matrix, the extracted material.* n = 9 *for each group. Mean ± SE.*

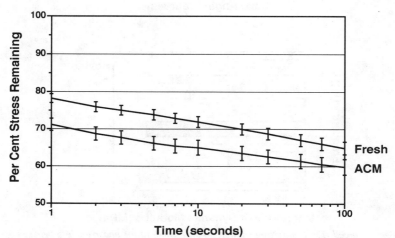

FIG. 16—*The stress relaxation behavior for bovine pericardium was the only mechanical parameter altered by the extraction process. The extracted material relaxed slightly but significantly more rapidly than did the fresh material (*$p < 0.05$*); however, the curve shape was retained. ACM = acellular matrix, the extracted material.* n = 9 *for each group. Mean ± SE.*

the concave upward shape of the stress-strain curve) and phase angle significantly increased at 10 Hz (compared to 0.1 or 1 Hz). However, in stress relaxation tests at either initial load, fresh tissues were more elastic than extracted tissues, showing 64.9 ± 1.7% stress remaining after 100 s compared to 59.9 ± 2.1% remaining in the extracted tissues ($p < 0.05$, Fig. 16). This slight change in relaxation behavior was the only mechanical effect of extraction that was observed.

Discussion

The results of the three studies presented in this paper present a consistent picture of the viscoelastic behavior of pericardial biomaterials. First, it is clear that these materials are substantially more viscoelastic in large deformations than was previously believed on the basis of low strain rate studies. Stress relaxation results showed that, if the loading time is reduced from 10 s to 0.1 s, then the percent loss of stress over 100 s increases from 17% to 33%. While in the former case we might consider the material to be reasonably elastic, we cannot hold this to be the case when the material loses fully one third of its initial stress over this relatively short period. The ability to load the samples in as little as 0.1 s is therefore critical. To appreciate the amount of relaxation that occurred over a single decade of time, one need only consider the vertical spacing between the curves in Fig. 8. The space between the curve for 0.1-s loading time and that for 1-s loading time shows that a significant amount of relaxation occurred during the extra 0.9 s required to reach maximum load in the latter experiment. Indeed, the importance of relaxation on a time scale of tenths of a second is confirmed by the large hysteresis loops seen in stress-strain studies at 10 Hz when compared to those at lower frequencies. In earlier stress relaxation studies (including our own [8,10,11]), where loading times were of the order of seconds, much of this relaxation behavior could not be observed; it occurred instead during loading and must have been expressed in the stress-strain curves as lower stress values at any given strain.

This viscoelasticity under large deformations must be contrasted with: (1) the quite elastic behavior under small deformations, and (2) the apparent independence of the stress-strain curve on strain rate (or loading time). In forced vibration, the phase angle ϕ is a good indicator of the degree of viscoelastic behavior since $\tan(\phi)$ is the ratio of the loss or viscous modulus E_L to the storage or elastic modulus E_S. The ϕ values seen in these studies were very small, lying in the range of 3 to 10°. This behavior is as elastic as that observed in the aorta [32]—a structure that we consider to be quite elastic. When compared to small vibrations, large deformations of the collagen/elastin network in these materials may produce greater shearing of the glycosaminoglycan matrix, and thus greater viscous losses. Alternatively, larger deformations of the fiber bundles themselves may have significant associated energetic losses. In either case, the extraction experiments have confirmed that the cellular components or loosely associated proteinaceous materials do not play a significant role. The independence of the stress-strain curves on strain rate—over time scales where significant relaxation behavior is observed—indicates that the viscoelastic behavior of these materials is not linear. The glycosaminoglycan hydrogel matrix surrounding the fibers likely displays both gel/sol transitional behavior (thixotropy) and decreasing viscosity with increasing shear rate (pseudoplasticity) [33]. Some combination of these behaviors would allow for both significant relaxation and hysteresis and for the observed strain rate independence.

In each of the stress relaxation curves presented, the curve on a $\log_{10}$ of time scale was nearly linear. In either linear or quasi-linear viscoelastic modeling [34], this curve shape is not describable using any discrete spring and dashpot model, including that suggested by Trowbridge in arguing that glutaraldehyde treated pericardium could be viewed as functionally elastic [8,35]. Discrete characteristic relaxation times produce discrete falls in the reduced relaxation function $G(t)$ (approximated in the present studies as $G(t) \approx \sigma(t)/\sigma_0$). Instead, the present curve must be described using a continuous relaxation spectrum with a constant spectral density $H(\log_{10}(t))$. In a quasi-linear model, and on a $\log_{10}$ time scale, the stress/time curve $\sigma(t)$ is related to the imposed strain/time curve $\varepsilon(t)$ through a convolution equation of the form

$$\sigma(t) = \int\limits_{\tau=0}^{t} G(t - \tau) \frac{d\sigma_E(\varepsilon)}{d\varepsilon} \frac{d\varepsilon}{d\tau} d\tau$$

where $\sigma_E(\varepsilon)$ is the assumed elastic stress-strain curve which would be observed under instantaneous loading and $d\varepsilon(t)/dt$ is the imposed strain rate, the derivative of $\varepsilon(t)$ [36]. The function $G(t)$ will in turn be linear when plotted against $\log_{10}t$ if the spectral density $H(\log_{10}(t))$ has the form of a box relaxation spectrum which has both constant density and minimum and maximum characteristic relaxation times τ_{min} and τ_{max}. From the present studies, there is no evidence of the flattening of the relaxation curve at long or short times; that is, no indications of the presence of end points to the spectrum. From other experiments, we know that relaxation continues to occur over at least 16 h, albeit very slowly. We must also assume that relaxation also occurs over time frames less than 0.1 s and that even the present relaxation data underestimate the viscoelastic character of these materials. Calculation of the viscoelastic strains resulting from strains applied to these materials remains difficult and must rely on box spectra which describe at least the experimental behavior.

Use of a servohydraulic testing system to measure the behavior of these materials at high strain rates posed several technical problems. First, the use of low load cells (250 g or 1 kg) on the Instron load frame introduced significant frame resonance noise into the load signal. While the 5th order Butterworth filter at 100 Hz provided a very sharp cutoff to the higher frequency noise, its use precluded decreasing loading times a further decade to 0.01 s. Second, the large phase angles and hysteresis losses which we first observed at 10 Hz were eventually reduced by correction for sequential sampling of displacement and load signals and for the phase shift from the Butterworth filter. However, before believing even the present data, we were forced to perform a variety of control experiments with more elastic materials, with and without the water bath, and with added masses to confound system resonances. We are now convinced that the increase in ϕ at 10 Hz is real. Third, experiments at 10 Hz precluded the use of video-based dimension measurements to measure central deflections in the specimen (as opposed to the grip-to-grip deflections measured with the LVDT). Video interlace is limited to 60 Hz, yielding only 6 data points per cycle and no hope of resolving phase differences. While we are currently experimenting with high frame rate modified video with an interlace of 240 Hz over one quarter of the screen, these units can still only resolve a phase shift of 15° at 10 Hz. Fortunately, from low strain rate experiments with microscopically imaged specimens on a micro-tensile tester, we have evidence to suggest that the central strains in our specimens do not differ significantly from the grip-to-grip mean strain and feel somewhat reassured about our strain data.

Other than the rapid deformations attainable, the present servohydraulic testing system offered another important advantage over the use of screw-driven equipment or even stepper motor type systems. Since the testing machine was controlled using an electronic waveform generator, it was possible to specify with precision the loading time or frequency of cyclic loading in each experiment. In our earlier experiments, the screw-driven systems operated at chosen deflection rates (cross-head speeds); e.g., 10 mm/min. This meant that an extensible glutaraldehyde treated specimen took much longer to extend the sample to an 80 g load than did a less extensible specimen of fresh tissue. This difference in loading times would distort the observed stress relaxation behavior—over and above the problems associated with overall slow loading. In the relaxation experiments presented here, all specimens were extended to their initial load in 0.1 s, regardless of extensibility, and this distortion was avoided.

In the present experiments, our testing protocol applied three types of deformation (large deformation cycling, stress relaxation, and forced vibration tests) in a set order, as opposed to a randomized order of application. It is well understood that in soft, viscoelastic materials, the mechanical properties of the material are functions of the loading history. Indeed, over ten years ago we made it clear that the stress-strain behavior of canine pericardium was necessarily altered during stress relaxation or creep experiments [35]. With this understanding, we feel that testing with a fixed order protocol produces the most reproducible results in the sense that, by duplicating the protocol, another worker could measure the same parameters in a material that was in the same state (in terms of loading history). Nonetheless, differences in mechanical behavior will exist between the material on first extension and that same material after extensive testing. This problem has been the subject of much discussion between those workers who favor preconditioning to establish a reproducible (but potentially artifactual) state in the tissue and those who favor examination only of materials with no previous extension history. It is fair to say that no consensus has been reached on this issue, but we prefer the definition of a conditioned specimen and have been careful to repeat the preconditioning step between tests.

A second advantage to the use of a fixed preconditioning and testing regime may be that it reduces the sample sizes required to reach statistically supportable conclusions. Randomization of the testing order may introduce added variations in mechanical parameters (due to differences in the state of the tissue during testing) increasing sample size requirements. In our experience with the present regimen, standard errors of approximately 10% of the mean can be achieved using sample sizes of 5 to 8. This variation is not substantially decreased by increasing the sample size to 20; indeed, nested analysis of variance has shown that our experimental scatter primarily reflects animal-to-animal differences in the tissue samples, over differences either measurement-to-measurement on the same specimen or specimen-to-specimen within the same animal. As a result, the power of our experiments is typically limited to detection of differences of about 20% in a given parameter, differences large enough to be distinguished despite interanimal variation.

While high strain rate studies have provided new insights into the large deformation/small deformation viscoelastic behavior of these materials, those characteristics have been surprisingly similar under crosslinking, across species, and after biochemical extraction. For instance, the mechanical results of Study 1 largely confirmed the conclusions reached by Pereira et al. [20] using low strain rates. Only the forced vibration results provided new insights since they were not part of the earlier protocol. Specifically, the decrease in relaxation produced by crosslinking was unaccompanied by any decrease in the forced vibration phase angle—a result expected under linear or quasi-linear viscoelasticity. Again, this observation emphasizes that the viscoelastic behavior of these materials is nonlinear and strongly influenced by the magnitude of the imposed deformations. The mechanical effect of crosslinking is apparently most strongly expressed in large deformations where significant unfolding of collagen crimp and collapse of the fiber network toward the direction of the applied stress would be expected.

In Study 2, high strain rate testing showed that the viscoelastic characteristics of the pericardia from the two species were strikingly similar. Stress relaxation and phase angles in forced vibration were not significantly different between species. These observations were in contrast to the hypothesis set forth by Lee and Boughner [11] that differences in thickness (at least between dogs and humans) were due to differences in collagen/water content, the thicker pericardia having more water and less collagen per unit volume. They felt that the increased water content would then be expressed in increased stress relaxation (as they observed with human tissue). In the present case, bovine and porcine pericardia were shown by Naimark and coworkers [31] to have equivalent water and collagen contents, and indeed the viscoelastic behaviors were nearly identical. The significant differences between species were found instead in the stress-strain curves and in the dynamic moduli under forced vibration; that is, in the characteristics best equated with elastic stiffness. Naimark et al. showed that these differences correlated best with differences in the content of crosslinked type III collagen—a result unpredicted in the literature. The role of high strain rate testing in these studies has clearly been only to disprove the former hypothesis regarding collagen/water content. The differences actually observed did not require new methods. While the dynamic modulus results were confirmatory, the difference in elastic stiffness between bovine and porcine pericardia would have been observable using low strain rate methods.

The gentle extraction of cellular components from the pericardium (as was performed in Study 3) similarly produced very little change in viscoelastic function, the sole exception being a slight increase in stress relaxation. We may infer that, since the linear stress relaxation curves in Fig. 16 are nearly parallel from one second onward, the difference in relaxation behavior occurred over yet shorter time periods. Again, the nonlinearity (magnitude dependence) of the viscoelastic behavior is confounding since we see no difference in phase angle ϕ at either 1 Hz or 10 Hz to confirm this inference. The overall retention of viscoelastic behavior through extraction strongly suggests that the structural elements which are important in determining viscoelastic function are either the fibers themselves or tightly enough bound to this network to resist an extraction process which Courtman et al. [26] showed removed the vast bulk of cellular components.

The high strain rate testing methods described in this paper and used in the three reviewed studies have provided new insights into the nature of the viscoelastic behavior of pericardial biomaterials. These materials are seen to be significantly viscoelastic in large deformations, but markedly elastic in small deformations. This contrast, in combination with the strain rate independence of the stress-strain curves, indicates that these materials possess nonlinear viscoelastic behavior. Description of the viscoelastic behavior is further complicated by the requirement for the use of a continuous relaxation spectrum, even in a simplified linear model. It is perhaps most interesting that these properties are preserved with crosslinking, across species, and after cellular extraction, and that many structural/mechanical linkages may be established in simpler experiments that do not require this more complicated experimental approach.

Acknowledgments

The authors wish to express their thanks to David Abdulla, Technical Coordinator, Centre for Biomaterials, for his invaluable technical help with apparatus design and construction. Thanks are also due to Dr. David Cheung, University of Southern California, and Dr. Hardy Limeback, University of Toronto for their guidance and collaboration in the biochemical analyses for comparison of bovine and porcine pericardia. Special thanks are extended to Villa Kashef and Donna McComb, The Hospital for Sick Children, for the biochemical analysis and extraction of the acellular pericardial materials, respectively. This work was supported by grants to Dr. Lee from the Natural Sciences and Engineering Research Council of Canada (NSERC), the Canadian Heart and Stroke Foundation, and the Ontario Centre for Materials Research (OCMR), and to Dr. Wilson from the Medical Research Council of Canada (MRC).

References

[1] Jünemann, M., Smiseth, O. A., Refsum, H., et al., "Quantification of Effect of Pericardium on LV Diastolic PV Relations in Dogs," *American Journal of Physiology,* Vol. 252, 1987, H963–H968.

[2] Gabbay, S., Kadam, P., Factor, S., and Cheung, T. K., "Do Heart Valve Bioprostheses Degenerate for Metabolic or Mechanical Reasons?" *Journal of Thoracic and Cardiovascular Surgery*, Vol. 95, 1988, pp. 208–215.

[3] Gonzalez-Lavin, L., Gonzalez-Lavin, J., Chi, S., et al., "The Pericardial Valve in the Aortic Position Ten Years Later," *Journal of Thoracic and Cardiovascular Surgery*, Vol. 101, 1991, pp. 75–80.

[4] Chauvaud, S., Jebara, V., Chachques, J. C., et al., "Valve Extension with Glutaraldehyde-Preserved Autologous Pericardium: Results in Mitral Valve Repair," *Journal of Thoracic and Cardiovascular Surgery*, Vol. 102, 1991, pp. 171–177.

[5] Salles, C. A., Puig, L. B., Casagrande, I. S., et al., "Early Experience with Crimped Bovine Pericardial Conduit for Arterial Reconstruction," *European Journal of Cardio-thoracic Surgery*, Vol. 5, 1991, pp. 273–278.

[6] Bunton, R. W., Zabregas, A. A., and Miller, A. P., "Pericardial Closure After Cardiac Operations: An Animal Study to Assess Currently Available Materials with Particular Reference to Their Suitability for Use After Coronary Artery Bypass Surgery," *Journal of Thoracic and Cardiovascular Surgery*, Vol. 100, 1990, pp. 99–107.

[7] Haluck, R. S., Richenbacher, W. E., Myers, J. L., et al., "Pericardium as a Thoracic Aortic Patch: Glutaraldehyde-Fixed and Fresh Autologous Pericardium," *Journal of Surgical Research*, Vol. 48, 1990, pp. 611–614.

[8] Trowbridge, E. A., Black, M. M., and Daniel, C. L., "The Mechanical Response of Glutaraldehyde-Fixed Bovine Pericardium to Uniaxial Load," *Journal of Materials Science*, Vol. 20, 1985, pp. 114–140.

[9] Wiegner, A. W., Bing, H. L., Borg, T. K., and Caulfield, J. B., "Mechanical and Structural Correlates of Canine Pericardium," *Circulation Research*, Vol. 49, 1981, pp. 807–814.

[10] Lee, J. M., Haberer, S. A., and Boughner, D. R., "The Bovine Pericardial Xenograft: I. Effect of Fixation in Aldehydes Without Constraint on the Tensile Viscoelastic Properties of Bovine Pericardium," *Journal of Biomedical Materials Research*, Vol. 23, 1989, pp. 457–475.

[11] Lee, J. M. and Boughner, D. R., "Mechanical Properties of Human Pericardium: Differences in Viscoelastic Response Compared with Canine Pericardium," *Circulation Research*, Vol. 55, 1985, pp. 475–481.

[12] Cohn, D., Younes, H., Milgarter, E., and Uretsky, G., "Mechanical Behavior of Isolated Pericardium: Species, Isotropy, Strain Rate, and Collagenase Effect on Pericardial Tissue," *Clinical Materials*, Vol. 2, 1987, pp. 115–124.

[13] Lee, M. C., Fung, Y. C., Shabetai, R., and LeWinter, M. M., "Biaxial Mechanical Properties of Human Pericardium and Canine Comparisons," *American Journal of Physiology*, Vol. 253, 1987, H75–H82.

[14] Vito, R. P., "The Mechanical Properties of Soft Tissues—I: A Mechanical System for Biaxial Testing," *Journal of Biomechanics*, Vol. 13, 1980, pp. 947–950.

[15] Missirlis, Y. F. and Armeniades, C. D., "Stress Analysis of the Aortic Valve During Diastole: Important Parameters," *Journal of Biomechanics*, Vol. 9, 1976, pp. 477–480.

[16] Gong, G., Ling, Z., Seifter, E., et al., "Aldehyde Tanning: The Villain in Bioprosthetic Calcification," *European Journal of Cardio-thoracic Surgery*, Vol. 5, 1991, pp. 288–299.

[17] Golomb, G., Schoen, F. J., Smith, M. S., et al., "The Role of Glutaraldehyde-Induced Cross-Links in Calcification of Bovine Pericardium Used in Cardiac Valve Bioprostheses," *American Journal of Pathology*, Vol. 127, 1987, pp. 122–130.

[18] Vesely, I., Boughner, D. R., and Song, T., "Tissue Buckling as a Mechanism of Bioprosthetic Valve Failure," *Annals of Thoracic Surgery*, Vol. 46, 1988, pp. 302–308.

[19] Imamura, E., Sawatani, O., Koyanagi, H., et al., "Epoxy Compounds as a New Cross-Linking Agent for Porcine Aortic Valve Leaflets: Subcutaneous Implant Studies in Rats," *Journal of Cardiac Surgery*, Vol. 4, 1989, pp. 50–57.

[20] Pereira, C. A., Lee, J. M., and Haberer, S. A., "Effect of Alternative Crosslinking Methods on the Low Strain Rate Viscoelastic Properties of Bovine Pericardial Bioprosthetic Materials," *Journal of Biomedical Materials Research*, Vol. 24, 1990, pp. 345–361.

[21] Van Gulik, T. M., Christiano, R. A., Broekhuizen, A. H., et al., "A Tanned, Sheep Dermal Collagen Graft as a Dressing for Split-Skin Graft Donor Sites," *Netherlands Journal of Surgery*, Vol. 41, 1989, pp. 65–67.

[22] Weadock, K., Olsen, R. M., and Silver, F. H., "Evaluation of Collagen Crosslinking Techniques," *Biomaterials, Medical Devices, and Artificial Organs*, Vol. 11, 1983–4, pp. 293–318.

[23] Milthorpe, B. K., True, K., Sun, L., and Schindhelm, K., "Quantitative Histological Evaluation of Crosslinked Kangaroo Tail Tendon: Progress and Problems," (abstract) *Proceedings of the 9th European Conference on Biomaterials*, 1991, p. 11.

[24] Malone, J. M., Brendel, K., Duhamel, R. C., and Reinert, R. L., "Detergent-Extracted Small-Diameter Vascular Prostheses," *Journal of Vascular Surgery*, Vol. 1, 1984, pp. 181–191.

[25] Wilson, G. J., Yeger, H., Klement, P., et al., "Acellular Matrix Allograft Small Caliber Vascular Prostheses," *Transactions of the American Society for Artificial Internal Organs,* Vol. 36, 1990, M340–M343.

[26] Courtman, D. W., Pereira, C. A., Kashef, V., et al., "Development of a Pericardial Acellular Matrix Biomaterial: Effects of Cell Extraction and Fixation," *Journal of Biomedical Materials Research,* in press.

[27] Haberer, S. A., Lee, J. M., and Pereira, C. A., "High Strain Rate Viscoelastic Properties of Bovine Pericardial Xenograft Materials: Effect of Fixation in Alternative Crosslinking Agents," submitted for publication in *Journal of Biomechanics,* 1992.

[28] Trowbridge, E. A. and Crofts, C. E., "The Standardization of Gauge Length: Its Influence on the Relative Extensibility of Natural and Chemically Modified Pericardium," *Journal of Biomechanics,* Vol. 19, 1986, pp. 1023–1033.

[29] Fentie, I. H., Allen, D. J., Schenck, M. H., and Didio, L.J.A., "Comparative Electron Microscopic Study of Bovine, Porcine, and Human Parietal Pericardium as Materials for Cardiac Valve Bioprostheses,"*Journal of Submicroscopic Cytology,* Vol. 18, 1986, pp. 53–65.

[30] Lauridsen, P., Jacobsen, J. R., and Wennevold, A., "Suitability of Stabilized Porcine Pericardium as Baffle in the Mustard Operation for Transposition of the Great Arteries," in *Biologic & Bioprosthetic Valves,* E. Bodnar and M. Yacoub, Eds., Yorke Medical Books, London, 1986, pp. 677–683.

[31] Naimark, W. A., Lee, J. M., Limeback, H., and Cheung, D. T., "Correlation of Structure and Viscoelastic Properties in the Pericardia of Four Mammalian Species," *American Journal of Physiology,* Vol. 263, 1992, H1095–1106.

[32] Imura, T., Yamamoto, K., Satoh, T., et al., "In vivo Viscoelastic Behavior in the Human Aorta," *Circulation Research,* Vol. 66, 1990, pp. 1413–1419.

[33] Finlay, J. B., "Thixotropy in Human Skin," *Journal of Biomechanics,* Vol. 11, 1978, pp. 333–342.

[34] Fung, Y. C., *Biomechanics: Mechanical Properties of Living Tissues,* Springer-Verlag, New York, 1981.

[35] Lee, J. M. and Boughner, D. R., "Bioprosthetic Heart Valves: Tissue Mechanics and Implications for Design," in: *Blood Compatible Materials and Devices: Perspectives Towards the 21st Century,* C. P. Sharma and M. Szycher, Eds., Technomic Publishing Co., Lancaster, 1991, pp. 167–188.

[36] Ward, I. M., *Mechanical Properties of Solid Polymers (2nd ed.),* John Wiley & Sons, Toronto, 1983, pp. 79–165.

S. H. Teoh,¹ S. C. Lim,¹ E. T. Yoon,¹ and K. S. Goh²

A New Method for *In-Vitro* Wear Assessment of Materials Used in Mechanical Heart Valves

REFERENCE: Teoh, S. H., Lim, S. C., Yoon, E. T., and Goh, K. S., "A New Method for *In-Vitro* Wear Assessment of Materials Used in Mechanical Heart Valves," *Biomaterials' Mechanical Properties, ASTM STP 1173,* H. E. Kambic and A. T. Yokobori, Jr., Eds., American Society for Testing and Materials, Philadelphia, 1994, pp. 43–52.

ABSTRACT: Accelerated life testing has been in use for a number of years to study the long-term *in-vitro* durability of heart valves. These tests were designed to test concurrently the durability of the materials and design of the heart valves. However, problems interpreting the results and relating them to actual clinical applications were encountered. Current view is that the life testing of mechanical heart valves can best be performed by partitioning the *in-vitro* wear assessment of the material separate from that due to the overall design of the heart valve. A new method, simulating the impact-cum-sliding action in mechanical heart valves, at a low frequency, was developed to test a variety of candidate materials: polyoxymethylene (Delrin), polyetheretherketone (PEEK), polyethersulphone (PES), and ultrahigh molecular weight polyethylene (UHMWPE). The results were compared with those reported earlier in published literature. The damage features seen on the different test specimens and the wear debris produced were similar to those found on an explanted heart valve of more than 17 years old, supporting that the present technique could simulate the wear conditions in mechanical heart valves. The technique saved time and was amenable to wear mechanisms study using the scanning electron microscope (SEM). The wear results showed that, in terms of maximum wear depth, UHMWPE wore the least followed by Delrin, PEEK, and PES. There does not appear to be any correlation between wear and the molecular weight of Delrin. The incorporation of 0.3% carbon did not improve the wear performance of Delrin. Both UHMWPE and PES produced debris that were significantly larger than the rest. Because of the possibility of dislodgement of large debris in the range of 100 μm or more, UHMWPE was not considered to be a good material for use as occluder in mechanical heart valves even though it wore the least. At present, Delrin is still considered to be the best occluder material examined. PEEK showed good potential but longer experiments need to be carried out in order to show its full potentiality. PES showed the worst wear characteristics.

KEYWORDS: wear, mechanical heart valves, accelerated life-test, impact-cum-sliding, Delrin, polyetheretherketone (PEEK), polyethersulphone (PES), ultrahigh molecular weight polyethylene (UHMWPE)

Accelerated life testing of prosthetic heart valves has been in use for a number of years to study the long-term *in-vitro* durability of cardiac valves [*1–3*]. This type of test is particularly useful in relative comparisons of performance of different cardiac valves where materials and design of the heart valves need to be evaluated together. However, many problems are encountered, most of which are related to interpreting the results and relating them to actual clinical applications. Often the equipment itself may fail due to fatigue fracture before the required cycles of testing are reached. A typical duration of test for an equivalent 10 years service life is

¹ Senior lecturers and research scholar, respectively, Mechanical and Production Engineering Department, National University of Singapore, Singapore 0511.
² R&D manager, St. Vincent's Meditech Pte. Ltd., Singapore Science Park, Singapore 0511.

about 8 months at 15 Hz. This is a long time to wait for material wear evaluation. One could increase the frequency of testing in order to speed up the process. However, recently [4] we have noted that this may not be good because the mechanism of wear has been changed drastically. Materials like titanium, which is a common metal used in cardiac valves, form a layer of protective film in the presence of oxygen and if this passive film is removed faster than it could form, the material will fail prematurely by a mechanism related to environmental stress cracking. Furthermore, a reasonable amount of time in between impacts for the polymer to relax just like an actual implanted occluder needs to be considered when one tries to simulate the actual wear in *in-vivo* situations for polymeric materials. The other problem is due to the fact that the area of wear is not constant throughout the duration of testing; hence, there is difficulty to specify a unique area for wear measurement. By examining the closing and opening of a mechanical heart valve it can be realized that there are two important mechanisms: one of impact of the occluder against the supports' strut and one of sliding between these two. We have therefore decided to assess the wear aspects of the material separately from the design of mechanical heart valves by designing an impact-cum-sliding mechanism of wear between the titanium and the disc occluder on a fix contact area and reducing the frequency of testing to well below 5 Hz to take into account the relaxation of the polymer and reduce the possibility of introducing other mechanisms when testing at a higher frequency.

Wear of Biomedical Polymers

In biomedical applications such as occluders in mechanical heart valves [5] and joint prostheses, wear of the biomedical polymers has been considered an important factor in determining the durability of the prostheses. Factors influencing the wear properties of ultrahigh molecular weight polyethylene (UHMWPE), which has been used in many hip joint prostheses, were examined by Trainor and Haward [6]. Their results indicated that a significant improvement in wear (using pin-on-plate or rotating shaft-on-plate system in a medium of distilled water) behavior was obtained by molding the UHMWPE between 190 and 200°C. The addition of some antioxidants also appeared to improve the wear resistance. Molding at higher pressures and increasing the molecular weight were reported to be detrimental. Nonetheless, there is a possibility that there could be an optimum processing condition and molecular weight distribution that could give the best wear characteristics. Work was carried out to study the wear and degradation of retrieved polymeric implants [7]. This interesting piece of work examined 30 implants ranging from UHMWPE to silicone occluders. Wear mechanisms related to abrasive wear and environmental stress cracking between the incompletely sintered UHMWPE powder were reported. For polymeric valve occluders, abrasive wear was predominant. Such conclusions were also reported for polyacetal (Delrin) [5–9] and pyrolytic carbon [5]. In a recent examination [5] of an explanted valve (Björk-Shiley Delrin Disc mechanical heart valve) which had been in a patient for more than 17 years (the longest reported *in-vivo* wear of a Delrin occluder), abrasive and static wear marks, arising from plastic deformation and surface material flow (Fig. 1) and polymer debris adhesion on the metallic struts were observed. The work by Clarke and McKellop [10] should also be mentioned. They compared the wear of Delrin 150 with UHMWPE, polyester, and Teflon® (PTFE). A pin (polymer)-on-disc (316 stainless steel) in bovine serum solution was used. Their results indicated that Delrin, polyester, and PTFE wear 60, 2576, and 4986 times more than UHMWPE, respectively. However, Shen and Dumbelton [11] reported that Delrin wore less than UHMWPE. Although no conclusive reason was offered then, it is highly possible that the UHMWPE used by each of them was different since a difference as high as 100 times in mean wear rate was reported for the different UHMWPE tested by Trainor and Haward [6]. Such differences prompted a detail specification for the processing UHMWPE (ASTM F 648, Specification for Ultra-High-Molecular-Weight-Polyethylene Powder and Fabricated Form for Surgical Implants).

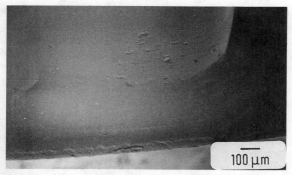

FIG. 1—*Scanning electron micrograph of an explanted Björk-Shiley Delrin Disc mechanical heart valve (17 yrs. 5 mos.) showing the static wear mark, surface material flow, deformation, and some debris in the worn area* [8].

The above findings indicated that wear of biomedical polymers is a complex problem and the mechanisms of *in-vivo* wear may be very different from those performed *in-vitro*. However, if the actual wear characteristics can be reproduced in the *in-vitro* experiments in terms of the environment and mode of deformation, then *in-vitro* experiments can prove to be very useful in cost and also in elucidating the actual wear mechanisms.

This paper reports on a new method of *in-vitro* wear assessment of materials used in mechanical heart valves by simulating the impact-cum-sliding action as experienced in the actual closing and opening of mechanical heart valves. Materials such as Delrin, UHMWPE, polyethersulphone (PES), and polyetheretherketone (PEEK) were tested. PES and PEEK are relatively new and are stiff polymers with high temperature durability and may prove useful in biomedical applications [12,13]. However, their wear properties relative to Delrin and UHMWPE need to be studied. Also of interest is the relationship between molecular weight of Delrin and its wear characteristics against titanium. The effect of incorporation of a small amount of carbon on wear in Delrin is also investigated.

Experimental Procedure

Materials

Four types of thermoplastic materials were used: Delrin, PEEK, PES, and UHMWPE. The Delrin was supplied by E.I. DuPont de Nemours & Co. Four different grades of Delrin were used, namely, Delrin 100, 500, 900, and BK602. Their molecular weights (except BK602) are shown in Table 1. BK602 is the same as Delrin 500 except it has 0.3% carbon incorporated in it. All the Delrin came in as pellets and were injection-molded into rectangular plates (21 by 124 by 2 mm) using fan gating system in an Arburg injection molding machine. Both PEEK and PES were supplied by ICI Advance Materials and coded as Victrex PEEK 450G (high

TABLE 1—*Molecular weights of different grades of Delrin.*

Polymer, M_w	Number Average, M_n	Weight Average
Delrin 900	30 000	60 000
500	40 000	80 000
100	70 000	140 000

molecular weight and high melt viscosity) and 4800G, respectively. These were supplied in square plates (125 by 125 by 3 mm). They were injection-molded using a flash gate system. The UHMWPE was supplied in 76.2 mm (3 in.) diameter rod form by Poly-Hi Menaha Corporation, USA and made to comply to ASTM F 648. The original raw powder was from Amer Hoescht and designated 415 GUR. For the counter surface, high-purity titanium (ASTM Grade 2) was used throughout the experiment.

Impact-Cum-Sliding Wear Test

In an effort to simulate the wear in the mechanical heart valves involving a tilting disc, an impact-cum-sliding wet wear test apparatus (Fig. 2a) was developed. The mechanism used to achieve this impact-cum-sliding action is illustrated in Fig. 2b. A specially designed cam was machined and this executed the impact-cum-sliding motion via a rotating shaft that was connected to a motor. The philosophy behind this design was that one can accelerate the wear by increasing the stiffness of the restraining spring without having to increase the frequency of the test. Important to note was that the area of contact was always constant for each cycle. The test assembly was housed in a perspex test chamber with deionized water at 37 ± 1°C to simulate the body temperature. The titanium plunger was made to slide over a short distance on

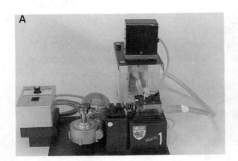
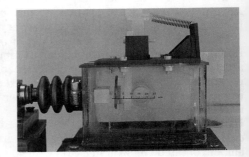

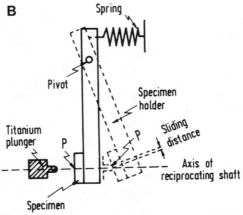

FIG. 2—(a) *Pictorial view of the impact-cum-sliding wear test rig used for material wear assessment in* mechanical heart valves. (b) *Schematic view of the impact-cum-sliding mechanism.*

the plastic test specimen after impact as a result of the movement of the specimen holder about its pivot. The restraining spring caused the specimen to swing quickly back to its original position after each impact. The restraining spring exerted an average force of 4 N. The titanium plunger was connected to a reciprocating arm rotating at a frequency of 3 Hz. The frequency of impact could be adjusted easily by the rotational speed of a cam which was designed specifically to give an impact-cum-sliding motion. It was ideal to have the tester work at 1 Hz; however, this would make the tests unduly lengthy. Too high an impact frequency would cause the specimen to stay almost permanently in the "swung-up" position, defeating the impact-cum-sliding mechanism. The final choice of 3 Hz was made after numerous trials until the wear features seen on the test specimens resemble closely the wear groove seen on the 17-year-old explanted valve. The rectangular (9 by 26 mm) titanium plunger was designed to have a line contact with a tip radius of 0.75 mm and protrusion of 2.5 mm. The plastic test specimen (10 by 15 by 3 mm) and the titanium plunger were first polished to a surface finish of 1 μm using diamond paste before securing (by two plastic screws) onto the wear test rig. Prior to each test, the specimens were flushed with running water and then put into an ultrasonic bath of alcohol for at least 30 min in order to remove any trace of polishing agents and dirt. They were then soaked in distilled water at 37 $\pm$ 1°C for about 24 h. At least three specimens of each candidate material were tested for the short duration wear tests. For the long-term wear test in excess of 23 million cycles only Delrin BK602 was tested. Because of the long duration, the last point was based on only one specimen.

Wear Measurement

The traditional way of determining wear by measuring the loss of mass was not used here mainly because of the very small amount of mass involved and, hence, the large amount of uncertainty associated with the measuring devices. Further complication arose because of the inability to accurately account for the amount of mass gained by the polymer, especially Delrin, due to water and moisture adsorption, although controlled specimens were used throughout the tests. Very often, wear occurred in the form of surface material flow as a result of the deformation of the polymer arising from the impact-cum-sliding action of the titanium plunger, with no detectable change of mass, although an obvious wear groove could be seen on the test specimen. It was therefore decided that the most meaningful method for wear measurement was done by measuring the shape of the wear groove on the plastic specimen using a profilometer (Talysurf 4). For each wear measurement, the wear test was interrupted and the duration of the test was recorded. After the profilometric measurement, the specimen was then carefully repositioned in the wear test rig so that the titanium plunger would keep hitting the same wear grove (simulating an occluder that did not rotate in service). In order to ensure that the surface profile was measured consistently along the same positions after each interruption of test which was required for each profilometry measurement, the face of each specimen was marked (away from the area of contact with the plunger) by a razor blade to act as a reference. Twelve traces, each spaced 1 mm from the next and measured in a direction perpendicular to the wear groove, were taken on every specimen. A sample trace is shown in Fig. 3. The maximum wear depth was recorded after each wear test. In this way, analysis of results will give a more conservative approach and can be compared to other results published earlier [1,5].

Scanning Electron Microscopy

After the completion of each wear test, the plastic specimens were examined under a scanning electron microscope (SEM) (Jeol JSM-T330A). Prior to SEM examination, the specimens were sputter gold coated in a vacuum evaporator (Jeol JEE-4X). In order to avoid exces-

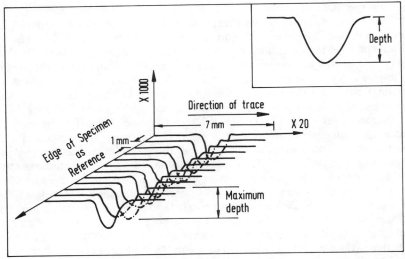

FIG. 3—*Surface contour plot of a worn material.*

sive radiation damage especially for the Delrin specimens, a low acceleration voltage of 10 kV was used. Micrographs were taken with the help of an image processing system (SEMICAP) developed by the Electrical Engineering Department, National University of Singapore.

Results and Discussion

Variation of Maximum Wear Depth Versus Log (Cycle)

Delrin BK602 is currently being used as the occluder material for the St. Vincent's mechanical heart valve [5]. This material was tested till 23.2 million cycles so as to compare to the results published earlier by Teoh et al. [5] and ascertain the usefulness of using the present impact-cum-sliding wear simulator to assess candidate materials for use in mechanical heart valves. The maximum wear depths were plotted against log (cycle) as shown in Fig. 4. Here the data points of the Björk-Shiley and St. Vincents' Delrin mechanical heart valves from earlier work [1,5] were incorporated for comparison. (In these earlier works the wear depths were also measured using a profilometer, thus making the present measurement amenable for comparison. Both *in-vivo* and *in-vitro* (accelerated life tester) wear results of mechanical heart valves of the tilting disc type were used.) Figure 4 shows that after an initial period of very low wear, the maximum wear depth of the Delrin BK602 specimen gradually increased with a trend similar to the other data points. The data from the two *in-vitro* tests and from the *in-vivo* (explanted) occluders exhibit a similar trend. The gradients of these lines are very similar especially to the three representing the *in-vitro* and *in-vivo* data for the Björk-Shiley Delrin tilting valves and the present impact-cum-sliding mechanical heart valve simulator. The present results, though coincidental as it may appear, do suggest that the simulator is able to reproduce wear characteristics that are comparable to those of commercially available accelerated life tester as well as the actual implanted valves. (The St. Vincents' design appears to be wearing at a lower rate since, as reported earlier [5], the contact stresses have been reduced relative to the Björk-Shiley design.) An interesting point also can be noted in Fig. 4: The impact-cum-sliding mechanical heart valve simulator actually produced wear faster than in an accelerated life-tester. This may be useful from the point of view of materials selection as it is now possible to produce a greater amount of wear in a shorter number of cycles. Furthermore, operating at a frequency of about 3 Hz (considerably slower than many life-testers), the simulator has an added advantage in that there is now a reasonable amount of time in between impacts for the polymer to relax just like an actual implanted occluder—a feature which the faster life-tester cannot emulate. Figure 4 also shows that there is a considerable period of time when the Delrin did not register any significant amount of wear: the wear grooves only became visible after about 10^5 cycles and the depth increases very gently until about 10^7 cycles where the gradient suddenly rises sharply. It may be concluded that an incubation period exists in the wear of Delrin BK602 against titanium. The observation that the other lines also intercept around 10^7 cycles meant that this incubation period can be taken to be a characteristic feature for Delrin under wet lubricating environment.

For the other candidate materials, because of the time factor, each was tested for a total duration of about 2 weeks (4×10^6 cycles). Their results are shown in Fig. 5. In the case of the four grades of Delrin tested, no significant differences exist among them, indicating that under the simulated impact-cum-sliding condition, the wear of Delrin on titanium is nearly inde- pendent of molecular weight and that the addition of 0.3% carbon (BK602) does not alter this conclusion. From Fig. 5, it is clear that PES suffered the most wear and UHMWPE has the least wear. PES began to wear quickly after 10^5 cycles, whereas the rest were still having neg- ligible wear. PEEK performs less satisfactorily when compared to Delrin over this short-term duration. However, longer tests need to be performed in order to confirm this trend.

Scanning Electron Micrographs

Using the present impact-cum-sliding wear simulator, wear grooves similar to those in Fig. 1 were observed on the seven candidate materials. Wear on the titanium plunger was negligibe (except for a few small scratches). No weight loss or severe deformation were detected on the titanium. The wear debris of Delrin, PEEK, PES, and UHMWPE are shown in Fig. 6. The wear debris (for Delrin Fig. 6*a*) were seen to have features similar to that of the explanted one reported earlier [8]. These striking resemblances are another strong indication that the impact- cum-sliding conditions experienced in the simulator are very close to those of the actual con- ditions experienced in implanted occluders. It can be seen from these micrographs that the

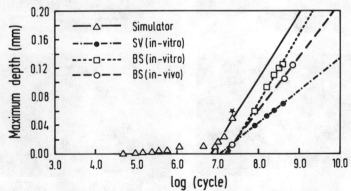

FIG. 4—*Comparison of the maximum wear depths of various Delrin occluders versus log (cycle). (SV: the St. Vincents' Design; BS: the Björk-Shiley Design.) The last data point from the simulator, marked with an asterisk, was only based on one specimen due to time constraints.*

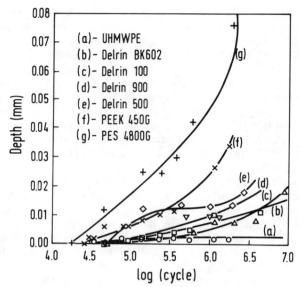

FIG. 5—*Wear depth versus log (cycles).*

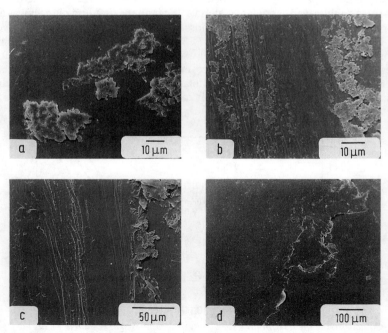

FIG. 6—*Scanning electron micrographs of the wear debris for* (a) *Delrin,* (b) *PEEK,* (c) *PES, and* (d) *UHMWPE.*

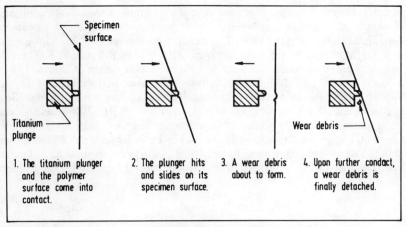

FIG. 7—*Proposed process of wear debris formation.*

wear debris produced generally adopted a flake-like morphology. Three observations were made on the size of the debris:

1. the wear debris of UHMWPE are mostly larger than 100 μm,
2. the wear of PES consistently produced debris of about 60 μm, and
3. the wear debris of the other five materials averaged about 30 μm.

The wear debris of UHMWPE and PES are considerably large and may not be suitable for heart valve applications as the large wear debris may give rise to complications when they enter the blood circulation system in the human body. The micrographs also show some flaky wear debris about to be detached from the sliding surface (see Fig. 6c). Such a manifestation suggests that the mechanism of wear debris formation may be described by the process illustrated in Fig. 7. When the titanium plunger hits the surface of the polymer the restraining springs exert a reactive force at the point of contact. As a result an indentation (groove mark) is formed. The plunger also slides on the surface of the specimen and this caused the polymeric material to flow on the surface. On repeated impact-cum-sliding, more and more material is made to flow on the surface. Evidently some will be compressed by the subsequent action of the plunger, hence producing flake-like features sticking on the surface of the polymer. Finally, a stage is reached when this material actually forms flake-like debris which becomes detached.

Conclusions

Accelerated life testing of mechanical heart valves can best be performed by partitioning the *in-vitro* wear assessment of the material separate from that due to the overall design of the mechanical heart valve. Since the opening and closing of the valve causes impact and sliding to occur on the occluder, a new method simulating the impact-cum-sliding action in mechanical heart valves was developed to test a variety of candidate materials: Delrin, PEEK, PES, and UHMWPE. The present results, though coincidental as they may appear, do suggest that the simulator is able to reproduce wear characteristics that are comparable to those of a commercially available accelerated life tester as well as the actual implanted valves [1,5]. The wear grooves and the debris morphology of the Delrin tested in this method were also similar to the one seen in an explanted mechanical heart valve using Delrin as the occluder. These results indicated that the present technique proved to be able to simulate the actual closing and open-ing conditions in mechanical heart valves. The technique saved time and was amenable to wear mechanisms study using the SEM. The wear results showed that, in terms of maximum wear depth, UHMWPE wore the least, followed by Delrin, PEEK, and PES. There does not appear to be any correlation between wear and the molecular weight of Delrin. The incorpo-ration of 0.3% carbon (BK602) did not improve the wear performance of Delrin. Both UHMWPE and PES produced debris that were significantly larger than the rest. Because of the possibility of large debris in the range of 100 μm or more, UHMWPE was not considered to be a good material for use as occluder in mechanical heart valves even though it wore the least. At present, Delrin is still considered to be the best occluder material. PEEK showed some potential but longer experiments need to be carried out in order to show its full potentiality. PES showed the worst wear behavior and may not be a good material for use in mechanical heart valves.

References

[1] Fettel, B. E., Johnston, D. R., and Morris, P. E., "Accelerated Life Testing of Prosthetic Heart Valves," *Medical Instruments,* Vol. 14, No. 3, 1980, pp. 161–164.

[2] Clark, E. R., Swanson, W. M., Kardos, J. L., et al., "Durability of Prosthetic Heart Valves," *The Annals of Thoracic Surgery,* Vol. 26, No. 4, 1978, pp. 323–335.

[3] Herold, M., Lo, H. B., Reul, H., et al., "The Helmholtz-Institute-Tri-Leaflet-Polyurethane-Heart Valve Prosthesis: Design, Manufacturing and First In-Vitro and In-Vivo Results," *Polyurethane in Biomedical Engineering II,* H. Plank, I. Syre', M. Dauner, and G. Eber, Eds., Elsevier Science Pub-lishers, Amsterdam, 1987, pp. 231–256.

[4] Teoh, S. H., Lim, S. C., Lee, K. H., et al., "Mechanical Heart Valves—Fracture, Wear and Computer Aided Design." *Digest of the World Congress on Medical Physics and Biomedical Engineering,* Vol. 29, No. 2, 1991, p. 880.

[5] Teoh, S. H., Martin, R. L., Lim, S. C., et al., "Delrin as an Occluder Material," *American Society for Artificial Internal Organs Transactions (ASAIO Trans.),* Vol. 39, No. 3, 1990, pp. M417–M421.

[6] Trainor, A. and Haward, R. N., "Factors Influencing the Wear Properties of High Molecular Weight Polyethylene for Prostheses," *Mechanical Properties of Biomaterials,* G. W. Hastings and D. F. Wil-liams, Eds., John Wiley & Sons Ltd., 1980, pp. 65–71.

[7] Gibbons, D. F., Anderson, J. M., Martin, R. L., and Nelson, T., "Wear and Degradation of Retrieved Ultrahigh Molecular Weight Polyethylene and Other Polymeric Implants," *Corrosion and Degra-dation of Implant Materials, ASTM STP 684,* B. C. Syrett and A. Archaya, Eds., American Society for Testing and Materials, Philadelphia, 1979, pp. 20–39.

[8] Teoh, S. H., Lim, S. C., Lee, K. H., et al., "Wear Studies in Mechanical Heart Valves," *Proceedings of the 6th International Conference on Biomedical Engineering,* J. C. H. Goh and A. Nather, Eds., National University of Singapore, 1990, pp. 453–459.

[9] Björk, V. O., "Delrin as an Implant Material for Valve Occluders," *Scandinavian Journal Thoracic Cardiovascular Surgery,* Vol. 6, 1972, pp. 103–107.

[10] Clarke, I. C. and McKellop, H., "The Wear of Delrin 150 Compared with Polyethylene, Polyester and PTFE," *Mechanical Properties of Biomaterials,* G. W. Hastings and D. F. Williams, Eds., John Wiley & Sons Ltd., 1980, pp. 27–37.

[11] Shen, C. and Dumbelton, J., "The Friction and Wear Behaviour of Polyoxymethylene in Connec-tion with Joint Replacement," *Wear,* Vol. 38, 1976, pp. 291–303.

[12] Klein, A., "Bioplastics and the Artificial Heart," *Proceedings of the 45th Annual Technical Confer-ence,* ANTEC '87, 4–7 May, Los Angeles, Society of Plastics Engineers, 1987, pp. 1205–1209.

[13] Wenz, L. M., Merritt, K., Brown, S. A., and Moet, A., "In-vitro Biocompatibility of Polyether-etherketone and Polysulphone Composites," *Journal of Biomedical Materials Research,* Vol. 24, 1990, pp. 207–215.

Hana Holubec,[1] Glenn C. Hunter,[1] Milos Chvapil,[1] Thomas A. Chvapil,[1] Victor M. Bernhard,[1] Ronald L. Misiorowski,[1] and Charles W. Putnam[1,2]

The Relationship Between PTFE Graft Ultrastructure and Cellular Ingrowth: The Influence of an Autologous Jugular Vein Wrap

REFERENCE: Holubec, H., Hunter, G. C., Chvapil, M., Chvapil, T. A., Bernhard, V. M., Misiorowski, R. L., and Putnam, C. W., **"The Relationship Between PTFE Graft Ultrastructure and Cellular Ingrowth: The Influence of an Autologous Jugular Vein Wrap,"** *Biomaterials' Mechanical Properties, ASTM STP 1173*, H. E. Kambic and A. T. Yokobori, Jr., Eds., American Society for Testing and Materials, Philadelphia, 1994, pp. 53–64.

ABSTRACT: Here, we report the differential effects on cellular ingrowth and healing caused by varying the internodal distance (IND) of polytetrafluoroethylene (PTFE) grafts. In addition, we examined whether cellular ingrowth could be enhanced by an additional source of endothelial cells. Both carotid arteries of greyhound dogs were replaced with 5-cm lengths of 4-mm-diameter PTFE grafts of varying IND (30, 40, 60 μm). The histologic characteristics of anastomotic and midgraft segments of grafts wrapped with autologous vein graft as a source of endothelial cells were compared to the contralateral unwrapped graft of identical IND. At five weeks the grafts were excised and examined histologically and the *in vivo* IND, cellular and microvessel ingrowth, and endothelialization of the luminal surface quantitated. All 30 μm grafts ($N = 8$) were occluded by anastomotic pannus ingrowth (PI). The anastomoses of 40 and 60 μm grafts were characterized by either intimal hyperplasia (IH) ($N = 10$) or healing with minimal intimal thickening (H) ($N = 4$). The mean reduction in IND at anastomoses was 68 to 75% for all grafts whereas midgraft IND was unaffected. The mean IND at anastomoses with PI was 7.0 $\pm$ 1.5 μm, IH 12.0 $\pm$ 2.5 μm, and 19.0 $\pm$ 2.0 μm for healed anastomoses. Midgraft cellular ingrowth was greater than that observed near anastomoses and varied with IND. The application of a vein wrap enhanced cellular and microvessel ingrowth and endothelialization of 40 and 60 μm grafts. These data suggest that alterations in PTFE ultrastructure likely resulting from surgical manipulation during implantation may adversely influence anastomotic healing.

KEYWORDS: polytetrafluoroethylene (PTFE), porosity, anastomotic healing

The useful life span of small diameter ($<$6 mm) polytetrafluoroethylene (PTFE) prosthetic grafts is usually terminated by thrombosis, the consequence of their inherent thrombogenicity, or the host responses manifest by intimal hyperplasia (IH) or pannus ingrowth (PI), occurring at the anastomoses. While the role of thrombogenicity can be diminished experimentally by preselecting animals with low thrombotic potential, by giving them antiplatelet drugs or by seeding the grafts with endothelial cells, therapeutic interventions to prevent or retard anastomotic stenosis from IH or PI have proven unsuccessful [1–4].

The etiology of IH is unknown. Contributing factors, however, include a mismatch in compliance, immune reactivity, physical or chemical injury, and vessel wall ischemia. To date, the

---

[1] Departments of Surgery and [2]Pharmacology, The University of Arizona Health Sciences Center, Tucson, AZ 85724.

influence of the spatial geometry, specifically the internodal distances of PTFE grafts, on anastomotic healing has not previously been addressed [5–8].

The fabrication of PTFE grafts results in a unique ultrastructure, consisting of solid nodes interconnected by longitudinally oriented fibrils. The node fibril array confers porosity (it is 80% air) which readily accommodates the cellular ingrowth vital to healing [9]. The extent of the cellular ingrowth is proportional to the IND of these grafts [10,11].

It should be mentioned that the node fibril structure is vulnerable to distortion and disruption through manipulation with surgical instruments or faulty suture technique [12].

This study was undertaken to evaluate the influence of alterations in PTFE ultrastructure and of providing an additional source of endothelial cells on anastomotic and midgraft healing.

Material and Methods

Animal Model

Eight adult, three-year-old greyhound dogs of either sex were used. The animals were cared for according to the "Principles of Laboratory Animal Care" (formulated by the National Society for Medical Research) and the "Guide for the Care and Use of Laboratory Animals" (NIH Publication No. 80-23, revised 1985).

Surgical Procedure

After an overnight fast, the animals were anesthetized with sodium methohexital and maintained on halothane by inhalation. Both carotid arteries were exposed through a midline incision and the right external jugular vein harvested and stored in a heparin-saline solution at room temperature. Each dog was then given 30 units/kg of heparin intravenously, prolonging the activated clotting time twofold. Five-cm segments of both carotid arteries were replaced by identical lengths of 4-mm-diameter 30 μm reinforced (Gore and Assoc., Flagstaff, AZ) or 30, 40, and 60 μm unreinforced (Impra Tempe, AZ) PTFE grafts. The grafts were anastomosed end to end using continuous 6.0 polypropylene suture, aided by loops (2.5×). Prior to implantation, one of the paired grafts was inserted into a sleeve of external jugular vein with the endothelial surface of the vein abutting the external surface of the graft.

After five weeks, the animals were anesthetized and anticoagulated with 100 units/kg of heparin intravenously. The grafts, plus a 2-cm segment of host artery adjacent to each anastomosis, were excised for analysis. The harvested specimens were gently rinsed in heparinized phosphate buffered saline (PBS), opened longitudinally, pinned on a board, photographed, and preserved in 10% buffered formalin for light microscopy. Patency was determined by inspection.

Light Microscopy

Each graft was bissected and processed for histology. Five-micron sections oriented longitudinally were stained with Hematoxylin and Eosin (H & E). Endothelialization of the luminal surface and interstitial cellular and microvascular ingrowth were evaluated. Endothelial cell coverage of each segment was determined in the longitudinal sections of both halves of the graft including proximal and distal anastomoses and was expressed as a percentage of the entire graft. Microvessels within the graft wall were counted and expressed per mm². Transmural cellular ingrowth from perigraft tissue was graded on a scale of 1 to 5, Grade 1 corresponding to less than 10% ingrowth and Grade 5 indicating that more than 50% of the graft wall was penetrated by cells. Each manufacturer provided preimplantation IND specifications; these were confirmed in our laboratory by SEM measurements. Postimplantation IND of representative sections from the entire segment was determined microscopically using a stage micrometer. The mean IND at selected anastomoses was evaluated and compared to the cognate midgraft section. All measurements of the physical and healing characteristics of the PTFE grafts were determined in duplicate. Selected specimens were stained with antibody to Factor VIII antigen (Dako Corp.).

Statistical Analysis

Differences between control and vein wrapped grafts and the relationship of IND to cellular and microvessel ingrowth were analyzed by Between-Within ANOVA.

Results

Patency

At five weeks all 40 and 60 μm grafts were patent. Every 30 μm graft, whether reinforced or unreinforced, was occluded.

Cellular Reaction at the Graft Interface

At harvest, the jugular vein wrap was almost completely resorbed. A cellular infiltrate, consisting of macrophages, granulocytes, and fibroblast-like cells, was present at the interface of the residual venous medial smooth muscle with the outer surface of the PTFE grafts (Figs. 1*a* through *d*). Transmural cellular penetration, originating from the vein wrap, was most marked in the 60 μm grafts. In contrast, cellular ingrowth into unwrapped 60 μm grafts was considerably less (Figs. 1*c* and *d*). A similar but less dramatic pattern of cellular infiltration was seen with wrapped versus unwrapped 40 μm grafts. However, both reinforced and unreinforced 30 μm grafts showed much less cellular infiltration, whether or not they were wrapped with vein (Figs. 1*a* and *b*).

Microvessel Ingrowth

Only occasional microvessels originating in the perigraft tissue or vein wrap were visible in the 30 μm grafts. Strikingly, the number of microvessels in the interstices of 40 and 60 μm grafts was significantly greater in wrapped than in unwrapped grafts (Table 1). While the greatest density of microvessels was observed at the vein-graft interface, several of the microvessels in vein wrapped 60 μm grafts reached the luminal surface. Microvessel ingrowth was evident within the pannus, when that was present.

Endothelization of Graft Luminal Surface

Because of overlying thrombus, endothelial cells (EC) could not be identified in 30 μm grafts (Fig. 2). The monolayer of endothelial cells lining the unwrapped 40 μm PTFE grafts lined 16.9 $\pm$ 7.8% of the graft sections compared to 33.1 $\pm$ 3.5% of the vein wrapped grafts of identical IND (Table 1). Endothelial cell ingrowth into unwrapped 60 μm grafts lined 20.4 $\pm$ 4.3% of the luminal surface, compared to 64.3 $\pm$ 2.5% of the vein wrapped grafts. The majority of

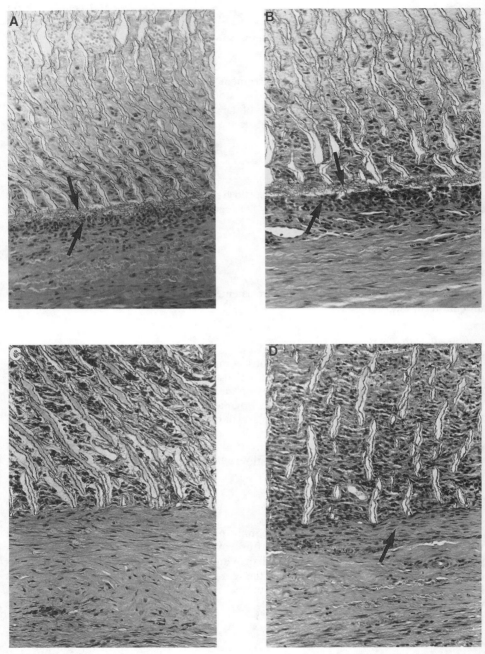

FIG. 1—*Histological sections of 30 μm reinforced and 60 μm grafts:* (a) *Unwrapped 30 μm graft showing PTFE membrane* (upper arrow) *with minimal inflammatory reaction and cellular ingrowth* (lower arrow); (b) *30 μm vein wrapped graft showing PTFE membrane* (upper arrow) *an inflammatory cell response* (lower arrow) *at the vein graft interface and some cellular ingrowth into the wall of the graft;* (c) *60 μm unwrapped graft showing a minimal perigraft inflammatory reaction with cellular infiltrate present within the wall;* (d) *60 μm vein wrapped graft showing the residual portion of the vein* (arrow) *with cellular and microvessel ingrowth into the interstices of the graft. H & E, 210×.*

TABLE 1—*Healing characteristics of 40 and 60 μm grafts at 5 weeks.*

Internodal Distance	40 μm		60 μm	
	Control	Vein Wrap	Control	Vein Wrap
N	2	2	2	2
Patency, %	100	100	100	100
Endothelialization, %	16.9 ± 7.8	$33.1 \pm 3.5^*$	20.4 ± 4.3	$64.3 \pm 12.5^*$
Microvessels, mm^2	1.2 ± 0.5	$6.8 \pm 2.1^*$	5.6 ± 5.8	$16.4 \pm 6.5^*$
Cellular Ingrowth	2.0 ± 1.4	$4.0 \pm 1.4^*$	3.0 ± 1.4	$4.5 \pm 0.7^*$

$^*p < 0.05$

cells lining the surface of 40 and 60 μm grafts stained positively for Factor VIII antigen indicating that they were of endothelial cell origin. The portions of the graft lined by EC were devoid of platelet or thrombus accumulation (Fig. 3), whereas thrombus was invariably present in grafts lacking an endothelial cell lining.

Anastomotic Changes

Three distinct anastomotic changes were observed: PI ($N = 8$), IH ($N = 10$), and H (with minimal or no intimal thickening) ($N = 4$). Anastomotic PI, organized thrombus invaded by fibroblasts and granulation tissue, produced a greater luminal narrowing and extended further from the anastomoses than did IH. Anastomotic IH, multi-layered smooth muscle cells lined by endothelium, was confined to a distance of 800 to 1200 μm from the proximal and distal anastomoses.

The anastomoses of all 30 μm grafts were occluded by PI (Fig. 4). Anastomotic intimal hyperplasia was characteristic of all 40 μm grafts and some 60 μm grafts (Fig. 5). Healing was observed in wrapped and unwrapped 60 μm grafts (Fig. 6).

Marked differences in internodal distance and hence the degree of cellular infiltration were seen at the anastomoses compared to the midportions of the same grafts. At the anastomotic sites, IND was markedly reduced. The lowest observed mean IND (7.0 ± 1.5 μm) was at the

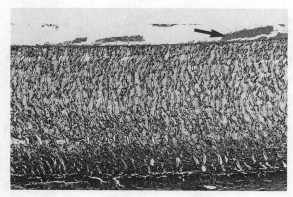

FIG. 2—*Histologic section demonstrating thrombus accumulation on the luminal surface of 30 μm rein-forced graft* (arrow) *with minimal cellular ingrowth limited to the outer third of the wall. H & E, 80×.*

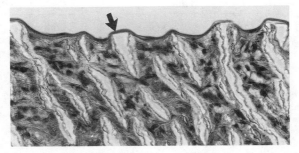

FIG. 3—*Histologic section showing endothelial cells (EC) lining the luminal surface of a 40 μm PTFE graft* (arrow). *No thrombus or platelet accumulation can be seen on the EC lined surface. H & E, 330×.*

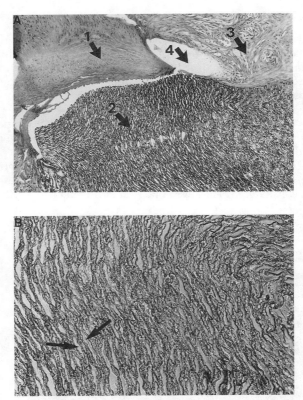

FIG. 4—*Histologic section demonstrating PI at the anastomosis of a 30 μm graft.*(a) *Arrows indicate:* (1) *carotid artery,* (2) *compressed graft,* (3) *pannus ingrowth, and* (4) *prolene suture. H & E, 80×.* (b) *Higher magnification of graft ultrastructure immediately adjacent to the anastomosis demonstrating a marked reduction in the internodal distance with no cellular growth* (arrows). *H & E, 210×.*

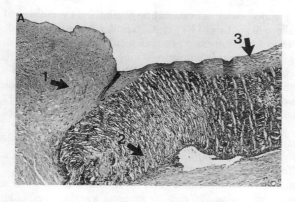

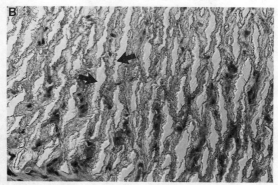

FIG. 5—*Histologic section of 40 μm graft demonstrating anastomotic intimal hyperplasia.* (a) *Arrows indicate:* (1) *carotid artery,* (2) *compressed graft, and* (3) *intimal hyperplasia 80×.* (b) *Higher magnification of graft ultrastructure showing a reduction in node fibril distance* (arrow)*with scattered cells within the interstices. H & E, 210×.*

anastomoses of 30 μm grafts (Fig. 4a). Few if any cells invaded the compressed portions of the grafts. The mean IND of 40 and 60 μm grafts immediately adjacent to anastomoses characterized by intimal hyperplasia was 12.0 ± 2.5 μm (Fig. 5a), whereas, 60 μm grafts with healed anastomoses had a mean IND of 19.0 ± 2.0 μm (Fig. 6a). The relationship between IND and anastomostic healing is shown in Fig. 7. The extent of cellular ingrowth varied with the degree of compression at the anastomoses; consequently, none of the grafts had as much cellular ingrowth at the anastomoses as in the midportions of the grafts. There were no observed differences in the healing between the proximal and distal anastomoses.

Discussion

Early failure of small diameter (<6 mm) PTFE grafts relates to technical errors or their inherent thrombogenicity, while late failures are usually attributable to anastomotic occlusion resulting from pannus ingrowth or intimal hyperplasia.

That PTFE grafts lack an endothelial lining is often cited as the principal reason for their failure. Experimentally, their thrombogenicity can be lessened by prior endothelial cell seeding, by enhancing endogenous endothelial migration, or by the use of anti-platelet drugs [2,3,11]. Endothelial cell seeding of PTFE grafts is hampered by weak adhesion of the cells to the graft surface even when adhesive proteins such as fibronectin are used. Similarly, anti-platelet drugs have not significantly improved long-term patency [13]. Recently, factors that might enhance endogenous endothelial cell ingrowth have received attention. Potential sources of endogenous endothelial cells include the circulating blood, migrating cells from the adjacent cut ends of arteries, or capillary ingrowth from perigraft tissue [11].

The node fibril ultrastructure of PTFE grafts appears to provide a suitable matrix for cellular ingrowth. While cellular ingrowth and endothelialization of the luminal surface readily occur in experimental animals, healing is slower and less complete in patients [14]. Nonetheless, animal studies provide insight regarding factors that facilitate healing, of which the internodal distance appears to be an important determinant [10,11].

The classical studies of Wesolowski et al. [15] demonstrated that Dacron® graft porosity exceeding 5000 mL/cm²/min at 120 mm Hg pressure was the threshold necessary to achieve a viable, metabolically active cellular lining. The relationship of IND to cellular ingrowth in

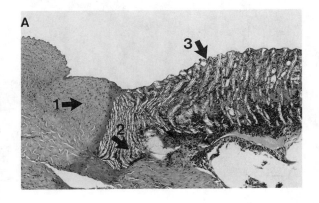

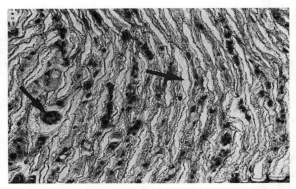

FIG. 6—*Histologic section of a 60 μm graft demonstrating anastomotic healing originated from the artery.* (a) *Arrows indicate:* (1) *carotid artery,* (2) *compressed graft, and* (3) *endothelial cells lining the surface. H& E, 80×.* (b) *Higher magnification of the compressed graft* (right arrow) *showing a reduction in the internodal distance with moderate cellular and microvessel ingrowth* (left arrow). *H & E, 210×.*

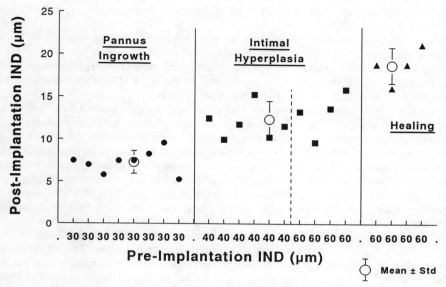

FIG. 7—*Relationship between internodal distance and anastomotic healing.*

PTFE grafts replacing segments of portal vein and vena cava was explored by Soyer et al. [16]. They found that cellular ingrowth was absent in grafts with IND of 0.5 to 2.5 μm in size. Surprisingly, Campbell et al. in dogs observed higher patency rates and less neointimal thickening in grafts with an average IND of 22 μm or less compared to grafts with internodal distances of 34 μm or greater [10]. Clowes et al. and Kogel et al. have recently reported improved healing of experimental grafts of 60 and 90 μm IND [11,17–19]. The disparity between the latter observations and those of Campbell et al. may relate to species differences in the animals used in them.

Commercially available PTFE grafts have an average node fibril distance range of 20 to 30 μm. The application of an external PTFE wrap to Gortex grafts, even though porous, may further compromise the ultimate IND by overlapping with the nodes and fibrils of the primary graft structure.

The IND of the graft immediately adjacent to the anastomosis was much less than observed preimplantation or in the midportion of the grafts at retrieval. This reduction in IND was most likely from the running suture technique and surgical manipulation despite taking great care to minimize compression by careful handling and precise suture technique. In view of the deformation of the node fibril structure observed at anastomoses using the running suture technique, a comparison between the running and interrupted suture technique is presently being undertaken.

Compression of the node fibril length at anastomoses correlated with the histologic findings. Pannus formation was evident when the IND was reduced to less than 10 μm, IH when the IND exceeded 12 μm, and anastomotic healing with INDs greater than 18 μm (Fig. 7). Cellular ingrowth from perigraft tissue adjacent to anastomoses was absent in grafts demonstrating pannus formation, minimal with IH and moderate in grafts with healed anastomoses. These findings are consistent with those of Kogel et al., who observed that cellular ingrowth and anastomotic healing only occurred in 60 and 90 μm PTFE grafts, whereas PI (with isolated islands of endothelial cells in the middle third of the grafts) characterized 30 μm PTFE grafts [18,19].

Cellular ingrowth and endothelization were more pronounced in the midportions than at anastomoses, but followed the same trends with regard to IND.

Using an external vein wrap as a source of endothelial cells with Dacron grafts has previously been described by Rosenberg et al. [20] and Graham et al. [21], and with small diameter polyurethane grafts by Sedlarik et al. [22], but not with PTFE grafts.

While at five weeks the vein surrounding the grafts was partially resorbed, a marked inflammatory cell reaction consisting of macrophages, fibroblast-like cells, and microvessels was seen at the vein-graft interface. When the vein wrap was used, significantly ($p < 0.05$) more cellular and microvessel ingrowth and endothelialization of 40 and 60 μm grafts were evident. Endothelialization of 40 and 60 μm grafts occurred more rapidly and covered a greater area of the flow surface. IND appeared to influence these changes, but not to a statistically significant degree. Microvessels, appearing to originate from the residual wall of the vein wrap, were more frequently observed in grafts with greater IND. These microvessels also underwent a phenotypic change from their tubular structure within the graft wall to a single layer of cells spreading over the luminal flow surface. These changes were more noticeable in the midportions of the grafts where the IND was unaltered than at the compressed anastomoses. The contribution of the inflammatory cell infiltrate to the healing of these grafts has not been fully elucidated. Macrophages, smooth muscle, and endothelial cells are known to produce a number of growth factors, including acidic and basic fibroblast growth factor, transforming growth factor β, and platelet derived growth factors, which may stimulate cellular proliferation, migration, and angiogenesis. Recently Zacharias [23] and Golden [24] have demonstrated that both smooth muscle and endothelial cells are capable of producing growth factors known to regulate SMC growth *in vitro*. Although these factors are best known for their angiogenic effects, their mitogenic potential may be a contributing factor to graft healing. The importance of the "intentionally" induced inflammatory reaction in promoting healing has been documented in previous work from our laboratory evaluating the effectiveness of various wound dressings to promote epithelization of skin wounds. Dressings inducing cellular reaction, classified as nonspecific inflammation, also enhanced healing and epithelization of the wound [25].

The cells lining the midportion of the grafts appeared to originate from perigraft microvessels, whereas those lining healed anastomoses appeared to arise from the adjacent artery. Whether endothelial cells derived from microvessels are capable of producing the anti- and pro-coagulant substances and growth factors produced by large vessel endothelial cells remains to be determined. It is interesting to note that thrombus only formed on the areas of the grafts devoid of endothelial cells, providing indirect evidence that these endothelial cells may possess some antithrombotic activity.

In other tissue implants (sponges, foams with continuing channels), the optimal porosity for cellular ingrowth was found to be 60 to 80 μm [26]; whereas a pore size of $>$ 120 μm was associated with reduced ingrowth, probably because of the smaller surface area available for cellular adhesion and locomotion.

The optimal IND necessary for cellular adhesion and migration appears to range between 60 and 90 μm. While cellular ingrowth and endothelization will occur more readily in grafts with larger internodal distances, they are subject to other complications. For example, unreinforced 60 μm PTFE grafts may develop circumferential creep and undergo aneurysm formation. Grafts with $\geq$ 90 μm IND will bleed through the wall and thus require preclotting. Wound seromas are more common with grafts of larger pore size.

Our study supports the observations of Clowes and others that the healing characteristics of PTFE grafts are related to their ultrastructure, cellular ingrowth occurring more rapidly in 60

μm grafts. Furthermore, healing of 40 and 60 μm grafts could be significantly enhanced by providing an additional source of endothelial cells. Surgical manipulation, especially near the anastomoses, results in permanent deformation of the graft ultrastructure. This reduction in IND may adversely influence anastomotic healing and, as a consequence, reduce the long-term patency rate of these grafts.

References

[1] Kaplan S., Marcoe K. K., Sauvage, L. R., et al., "The Effect of Predetermined Thrombotic Potential of the Recipient on Small-Caliber Graft Performance," *Journal of Vascular Surgery,* Vol. 3, No. 2, February 1986, pp. 311–321.

[2] Douville, E. C., Kempczinski, R. F., Birinyi, L. K., and Ramalanjaona, G. R., "Impact of Endothelial Cell Seeding on Long-term Patency and Subendothelial Proliferation in a Small-Caliber Highly Porous Polytetrafluoroethylene Graft," *Journal of Vascular Surgery,* Vol. 5, 1987, pp. 544–550.

[3] Nordestgaard, A. G. and Wilson, S. E., "Neoendothelialization of Small-Diameter Polytetrafluoroethylene Arterial Grafts Is Not Delayed by Aspirin and Dipyridamole," *Journal of Vascular Surgery,* Vol. 7, 1988, pp. 93–98.

[4] Foxall, T. L., Auger, K. R., Callow, A. D., and Libby, P., "Adult Human Endothelial Cell Coverage of Small-Caliber Dacron and Polytetrafluoroethylene Vascular Prostheses *in Vitro,*" *Journal of Surgical Research,* Vol. 41, 1986, pp. 158–172.

[5] Hoepp, L. M., Elbadawi, A., Cohn, M., et al., "Steroids and Immunosuppression," *Archives of Surgery,* Vol. 114, March 1979, pp. 273–276.

[6] Brody, W. R., Josek, J. C., and Agneli, W. W., "Changes in Vein Grafts Following Aorto-coronary Bypass Induced by Pressure and Ischemia,"*Journal of Thoracic and Cardiovascular Surgery,* Vol. 64, 1970, p. 847.

[7] Walden, R., L'Italien, G. J., Megerman, J., and Abbott, W. M., "Matched Elastic Properties and Successful Grafting," *Archives of Surgery,* Vol. 115, 1980, pp. 1166–1167.

[8] Lyman, D. J., Fazzio, F. J., Robinson, G., and Albo, D. Jr., "Compliance as a Factor Effecting the Patency of a Copolyurethane Vascular Graft,"*Journal of Biomedical Materials Research,* Vol. 12, 1978, pp. 337–345.

[9] Boyce, B., "Physical Characteristics of Expanded Polytetrafluoroethylene Grafts," in *Biologic and Synthetic Vascular Prostheses,* J. C. Stanley, Ed., Grune & Stratton, New York, 1982, pp. 553–561.

[10] Campbell, C. D., Goldfarb, D., and Roe, R., "A Small Arterial Substitute," *Annals of Surgery,* Vol. 182, 1975, pp. 138–143.

[11] Clowes, A. W., Kirkman, T. R., and Reidy, M. A., "Mechanisms of Arterial Graft Healing," *American Journal of Pathology,* Vol. 123, 1986, pp. 220–230.

[12] Holubec, H., Hunter, G. C., Putnam, C., et al., "Surgical Manipulation of PTFE Grafts Effects Microstructural Properties and Healing Characteristics," *The American Journal of Surgery,* Vol. 164, 1992, pp. 512–516.

[13] Budd, J. S., Allen, K. E., Bell, P. R. F., and James, R. F. L., "The Effect of Varying Fibronectin Concentration on the Attachment of Endothelial Cell to Polytetrafluoroethylene Vascular Grafts," *Journal of Vascular Surgery,* Vol. 12, 1990, pp. 126–130.

[14] Formichi, M. J., Guidoin, R. G., Jausseran, J-M., et al., "Expanded PTFE Prostheses as Arterial Substitutes in Humans: Late Pathological Findings in 73 Excised Grafts," *Annals of Vascular Surgery,* Vol. 2, 1988, pp. 14–27.

[15] Wesolowski, S. A., Fries, C. C., Karlson, K. E., et al., "Primary Determinant of Ultimate Fate of Synthetic Vascular Grafts," *Surgery,* Vol. 50, 1961, p. 91.

[16] Soyer, T., Cooper, P., Norton, L., and Eiseman, B., "A New Venous Prosthesis," *Surgery,* Vol. 72, 1972, pp. 864–872.

[17] Golden, M. A., Hanson, S. R., Kirman, T. R., et al., "Healing of Polytetrafluoroethylene Arterial Grafts Is Influenced by Graft Porosity,"*Journal of Vascular Surgery,* Vol. 11, 1990, pp. 838–845.

[18] Kogel, H., Vollmar, J. F., Stenzenberger, G., et al., "Morphologic Analysis of Artificial Blood Conduits in the Short-Term Carotid Artery Test," *Vascular Surgery,* Vol. 24, June 1990, pp. 297–306.

[19] Kogel, H., Amselgruber, W., and Frösch, D., "New Techniques of Analyzing the Healing Process of Artificial Vascular Grafts, Transmural Vascularization, and Endothelialization," *Research in Experimental Medicine,* Vol. 189, 1989, pp. 61–68.

[20] Rosenberg, J. C., Savarese, R. P., McCombs, P. R., and DeLaurentis, D. A., "Endothelial Infiltration and Lining of Knitted Dacron Arterial Grafts," *Surgical Forum,* Vol. 32, 1981, p. 336.

[21] Graham, L. M., Harrell, K. A., Sell, R. L., et al., "Enhanced Endothelialization of Dacron Grafts by External Vein Wrapping," *Journal of Surgical Research*, Vol. 38, 1985, pp. 537–545.
[22] Sedlarik, K. M., van Wachem, P. B., Bartel, H., and Schakenraad, J. M. "Rapid Endothelialization of Microporous Vascular Prostheses Covered with Meshed Vascular Tissue: A Preliminary Report." *Biomaterials*, Vol. 11, 1990, pp. 4–8.
[23] Zacharias, R. K., Kirkman, T. R., Kenagy, R. D., et al., "Growth Factor Production by Polytetrafluoroethylene Vascular Grafts," *Journal of Vascular Surgery*, Vol. 7, 1988, pp. 606–610.
[24] Golden, M. A., Tina Au, Y. P., Kenagy, R. D., and Clowes, A. W., "Growth Factor Gene Expression by Intimal Cells in Healing Polytetrafluoroethylene Grafts," *Journal of Vascular Surgery*, Vol. 11, 1988, pp. 580–585.
[25] Chvapil, M., Holubec, H., and Chvapil, T., "Inert Wound Dressing Is Not Desirable," *Journal of Surgical Research*, Vol. 51, 1991, pp. 245–252.
[26] Clark, R. E., Boyd, J. C., and Moran, J. F., "New Principles Governing the Tissue Reactivity of Prosthetic Materials," *Journal of Surgical Research*, Vol. 16, 1974, pp. 510–522.

A. Toshimitsu Yokobori, Jr.,[1] *Toshihide Maeyama,*[2] *Sumio Kuroda,*[3]
Takeo Yokobori,[4] *and Hiroshi Ohuchi*[5]

The Effect of Tissue Adhesion Due to Encapsulation on Anastomosis Strength and a Comparative Study of Vascular Substitute

REFERENCE: Yokobori, A. T. Jr., Maeyama, T., Kuroda, S., Yokobori, T., and Ohuchi, H., **"The Effect of Tissue Adhesion Due to Encapsulation on Anastomosis Strength and a Comparative Study of Vascular Substitute,"** *Biomaterials' Mechanical Properties, ASTM STP 1173,* H. E. Kambic and A. T. Yokobori, Jr., Eds., American Society for Testing and Materials, Philadelphia, 1994, pp. 65–74.

ABSTRACT: The anastomosis strength of vascular substitute and blood vessel is supported not only by the suture thread but also by tissue adhesion due to encapsulation of vascular substitute. In this paper, the *in vitro* and combined *in vivo* and *in vitro* mechanical tests were carried out to estimate the anastomosis strength between a vascular substitute and a blood vessel; good encapsulation of inner wall of the vascular substitute around the anastomosed part was found to be effective to enhance anastomosis strength. Furthermore, these results were compared with the experimental result of the anastomosis being performed by using suture thread only. Concerning the problem of the anastomosed part of the blood vessel with the vascular substitute, both effects mentioned above were found to be important requisites for the design of good functional vascular substitutes suitable for anastomosis. Finally, the significance of the *in vitro* and combined *in vivo* and *in vitro* mechanical tests are discussed.

KEYWORDS: mechanical test, *in vitro* test, *in vivo* test, vascular substitute, anastomosis strength, tissue adhesion, encapsulation

The anastomosis strength of a vascular substitute and a blood vessel is supported not only by the suture thread but also by tissue adhesion due to encapsulation of vascular substitute. In this paper, *in vitro* and combined *in vivo* and *in vitro* mechanical tests were carried out to estimate the anastomosis strength between a vascular substitute and a blood vessel.

From the experimental results obtained by these mechanical tests, the effects of encapsulation of the inner wall of a vascular substitute and suture thread on the anastomosis strength are described. Concerning the problem of the anastomosed part of the blood vessel with the vascular substitute, both effects mentioned above were found to be important requisites for the design of good functional vascular substitute suitable for anastomosis.

Finally, the significance of the *in vitro* and combined *in vivo* and *in vitro* mechanical tests is discussed.

[1] Department of Mechatronics and Precision Engineering, Tohoku University, Aramaki Aoba Aobaku, Sendai, Japan.
[2] Sendai Social Insurance Hospital, Dainohara Aoba-ku, Sendai, Japan.
[3] Sumitomo Metal Industries, Ltd., 1-1-3, Otemachi, Tokyo, Japan.
[4] School of Science and Engineering, Teikyo University, Utsunomiya, Tochigi, Japan.
[5] Sendai JR Hospital, Itsutsubashi, Aoba-ku, Sendai, Japan.

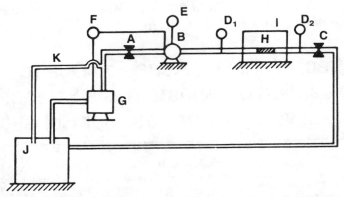

FIG. 1—*Schematic illustration of the apparatus which simulates the actual artery system. (A) valve; (B) apparatus for generating and regulating pulsatile flow; (C) valve; (D₁ and D₂) pressure gage; (E) counter; (F) apparatus for controlling the present system; (G) pump; (H) specimen (blood vessel or vascular substitute) for test; (I) container; (J) tank; (K) bypass.*

Methods

Mechanical Test Method

The methods for mechanical testing and estimation of the anastomosis strength between a vascular substitute and a blood vessel by using a pulsatile pressure flow testing machine were previously published by our group [1–3]. In this paper the same methods were adopted.

The schematic illustration of the apparatus is shown in Fig. 1. The pulsatile pressure through-flow is generated and regulated by the generator **B** with rotary valve driven by the motor whose speed is continuously changeable electrically. The motor is connected to the autocounter **E** which counts the number of pulsatile pressure flow cycles. The frequency rate was adjusted to 54 cycles/min, which is similar to the condition of human blood flow. The amount of the flow through the specimens (vascular substitute and thoracic aorta were used) can be regulated with valve **A**. The dynamic pressure is measured with the pressure transducer D_1 and D_2. The resistance to the flow is exerted with valve **C**, which corresponds to the peripheral resistance. The container **I** is installed so that the test can be made under the condition of the specimens dipped in Ringer liquid. The apparatus was described in detail previously [4]. It has been shown to simulate the artery system sufficiently [4].

Estimation Method on Anastomosis Strength [1–3]

In order to reduce the effect of the variability of the data caused by the difference between blood vessels of different individuals as much as possible, the following method was proposed. A natural blood vessel was anastomosed by suture thread at both ends, with the two different kinds of vascular substitutes to be tested as shown in Fig. 2.

We named this system the double anastomosed specimen (DAS). The natural blood vessel used was the canine thoracic aorta. The vascular grafts used were (1) woven polyester vascular substitute (Nakao Filter Ltd., Japan) and (2) double velour polyester vascular substitute (Cooley, Meadox International Ltd., USA). DAS was fixed to the chuck of the testing apparatus and subjected to repeated pulsatile internal pressure flow through circulating flow. The anastomosis site was sutured surgically by a two-point support continuous suture method using 4-

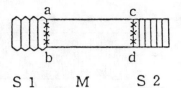

a-b, c-d: anastomotic site

S 1 : Vascular substitute

S 2 : Vascular substitute

FIG. 2—*Double anastomosed test method.*

0 Tev-dec threads. Ringer's solution was used as the circulating fluid. Each length of S_1, M, and S_2 in Fig. 2 is 15 mm.

By using the DAS method, it was possible to make a comparative estimation of the anastomosis strength of blood vessel and vascular substitute under conditions which reduced the scatter of data due to individual variation of the natural blood vessel. The reasons for the reduction in data scatter can be outlined as follows.

If we use the usual single anastomosed specimen, it contains four variables: S_1, S_2 (vascular substitute), M_1, and M_2 (blood vessel of canine).

On the other hand, the DAS method contains three variables: S_1, S_2, and M. Thus by taking the ratio $\sigma_{puls(S_1-M)}/\sigma_{puls(S_2-M)}$, that is, the ratio of anastomosis strength, we can control the difference due to the individuality of the canines and make a comparative estimation of the degree of degradation of anastomosis strength after subjection to repeated pulsatile pressure, thus usually reducing the scatter of the data induced by the difference between the canines within the range of 15% [2]. Each individual anastomosis strength, σ_{puls}, S_1, and σ_{puls}, S_2 causes 2.5 times scatter band as compared with that obtained from our proposed DAS method. Therefore, we can perform this experiment with a small number of sacrificed canines by using the DAS method.

Specimen

Specimens were prepared as A and B groups.

A Group—Woven (Nakao Ltd.) and Double velour (Cooley) polyester vascular substitutes (hereafter named W. polyester and D. polyester substitute, respectively) were implanted at the site of canine aorta by the double anastomosed method as shown in Fig. 2 [1–3]. After three months, this specimen was removed and subjected to the following two types of tests:

(1) The tensile anastomosis strength of both substitutes were measured (A1).
(2) The *in vitro* pulsatile flow through pressure test was carried out on this specimen under the fluctuating pulsatile pressure flow condition up to 2×10^4 cycles as shown in Fig. 3a; that is, $\Delta p_1 = 110$ mmHg and the number of pulsatile pressure is 2290 cycles. $\Delta p_2 = 147$ mmHg, $\Delta p_3 = 184$ mmHg, $\Delta p_4 = 220$ mmHg, $\Delta p_5 = 258$ mmHg and each pulsatile pressure process takes 260 cycles. Δp_6 is 294 mmHg and equals the constant pulsatile pressure amplitude in Fig. 3b; this process takes 3332 cycles. These processes were iterated up to 2×10^4 cycles. The pulsatile pressure flow condition of this type is the most severe and causes deterioration of the blood vessel [5]. After this test, the tensile strength of the anastomosis was measured (A2).

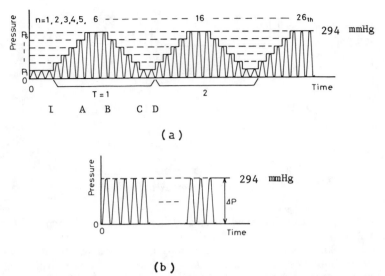

(a)

(b)

FIG. 3—*Pulsatile pressure flow conditions:* (a) *fluctuating amplitude* (b) *constant amplitude. n: total number of steps applied; each step consists of pulse group of equal amplitude. T: number of duplications of series consisting of step groups.*

B Group—Identical double anastomosed specimens (Fig. 2) without having been implanted were also in Tests 1 and 2 described for the A group (B1, B2a). These were performed to compare the results from the A group which have the added effect of tissue adhesion due to encapsulation.

The appearance and the dynamic behavior of the blood vessel and vascular substitute subject to the *in vitro* pulsatile pressure for the B group was shown in Fig. 4.

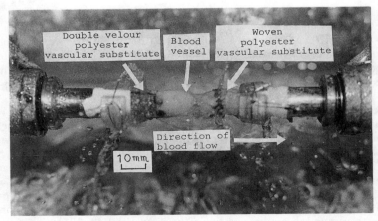

FIG. 4—*Actual global dynamic behaviors of the blood vessel-vascular substitute system (B groups).*

Results

Anastomosis Strength

The ratio of the anastomosis strength of D. polyester substitute with blood vessel to W. polyester substitute with blood vessel is shown in Fig. 5. The results are plotted against pulsatile pressure amplitude for the A group (□) and B group (○) for tests for 1 and 2. Furthermore, the results of the B group under constant through flow pulsatile pressure amplitude [*1–3*] (Fig. 3*b*) are also indicated in Fig. 5 (B2b, ●). The value at 0 mmHg in the abscissa corresponds to the results for Test 1. The pulsatile pressure amplitude in the abscissa represents the maximum pressure amplitude under the condition of pulsatile pressure flow as shown in Fig. 3.

From these results, for the B group, (i.e., the unimplanted), the anastomosis strength of D. polyester substitute with blood vessel is almost equal to that of W. polyester substitute with blood vessel.

On the other hand, for the A group, which *has* been implanted, the anastomosis strength of D. polyester substitute with blood vessel is much higher (almost 2.5 times higher) than that of W. polyester substitute with blood vessel. This ratio becomes larger under the fluctuating pulsatile pressure flow condition as compared with that under 0 mmHg. The enhanced effect on anastomosis strength by tissue adhesion due to encapsulation of D. polyester substitute described in Fig. 5 is more clearly shown in Fig. 6 which is plotted against the implant period.

Observation of the Inner Wall Around the Anastomosed Section of the Vascular Substitute

The inner wall of the anastomosed section of D. polyester and W. polyester substitutes with blood vessel are shown in Figs. 7*a* and 7*b*. The same results observed by scanning electron microscope (SEM, Hitachi Ltd. S415) were shown in Figs. 8*a* and 8*b*. From these results, the inner wall of the anastomosed section of D. polyester substitute with blood vessel was found to be well encapsulated as compared with that of W. polyester substitute with blood vessel,

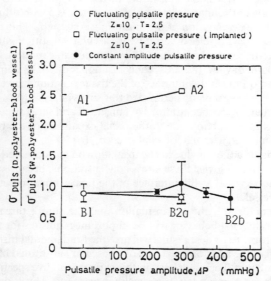

FIG. 5—*Anastomosis strength of D. polyester vascular substitute-blood vessel and W. polyester vascular substitute-blood vessel after being subjected to a pulsatile pressure up to 2×10^4 cycles.*

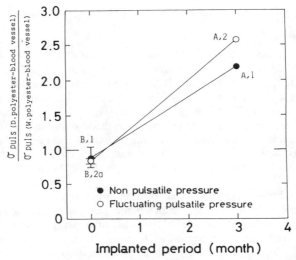

FIG. 6—*The effect of implant period on anastomosis strength.*

although the outer wall of the latter one is thickened. The suture threads were not well encapsulated when used with the W. polyester substitute.

Discussion

From these results, good encapsulation of the inner wall of anastomosed section was found to be very effective in enhancing the anastomosis strength. In previous work [1–3], we reported that if the anastomosis is performed using suture thread only, it is more useful to limit the dynamic pulsatile motion of the anastomosis system as much as possible during each pulsatile cycle in order to avoid the degradation of the anastomosis strength. This means that rigidity around the anastomosed part of blood vessel with vascular substitute is necessary to avoid stress concentrations at the suture thread due to dynamic pulsatile motion. On the other hand, from the mechanical point of view, the stress concentration induced by compliance mismatch at the anastomosed part occurs at the interface of the tissue junction between vascular substitute and blood vessel. We have already performed this stress analysis [6].

Our analysis shows that large concentrations of tangential and shear stress ($\sigma_{\theta\theta}$ and $\tau_{r\theta}$) occur at the interface of the tissue junction due to the radial expansion of the blood vessel by the internal pressure as compared with that of axial stress σ_{xx} [6].

Enhanced effect of tissue adhesion due to encapsulation on anastomosed strength described in this paper will be useful to lower these stress concentrations, because this effect restricts radial expansion of blood vessel at the interface of the tissue junction between the vascular substitute and blood vessel.

Therefore, the effects of both the encapsulation and the suture thread on anastomosis strength and on its mechanical behavior will be important requisites for the design of good functional vascular substitutes. These results will give the fundamental insights into the problem of the degradation of the anastomosed part of a vascular substituted blood vessel [7–10].

Concerning the number of specimens used in this experiment, five specimens were used for the B group test. But in the A group test, one specimen was used. This is due to the following.

In the B group test, aortae can be available from many canines sacrificed for various other experiments performed in the hospital which were not concerned with our experiment. But in the A group test, to investigate the effect of tissue adhesion on anastomosis strength, canines must be sacrified only for our experiment because of the necessity of the implant and its removal from canine.

However, it is very difficult to sacrifice many canines solely for the purposes of this experiment under the condition of preventing cruelty to animals.

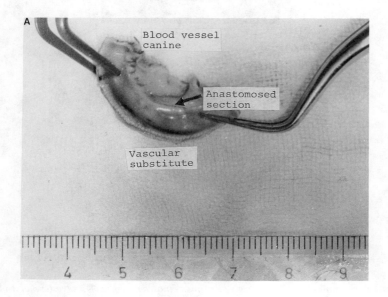

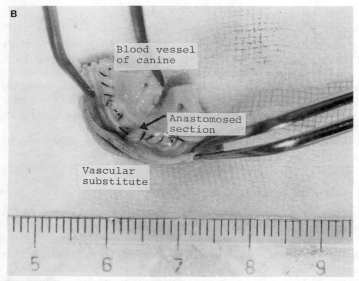

FIG. 7—*Inner wall of anastomosed part of* (a) *D. polyester and* (b) *W. polyester substitutes with blood vessel.*

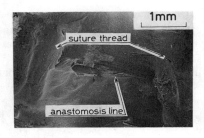

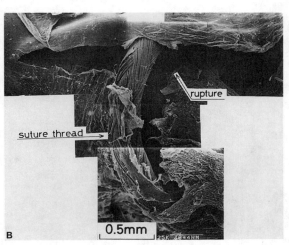

FIG. 8—*Photographs by SEM of inner wall of anastomosed part of* (a) *D. polyester and* (b) *W. polyester substitutes with blood vessel.*

The main purpose of our proposed method, that is, DAS, comes from this situation. Our method proved the data scatter on the anastomosis strength can be remarkably reduced [2]. The ability on the accuracy of the estimation by our testing method assures the significant difference on the anastomosis strength between the A and B groups as shown in Fig 5, because even though we consider that the maximum scatter in the B group test occurs also in the A group test, the anastomosis strength of the A group is significantly higher than that of the B group.

Therefore, this test method has an advantage in that it is compatibile with the demand for the prevention of cruelty to animals.

The Significance of the *In Vitro* and *In Vivo* Tests

The significance of *in vivo* and *in vitro* tests is shown in Fig. 9. Concerning the dialyzer used for hemodialysis, it operates under the *in vitro* condition. Therefore, the *in vitro* mechanical test will directly indicate the safety and strength of the system [3,11].

In the case of vascular substitutes which are accompanied with encapsulation, the *in vitro* test enables one to estimate the virgin strength of vascular substitute itself [1–3], but enhanced effect on its strength by encapsulation makes it difficult to predict its safety strength by only *in vitro* testing. By combining the *in vivo* and the *in vitro* mechanical test as described in this

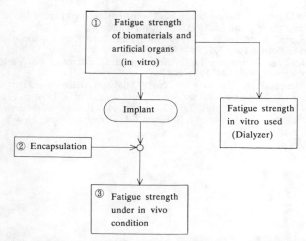

FIG. 9—*Stand points of in vitro and in vivo mechanical test methods.*

paper, this enhanced effect on its strength due to tissue adhesion and the resultant encapsulation will be clarified as shown in Figs. 5 and 6.

Therefore, *in vitro* and combined *in vivo* and *in vitro* tests will be useful in clarifying the mechanical characteristics of biomaterials and tissue material systems which are involved in interactions with physiological factors.

Conclusion

1. In this paper, *in vitro* and combined *in vivo* and *in vitro* mechanical tests were carried out to estimate the anastomosis strength between a vascular substitute and a blood vessel. From these experiments the effects of both of the encapsulation and suture thread on anastomosis strength and its mechanical behavior were investigated.
2. The significance of *in vitro* and the combined *in vivo* and *in vitro* mechanical tests was discussed.

References

[*1*] Yokobori, A. T. Jr., Ohuchi, H., Maeyama, T., et al., "Comparative Test Method for Anastomotic Part of Natural Blood Vessel and Vascular Substutite," *Transactions of the Society for Biomaterials,* Vol. 5, 1982, p. 129.
[*2*] Yokobori, A. T. Jr., Maeyama, T., Ohuchi, H., et al., "Testing Method of Anastomosis Strength and a Comparative Study of Vascular Graft Materials," *Clinical Materials,* Vol. 4, 1989, pp. 41–59.
[*3*] Yokobori, A. T. Jr. and Yokobori, T., "The Mechanical Test Method of Cardiovascular and Related Biomaterials," *Bio-Medical Materials and Engineering, An International Journal,* Vol. 1, 1991, pp. 25–43.
[*4*] Yokobori, A. T. Jr., Yokobori, T., Ohuchi, M., and Sasaki, H., *The Experimental Simulation of Elastic Model of Artery System; Fracture Mechanics and Technology,* Vol. 1, G. C. Sih, Ed., Sigthuft, Novidhoff International Publishers, 1977, pp. 623–638.
[*5*] Yokobori, A. T. Jr., Maeyama, T., Ohkuma, T., et al., "Bio-Mechanical Behaviour of Natural Artery Blood Vessel Under Constant and Variable Internal Pulsatile Pressure Flow Test In Vitro," *Transactions, ASME, Journal of Biomechanical Engineering,* Vol. 108, 1986, pp. 295–306.
[*6*] Yokobori, A. T. Jr. and Chunyun J., "Stress Analysis Around the Anastomotic Site Between Vascular Substitute and Blood Vessel," *Journal of Japanese Society for Biomaterials,* Vol. 10, No. 2, 1992, pp. 59–65.

[7] Sasaki, H. and Ohara, I., "Experimental Study on Anastomosed Part of Blood Vessel," *Journal of Artery and Blood Vessel,* Vol. 15, 1975, p. 11 (in Japanese).

[8] Summer, D. S. and Strandness D. E. "False Aneurysms Occurring in Association with Thrombosed Prosthetic Grafts," *Arch Surg,* Vol. 94, 1967, p. 360.

[9] Hokanson, D. F. and Strandness, D. E. "Stress-Strain Characteristics of Various Arterial Graft," *Surg. Gynecol, Obstet.,* Vol. 124, 1967, p. 1267.

[10] Kumada, J., Motohashi, H., Takemiya, S., et al., "Study on Anastomosed Part of Blood Vessel with Vascular Substitute," *Japanese Journal of Artificial Organ,* Vol. 1, 1972, p. 128 (in Japanese).

[11] Yokobori, A. T. Jr. and Yokobori, T., "Cellophane as a Biomedical Material," *Encyclopedia of Material Science and Engineering,* M. B. Bever, Ed., Pergamon Press, New York, 1986, pp. 557–559.

Adhesive Films and Plastics

S. H. Teoh[1]

Predicting the Life and Design Stresses of Medical Plastics Under Creep Conditions

REFERENCE: Teoh, S. H., **"Predicting the Life and Design Stresses of Medical Plastics Under Creep Conditions,"** *Biomaterials' Mechanical Properties, ASTM STP 1173*, H. E. Kambic and A. T. Yokobori, Jr., Eds., American Society for Testing and Materials, Philadelphia, 1994, pp. 77–86.

ABSTRACT: Polymers are finding increasing use in biomedical engineering applications. One of the major problems in designing with polymers is predicting when the material will fail and what stress values should be used in the design of components in order that the material will not fail prematurely. Recent work on modeling the creep rupture behavior of more than 15 polymers has produced a breakthrough in predicting the failure times as well as the upper stress and lower stress limits of the polymers [1,2]. The upper stress relates to the maximum stress that can be applied to the material before instantaneous fracture. The lower stress limit relates to the minimum stress that can be sustained by the material without failure and, in some cases, this also corresponds to the fatigue endurance limit of the polymer. The creep rupture times of some medical plastics such as high density polyethylene (HDPE), polycarbonate (PC), polypropylene (PP), polyoxymethylene (POM), polyvinylchloride (PVC), polysulphone (PSU), and polymethylmethacrylate (PMMA) were analyzed at 20°C in air. In order to optimize the parameters for creep rupture prediction, a nonlinear regression analysis program was used [1]. Special attention was made for Delrin (POM from Du Pont) which is of interest in cardiovascular applications related to wear of mechanical heart valves [3]. This material was tested in air at 37, 60, and 80°C. The effect of saline solution was also studied. Here, the lower stress limit was reduced from 20 MPa to 5 MPa. All the specimens brittle fractured. This may account why Delrin used in the artificial hip joint prosthesis [4] where the contact stresses exceed this limit was known to wear severely. However, in the disc of the mechanical heart valve [3] no failure occurs because the stresses were probably below the lower stress limit.

KEYWORDS: failure prediction, design stresses, medical plastics, creep, upper stress limit, lower stress limit, creep rupture modeling

Polymers such as polyethylene, polysulphone, polyoxymethylene, polyurethane, and polymethylmethacrylate are finding increased usage in biomedical engineering applications. For example Delrin, a homo-polymer polyoxymethylene produced by Du Pont, has an *in-vivo* experience of more than 17 years in the tilting disc Björk-Shiley mechanical heart valves [3]. Polyurethane is now used in the production of left ventricular assist devices. One of the major problems in designing with polymers used in the biomedical field is the prediction of when the material will fail and what stress values should be used in the design of components in order that the material will not fail prematurely. Figure 1 illustrates a typical example on the artificial knee ligament (anterior cruciate ligament) where the designer has to determine the size of the artificial ligament to withstand a certain dead load for a certain lifetime. Conventionally this is done by trial and error since predictive methods have not been very satisfactory. However,

---

[1] Senior lecturer, Mechanical and Production Engineering Department, National University of Singapore, Singapore 0511.

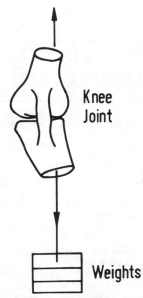

FIG. 1—*Schematic illustration of a knee ligament subjected to a uniaxial load.*

recent work on modeling the creep rupture behavior of more than 15 polymers has produced a breakthrough in predicting accurately the failure times as well as the upper stress and lower stress limits of the polymers [3,4].

This paper reports on the application of the creep rupture modeling to obtain design stresses for some medical plastics such as polyethylene, polycarbonate (PC), polypropylene (PP), polyoxymethylene (POM), polyvinylchloride (PVC), polysulphone (PSU), and polymethyl-methacrylate (PMMA). Special attention, in terms of creep testing and modeling at different temperatures, was made for Delrin since this material is currently under research in cardio-vascular applications related to wear in the design of mechanical heart valves [3]. The effect of saline solution was also investigated for this material.

Design Stress Prediction

Conventionally, design stresses were obtained from short-term tests such as from the constant strain rate test where safety factors were applied to the yield or proof stresses. This method may work for metals and ceramics, but in the case of plastics, because of viscoelasticity and time-dependent fracture, long-term tests need to be carried out in order to determine the design stresses. Creep rupture tests where the material is subjected to constant load and temperature (ASTM D 2990, Test Methods for Tensile, Compressive, and Flexural Creep and Creep Rupture of Plastics) are used frequently for long-term tests to evaluate the design stresses. The two important design stresses are the upper and lower stress limits. The upper stress relates to the maximum stress that can be applied to the material before instantaneous fracture. The lower stress limit relates to the minimum stress that can be sustained by the material without failure.

Creep rupture data involving rupture stress and time are often represented by log-log or semi-log graphs and the upper stress limit is defined by the intercept at the log time-axis of a straight line of best fit drawn across the data points using linear regression analysis [5]. However, the determination of the lower stress limit is not amenable to such a simple technique and since most components are designed to withstand a life of ten years, extrapolation of the stress to this period is taken as the lower stress limit. This may not be adequate for implant medical plastics. Application of plastics to biomedical use demands a more stringent and reliable method to predict both the upper and lower stress limits. The extensive creep rupture work on a variety of polymers by Gotham [6] and Teoh [1] indicated the existence of some stress limits where the specimen did not fail for a long time. Recently, Teoh [1] has published a model that could predict both the upper and lower stress limits and give some physical meaning to the elements used in the model [2]. Such modeling gives the designer a better understanding into the mechanisms that lead to fracture. For example, the lower stress limit has been shown to be a function of the cohesive energy density of the polymers indicating that the elastic and anelastic modulus in the model can be thought of as due to elastic stretching of main chain C-C segments and to the secondary Van der Waals forces acting between the chains, respectively [2].

Creep Rupture Model

Historically, plastic yielding was believed to be due to a temperature increase as a result of adiabatic strain energy conversion. The failure of such criterion to adequately predict the plastic yielding of polymers has led to a number of models ranging from free volume to rate-activated processes. Some of these models are too complex and involve numerous parameters to adjust. Questions arise as to the physical meaning of these parameters.

The creep rupture model used here involves a simple three-element mechanical model and a critical elastic stored energy criterion. As shown in Fig. 2a, this model incorporates two linear springs. One of these is paralleled by a nonlinear (Eyring) rate activated dashpot element and is characterized by a modulus E_a which in this paper, because it represents the elastic component of the anelastic (time-dependent) deformation, is termed the anelastic modulus. The second spring is characterized by a modulus E_e which, because it represents the instantaneously elastic deformation of the polymer, is termed the elastic modulus. These springs moduli can be thought of to represent the deformation of molecular domains in chain segment direction (E_e) and perpendicular to it (E_a) (Fig. 2b). The important result of this model is that it can be used to predict the lower stress limit (SN) at which the material sustains the load

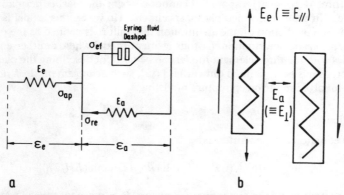

a   b

FIG. 2—(a) *A simple three-element model and* (b) *its physical interpretation used for creep rupture modeling.*

indefinitely and the upper stress limit (SX) at which the material fractures immediately on loading. These limits depend only on the elastic constants and on the resilience of the material.

The critical elastic stored energy criterion used in the creep rupture modeling follows that of the Reiner-Weissenberg theory [7] which assumes that failure depends upon a maximum value of the intrinsic free energy that can be stored elastically in the volume of a material. According to this criterion, failure will occur when the conserved work (W_e) in the elastic elements reaches a critical value R which is the resilience of the material. From thermodynamics, the conserved work is equal to the difference between the input (W) and the dissipated (D) work. The sum of their difference with respect to time can be expressed as

$$\dot{W_e} + \dot{D} - \dot{W} = 0.$$

Hence, the Reiner-Weissenberg failure criterion can be stated as:

$$W_e = \int_0^{t_f} (\dot{W} - \dot{D})\, dt = R$$

where t_f is the time to failure. One of the important aspects of this equation is that it shows that failure is dependent upon the loading history. The first verification of the Reiner-Weissenberg theory of strength was performed by Foux and Brüller [8] on the limit of linear viscoelastic behavior of perspex and epoxy resin. They found that the resilience values of the two materials were independent of strain rates. For the prediction of crazes or fractures, a modified version relating only to the energy associated with viscous flow process in polymers was found to be appropriate [9].

Applying the Reiner-Weissenberg failure criterion to simple mechanical models such as the Kelvin and Maxwell models under constant load gives the following interesting conclusions. A Kelvin solid fails when the strain reaches a critical limiting value and a Maxwell solid fails when the stress reaches a critical limiting value. When applied to the model as shown in Fig. 2a, under creep condition different critical stress limits can be obtained. These limits relate to the upper and lower stress limits, as derived in a previous publication [1]. The model shows only one retardation time. However, Fig. 2 should be viewed as a simplified model and if one incorporates similar multiple units in series or parallel with each other, a spectrum of retardation times can be realized. For the sake of simplicity and ease of computation, such arrangements have not been adopted. Although the model shown in Fig. 2 can describe the elastic and the anelastic (time-dependent) response, it cannot describe the plastic (permanent) response which is present in many deformed plastic specimens. However, this model is adequate for creep rupture time prediction on the assumption that failure is defined as the onset of large-scale permanent plastic deformation. (A four-element model where another dashpot is connected in series with the three-element model can be used for describing the plastic deformation. However, as has been pointed out earlier [1,2], such arrangement does not change the mathematics involved in the creep rupture modeling.)

Model Equation

The model equation can be written as

$$\ln t_f = \ln \{1/(CB) \ln [\tanh (B\sigma_{ap}/2)/\tanh (BH/2)]\} \tag{1}$$

where C = constant related to the activation energy, B = constant related to the activation volume, E_a = anelastic modulus, E_e = elastic modulus, R = resilience of the material (defined as the maximum elastic stored energy before fracture), σ_{ap} = applied stress, and $H = \sigma_{ap} - [2E_a(R - \sigma_{ap}^2/E_e)]^{1/2}$.

It can be seen that when the applied stress equals $(E_e R)^{1/2}$, immediate fracture occurs and when it equals $[R/(1/E_e + \frac{1}{2}E_a)]^{1/2}$, the material sustains the load indefinitely. The upper stress limit, SX, can be denoted as

$$SX = (E_e R)^{1/2} \tag{2}$$

and the lower stress limit, SN as

$$SN = [R/(1/E_e + \frac{1}{2}E_a)]^{1/2} \tag{3}$$

From Eqs 2 and 3, the local mechanical anisotropy can be derived as

$$E_e/E_a = 2[(SX/SN)^2 - 1] \tag{4}$$

Experimental Procedure

The materials examined were PSU, PC, PMMA, PVC, high density polyethylene (HDPE) (made under air cooling), POM, and PP. The creep rupture data of some of these materials such as PSU, PMMA, and PC were obtained from published literature [6]. These materials were either injection-molded, cast- or compression-molded. The full details of the fabrication methods of the other materials have been reported earlier [10,11].

The creep rupture experiments in air were performed at 20 ± 1 °C and $65 \pm 5\%$ RH, except for POM (Delrin 500 from Du Pont) which was also carried out at 37, 60, and 80 ± 1 °C. Dead weights were hung onto the specimens in a uniaxial direction with the help of a hydraulic jack. The creep rupture time was automatically recorded by a clock timer. The duration of the tests varied from a few seconds to more than three years. If the specimens did not break, the time taken for the elongation to reach the limit of the test rig (about 300% extension) was taken as the time to failure. The long-time creep rupture tests were necessary in order to confirm the lower stress limit predicted by Eq 1. All applied stress was calculated by dividing the applied load by the original cross-sectional area.

The specimen shape used by Gotham [6] does not have a constant width along the gage length of the specimens but has reduced cross-sections having a theoretical stress intensity factor of about 1.01. This is deemed insignificant when compared to the 10% experimental inaccuracy allowed for creep rupture experiments. All other specimens reported here have uniform cross-section along the gage length and conform to ASTM D 638 (Test Method for Tensile Properties of Plastics) Type II.

To study the effect of salt solution, the Delrin specimens were soaked in saline solution (0.9% NaCl) in glass tubes sealed on one end with silicone rubber and tested at 37 ± 1 °C till rupture. They were all subjected to at least 48 h in saline solution at room temperature before creep rupture testing. Occasionally, distilled water was added to the original level when the saline solution was found to have evaporated.

An IBM 3090 with SAS-NLIN nonlinear regression optimization was used to analyze the creep rupture data. From Eq 1 it can be realized that the function is nonlinear and optimizing the parameters (SX, SN, B, and C) will be highly sensitive to the initial estimates given to the parameters. The advantage of using SAS NLIN when compared to other statistical packages available commercially is that it performs an initial grid search of the parameters and uses the best set for the initial trial estimates. This eliminates a significant amount of time in obtaining

TABLE 1—*Parameters in creep rupture modeling of some medical plastics at 20°C in air.*

Plastics	SX (MPa)	SN (MPa)	B (MPa^{-1})	C (s^{-1})	E_e/E_a
POM (H)[a]	75	30	0.17	2.65E-7	9.5
POM (C)[b]	66	29	0.26	9.90E-8	8.4
HDPE	32	8	0.46	2.00E-6	30
PC	64	47	0.31	4.30E-7	1.7
PMMA	89	34	0.21	1.00E-7	11.7
PP (H)[a]	30	10	0.54	4.47E-8	16
PP (C)[b]	24	10	0.66	4.45E-6	9.5
PSU	81	42	0.29	1.67E-7	2.9
PVC	68	35	0.27	6.40E-7	5.5

[a] Homo-polymer.
[b] Co-polymer.

initial estimates of the parameters by trial and error method. For most consistent results, the Marquardt option in SAS NLIN is the best. This option is a compromise between the Gauss-Newton and Steepest Descent method and has been proven to be very reliable in practice and, in several cases, faster than other methods especially when the parameter estimates are highly correlated. Meaningful estimates can only be achieved if reasonable bounds were imposed on the parameters. The detailed computational procedures were reported earlier [1].

Results and Discussion

Table 1 shows the results of the creep rupture modeling at 20°C. The results of the effect of temperature and saline solution on Delrin are shown in Table 2. Figure 3 shows the creep rupture data fitted with Eq 1 for the nine medical plastics. The creep rupture modeling at various temperatures for Delrin is illustrated in Fig. 4. Figure 5 shows the effect of saline solution at 37°C on the creep rupture behavior of Delrin.

Generally, a good fit can be noticed for all the experimental points using Eq 1. This shows that the present model for creep rupture does apply for the medical plastics. An exception perhaps is PMMA where the fit at high stresses is less convincing. This may be due to the fact that the experimental data at high stresses are subjected to errors since fast fracture and localized heating can occur. It is interesting to note that the fit to all the experimental data is independent of the different creep fracture phenomena that have been observed [10,11]. For polyethylene and Delrin three regions corresponding to low, intermediate, and high stresses were identified with respect to the occurrence of stress whitening and brittle or ductile fracture, or

TABLE 2—*Parameters in creep rupture modeling of Delrin (POM).*

SX (MPa)	SN (MPa)	B (MPa^{-1})	C (s^{-1})	E_e/E_a	Test Conditions
75	30	0.17	2.65E-7	9.5	20°C/air
72	20	0.16	2.40E-7	23.9	37°C/air
61	10	0.24	2.60E-7	72.4	60°C/air
57	4	0.24	1.00E-7	404.1	80°C/air
72	5	0.24	2.51E-7	412.7	37°C/saline

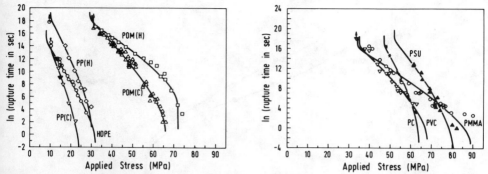

FIG. 3—*Creep rupture modeling of some medical plastics. (C = co-polymer, H = homo-polymer).*

both. The model proposed here is concerned with molecular fracture in a microscopic scale while the fracture phenomena observed are related to macroscopic events. The occurrence of permanent stress whitening or macro-necking [*10*] usually occurs toward the latter stages of creep (during tertiary creep). The time taken for fracture spans from primary, secondary, to tertiary creep. Hence when one uses fracture time as a modeling parameter, as in the present case, one would not expect macroscopic events which occur only at the end of a creep experiment for a short period to have any significant influence on the analysis of the results.

In a number of cases such as PVC, HDPE, and POM, the lower stress limits predicted by Eq 1 are close to the experimental results where the specimens did not fracture even after 3 years of testing (indicated by arrow heads in Fig. 3). Interestingly, the British Standard Institute (Code of practice 312) has designated a safe design stress of 5 MPa for long-term usage of polyethylene, and assuming a reasonable safety factor of 2, it can be realized that the computed SN for HDPE can be considered to be a good estimate of the lower stress limit before the application of the safety factor. Similarly, Riddell [*12*] reported the fatigue endurance limit for PP as 10 MPa which is obtained here. The SN values for the POM homo-polmyer, and co-poly-

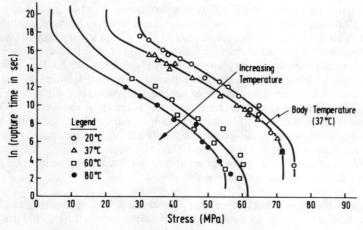

FIG. 4—*Creep rupture modeling of Delrin at various temperatures.*

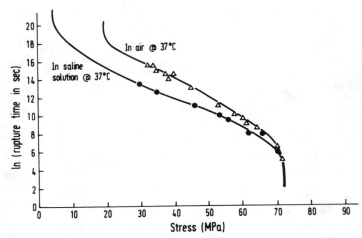

FIG. 5—*Creep rupture modeling of Delrin at 37°C showing the effect of saline solution.*

mer are 30 and 29 MPa, respectively (Table 1). These values are also very close to the endurance fatigue limit for Delrin reported by Du Pont [*13*].

Some plastics such as POM and PP can come in the form of homo- or co-polymer. From Table 1 evidently SX is lower for the co-polymers. However, SN is seen to be independent on the type of polymer. The parameter B is related to the activation volume (product of the area swept and the distance moved by a molecular flow unit) and the results indicate that the co-polymers have higher values. The E_e/E_a ratio is an indication of the local anisotropy [*2*]. Here, the results show that the POM is not greatly affected by the type of polymer but for PP, marked differences can be seen. PP homo-polymer has a higher local anisotropy when compared to PP co-polymer.

The effect of temperature on Delrin (Table 2 and Fig. 4) is to reduce both SX and SN. The local anisotropy increases dramatically with increase in temperature. This is more so for POM tested in saline solution where E_e/E_a ratio is even higher than that at 80°C and SN drops from 20 to 5 MPa. The effects of temperature (within this range of 20 to 80°C) and saline solution do not have significant contribution on the other parameters B and C. On measuring the strain to fracture, all the POM tested in saline solution has a strain to fracture less than 5% while those tested in air at the same temperature exceed 20% except at very high stress and stresses below 30 MPa where the strain to fracture is about 10% [*11*]. The fracture surfaces revealed a brittle failure mechanism where the plane of fracture is perpendicular to the tensile axis. This may account why Delrin used in the artificial hip joint prosthesis [*4*] where the contact stresses would have exceeded this limit was known to wear severely, while in the disc of the mechanical heart valves [*3*] no failure occurs because the stresses were probably below the lower stress limit. It is noteworthy that SX is not affected by saline solution. This meant that where applications involving only short loading time using only SX, such as in snap fits in the joints of catheters, the values of SX tested in air may be good enough.

For Delrin tested at elevated temperatures and in saline solution, the increase in the E_e/E_a ratio can be visualized as due to three possible effects:

1. Increase in the main chain stiffness due to work hardening or structural change, or both (example, due to change from spherulitic structure to fibrils during cold drawing).

2. Increase in the perpendicular distance between chain segments (see Fig. 2b) (example, due to a swelling agent).
3. Decrease in the secondary forces of attraction between chain segments (example, due to physical aging).

The first effect would increase E_e while the last two effects would decrease E_a. The observation that pre-rupture phenomena such as stress whitening, necking, and cold drawing usually occur towards the end of the creep rupture experiments and that the model Eq 1 uses the total time to failure, suggests that it will be unlikely due to an increase in E_e to account for the increase in the local anisotropy as seen in Table 2. It will be more probable that it is due to 2 and 3 above, since at higher temperatures the chain segments are more thermally activated and physical aging does increase with increase in temperature. The effect of saline solution can also be attributed to 2 and 3.

Conclusion

The creep rupture times of some medical plastics such as HDPE, PC, PP, Delrin, PVC, PSU, and PMMA were modeled accurately using an elastically stored energy criterion in conjunction with a simple three-element mechanical model. This model also predicted the upper and lower stress limits which are useful for design purposes in biomedical applications. In some cases, the predicted lower stress limits also corresponded to the published endurance fatigue limit. The assignment of physical elements in the molecular scale particularly in the interpretation of the local mechanical anisotropy made this creep rupture model useful in interpreting the mechanisms that might have contributed to the change in the stress limits. For Delrin it was noted that the lower stress limit drops from 20 to 5 MPa in the presence of saline solution. This may account for the reason why a number of implant prostheses using Delrin such as in the hip joint prostheses [4] where the contact stresses exceeded the lower stress limit in saline solution wear severely. However, those in heart valves occluders [3] have an *in-vivo* experience exceeding 17 years and still no failure since the contact stresses are generally very small. The creep rupture modeling work underscores the importance of accurately determining the design stresses and predicting the rupture time in body fluid of medical plastics. It also represents a significant improvement over conventional creep rupture stress prediction.

References

[1] Teoh, S. H., "Computational Aspects in Creep Rupture Modelling of Polypropylene Using an Energy Failure Criterion in Conjunction with a Mechanical Model," *Polymer,* Vol. 31, 1990, pp. 2260–2266.
[2] Teoh, S. H., Cherry, B. W., and Kausch, H. H., "Creep Rupture Modelling of Polymers," *International Journal of Damage Mechanics,* Vol. 1, 1992, pp. 245–256.
[3] Teoh, S. H., Martin, R. L., Lim, S. C., et al., "Delrin as an Occluder Material," *American Society of Artificial Internal Organs, Transactions,* Vol. 36, 1990, pp. M417–M421.
[4] Dumbleton, J., "Delrin as a Material for Joint Prosthesis—A Review,"*Corrosion and Degradation of Implant Materials, ASTM STP 684,* B.C. Syrett and A. Acharya, Eds., American Society for Testing and Materials, Philadelphia, 1979, pp. 41–60.
[5] Barton, S. J. and Cherry, B. W., "Predicting the Creep Rupture Life of Polyethylene Pipe," *Polymer Engineering Science,* Vol. 19, No. 8, 1979, pp. 590–595.
[6] Gotham, K. V., "Long-Term Strength of Thermoplastics—The Ductile-Brittle Transition in Static Fatigue," *Plastics and Polymers,* Vol. 40, 1972, pp. 59–64.
[7] Reiner, M., "A Thermodynamic Theory of Strength," *Fracture Processes in Polymeric Solids,* B. Rosen, Ed., Interscience, New York, 1964, pp. 517–527.

[8] Foux, A. and Brüller, O. S., "Limit of Linear Viscoelasticity Behaviour—An Energy Criterion," *Proceedings of the International Conference on Mechanical Behaviour of Materials, Kyoto,* Vol. 1, 1971, pp. 237–244.

[9] Brüller, O. S., "Energy-Related Failure Criteria of Thermoplastics,"*Polymer Engineering and Science,* Vol. 21, No. 3, 1981, pp. 145–150.

[10] Teoh, S. H. and Cherry, B. W., "Creep Rupture of a Linear Polyethylene—Part I: Rupture and Pre-Rupture Phenomena," *Polymer,* Vol. 25, 1984, pp. 727–734.

[11] Teoh, S. H. and Michaeli, W., "Creep Rupture Modelling of Polyacetal,"*Proceedings of the Joint FEFG/ICF International Conference on Fracture of Engineering Materials and Structures, Singapore,* S. H. Teoh and K. H. Lee, Eds., Elsevier Science Publisher, Barking, England, 1991, pp. 243–250.

[12] Riddell, M. N., *Plastics Engineering,* Vol. 30, No. 4, 1972, p. 71.

[13] *Design Handbook for Du Pont Engineering Plastics,* Module III, Delrin, Du Pont, Wilmington, DE 19880-0018.

Peter C. Moon,[1] Jeffrey W. Moxley,[2] Thomas W. Haas,[3] and Young H. Chang[2]

Mechanical Properties of Hard Tissue Adhesive Films

REFERENCE: Moon, P. C., Moxley, J. W., Haas, T. W., and Chang, Y. H., "**Mechanical Properties of Hard Tissue Adhesive Films,**" *Biomaterials' Mechanical Properties, ASTM STP 1173,* H. E. Kambic and A. T. Yokobori, Jr., Eds., American Society for Testing and Materials, Philadelphia, 1994, pp. 87–95.

ABSTRACT: Improved dental adhesives for bonding to the dentin of teeth have been introduced that may have the potential of bonding to bone. The properties of these materials have not been characterized. The purpose of this study was to measure the mechanical properties of three of these adhesive resins, Universal Bond II (UB2), Scotchbond II (SB2), and Tenure (Ten). These measurements were used to determine if the bond strengths approached the cohesive strengths of the materials and for finite element evaluation of polymerization shrinkage bond stress. Thin resin films (130 ± 5 μm) were cast and cured between microscope slides. The films ($N = 6$) were tested using an Instron tensile test at 2.5 mm/min and a Rheometric Solids Analyzer (1 Hz) after 24 hours in air. The breaking strength and maximum strain of TEN, SB2, and UB2 were 19.0 ± 2.8, 17.4 ± 3.7, 10.7 ± 1.0 MPa, and 8%, 6%, and 32%, respectively. The strength of UB2 was significantly different at $P < 0.05$. Rheometric analysis gave the dynamic (1 Hz) and static elastic modulus, $\tan d_{max}$, and T_g for TEN, SB2, and UB2 as follows: 1100, 1000, 600 MPa; 620, 530, 370 MPa; 0.20, 0.67, 0.21; and 75°C, 79°C, 84°C, respectively. The measurements were the first reported for properties of these materials.

The use of the measured mechanical properties in the finite element models to calculate the interfacial stress of bonded composite restoration demonstrated that the maximum shrinkage stresses were reduced below the bond strengths by using thick resin bonded films of 125 μm to allow stress relaxation. The finite element models indicated that variations in the maximum shrinkage stress and its location occurred depending on the curing conditions. These finite element analyses were the first models of curing shrinkage applied to dental bonding.

KEYWORDS: dentin bonding agents, mechanical properties, finite element analysis, shrinkage stress, thick bond films, composite resins

Dentin bonding agents have been available for about seven years for bonding dental composites to the dentin part of the tooth. Recent modifications have improved their bond strength and reduced microleakage around dental restorations [1]. However, the shrinkage stress of the curing composite resin was still sufficient to open a marginal gap and to allow reduced microleakage [2]. The newest dentin bonding agents used a primer for the dentin containing mild acids with wetting agents, and a visible light cured (VLC) adhesive resin [3]. The acid removed or modified the dentin smear layer to open the dentinal tubules. The wetting

[1] Director, Dental Materials Science, Medical College of Virginia, Biomedical Engineering Program, Virginia Commonwealth University, Richmond, VA 23298.

[2] A. D. Williams Research Fellow and Research Assistant, respectively, Medical College of Virginia Dental School, Richmond, VA 23298.

[3] Director, Engineering Program, Virginia Commonwealth University, Richmond, VA 23298.

agents wetted into the tubules so the hydrophobic dentin adhesive resin flowed into the tubules and locked into them when light-cured [4]. The visible light-curing adhesive films were generally more completely cured and crosslinked than the earlier generation of self-curing films [5]. The purpose of this study was to measure the mechanical properties of these adhesive films to determine if the bond strength was limited by the cohesive strength of the films and to characterize their mechanical properties to determine if differences in their performance were explained by their properties. In addition, the elastic properties measured were used in two-dimensional finite element analysis models to determine how film thickness (0, 125, 250, and 500 μm) and curing mode (visible light cured versus self-cure) affected the stress at floor and wall of bonded composite resin restorations placed in dentin root surfaces. Also, these bonding agents may have the potential for bonding to bone which has a composition similar to dentin but a different structural organization [6].

Materials and Methods of Mechanical Property Measurement

The materials used to form the adhesive films were marked in Table 1 with an asterisk. The compositions from the table were obtained from the respective companies. The tension specimens and solids analyzer specimens were formed by placing double-sided Scotch tape along the length of each edge on one side of a microscope slide so that a parallel channel approximately ⅜-in. (9.5-mm) wide was formed down the center, the length of the slide. Four drops of liquid for the adhesive film to be formed were dispensed near one end of the slide in the channel formed by the double-sided tape. A second glass microscope slide was rotated to contact the tape on the first slide starting at the end of the first slide where the liquid was dispensed.

TABLE 1—*Composition of dentin bonding agents.*

Tenure (Den Mat Inc.)	Primer	2.5% Nitric Acid 3.5% Aluminum Oxylate Aquas solution
	Solution A*	5% N-tolylglycine-glycidyl methacrylate in acetone
	Solution B*	10% pyromellitic acid dehydrid in acetone
	Visar Seal*	BisGMA[a] + VLC catalyst
Scotch Bond II (3M Co.)	Primer	5% Maleic Acid 55% Hema[b] 40% H₂0
	Adhesive*	60% BisGMA 40% Hema 1% Camphorquinone
Universal Bond II (Dentsply, Inc.)	Primer	34% Hema 6% Penta[c] in Ethanol
	Adhesive*	5% Penta .45% Glutaraldahyde 50+% Urethane Dimethacrylate BisGMA TEGMA[d] VLC Agents

* Used to make thin films.
[a] Bisphenol A Methacrylate.
[b] Hydroxy Ethyl Methacrylate.
[c] Dipenta Erythritol Pentacrylate Phosphate.
[d] Tetra Ethyl Glycidyl Methacrylate.

This rotating motion caused the liquid to flow down the channel without trapping air as the second slide adhered to the double-sided tape trapping the adhesive liquid between the tape channel and the glass slides to form a mold. If gross bubbles or clusters of fine bubbles were trapped during forming of the films, the films were not tested. All very small bubbles could not be eliminated. The adhesive liquids were cured into solid films of approximately 130 ± 5 μm thick by shining a Prismetics curing light (Caulk Co.) through the slides for 3 min moving it evenly to cover the film area. The films were separated from the slides by placing them in water for 20 min. The first slide was pried off and the film was slowly peeled from the second slide. Six tension tests were run for each adhesive film material to measure an average tensile strength in an Instron testing machine at a cross-head speed of 2.5 mm/min. The cross-sectional area of the films was calculated by multiplying the thickness times the width. The thickness and width were measured using a Mitutoyo digital micrometer which measured to 1 μm. The films were held during testing by pneumatic grips (Instron, Inc.) with a maximum load capacity of 90 kg and a flat metal gripping surfaces. The air pressure that actuated the pneumatic grips was set for a lower value of approximately 0.2 MPa. If any films broke at the grips, the value was not recorded and new films were made and tested. The static modulus, dynamic modulus (1 Hz), loss modulus, loss tangent maximum and loss tangent peak temperature (T_g — glass transition temperature) were measured on the films using a Rheometrics Inc. Solids Analyzer.

Materials and Methods for Computer Finite Element Modeling

The properties used to calculate the shrinkage stress for the Class 5 composite resins restorations found in tooth root surfaces of dentin are listed in Table 2. Algor, Inc. software was run on a 386 IBM Clone PC with a math coprocessor to calculate the finite element stress values. The composite restoration was modeled as a two-dimensional composite restoration 2-mm-deep and 4-mm-across with 2 mm of dentin thickness under the restoration and 2 mm dentin thickness at the preparation walls modeling the tooth. The tooth and restoration were meshed into 125 μm square elements. Symmetry allows the number of elements to be reduced by half. The node stress perpendicular to the walls and floor of the preparation were calculated by simulating the polymerization shrinkage by choosing a coefficient of thermal expansion and node temperature change for the composite resin elements to produce a thermal shrinkage equivalent to the polymerization shrinkage. Thus, the thermal residual stress represented the composite polymerization total volume shrinkage residual bond stress. The following curing conditions were simulated by using the order of the composite resin element temperature change and stress superposition to represent the reaction dynamics:

1. The self-cured reaction is simulated by allowing all composite resin elements to change temperature at the same time and the resultant stress calculated.

TABLE 2—*Material properties used for finite element analysis.*

	Elastic Modulus, GPa	Poisson's Ratio	Linear Shrinkage, %
Composite Resin P-50 (3M Co.)	15.0	0.216	0.83
Dentin Bonding Adhesive UB-2 (L. D. Caulk)	0.336	0.40[a]	0[b]
Dentin	13.0	0.30	

[a] Used Pmma.
[b] Precured; assumed 0.

2. The bulk visible light cure is simulated from the top of the restoration down to the floor by having the restoration cure in 500-μm layers (i.e., 4 elements thick) from the top down by changing the temperature of each layer separately, solving for the bond stresses of each layer and adding results at the nodes. If the 500-μm layers are numbered 1, 2, 3, and 4 starting from the top surface, they are cured in the same order.

3. The two-step light cured restoration was simulated by packing the composite resin in two increments of 1000 μm and curing after packing an increment. Each increment is cured as two 500-μm layers by changing the temperature for each 500-μm layer separately and superimposing the stress calculated at the interfacial nodes. Using the same layer numbering from 1 at the top surface to 4 at the floor of the restoration, the order of curing of the layers was 3, 4, 1, and 2.

4. The bulk light cure from the bottom of the restoration up, as would be represented by shining the curing light through the tooth, was simulated by having the 500-μm layers cured from the bottom to the top in the layer order 4, 3, 2, and 1 and superimposing the stresses from these individual solutions to approximate the resultant stress of the dynamic curing condition.

These conditions assumed that the adhesive bond film's thickness was zero so the maximum residual bond stress was high. Experimental adhesive films have been reported to be 10 to 30 μm in thickness [7,8]. Elements of this size would have increased the degrees of freedom of the model beyond the capacity of our software and hardware to analyze a solution. It was believed as the strain capacity of a 10-μm film was limited, a zero thickness film stress analysis was a good but slightly high approximation to the stress present in commercially available products. However, increments of resin thickness of 0, 125, 250, and 500 μm were accommodated easily by the model by changing the appropriate interfacial element properties (i.e., elastic modulus and Poisson's ratio). These calculations allowed the effect of thick resin adhesive film layers on the residual bond stress to be evaluated and the potential for the elastic strain capacity of thick films to reduce the shrinkage bond stresses to be determined.

Results of the Mechanical Tests of Dentin Bond Adhesives

Measurements of the different mechanical tests are listed in Table 3. From Table 3 and Fig. 1, it was evident that the mechanical properties of Tenure and Scotchbond-2 are higher than Universal Bond-2, except Universal Bond-2 is much more ductile with a 32% elongation compared to the 6% and 8% of Scotchbond-2 and Tenure, respectively. The increased ductility and lower yield stress have advantages in allowing stress relaxation in Universal Bond-2 bond lay-

TABLE 3—*Mechanical properties of dental adhesive films.*

Property	Tenure	Scotch Bond II	Universal Bond II
Average Tensile Strength	19.0 ± 2.8 MPa	17.4 ± 3.7 MPa	10.7 ± 1.0 MPa
Yield Stress (.6% offset)	13.3 MPa	14.3 MPa	5.1 MPa
Elastic Modulus Static	620 MPa	530 MPa	370 MPa
Elastic Modulus Dynamic (1 Hz)	1100 MPa	1000 MPa	600 MPa
Loss Modulus (25°C and 1 Hz)	120 MPa	210 MPa	90 MPa
Loss Tangent Peak Temperature (1 Hz)	75°C	79°C	84°C
Loss Tangent Maximum	.20	.67	.21
Bond Strength (Shear)	18.6 MPa	13.8 MPa	10.3 MPa

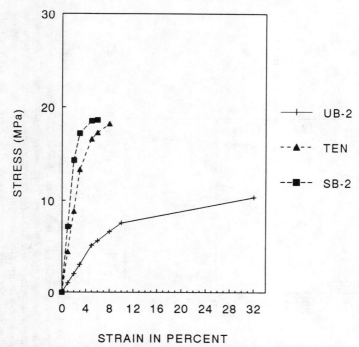

FIG. 1—*Representative stress-strain curves of dentin adhesive films that exhibited the maximum strain capacity.*

ers which may compensate for its lower bond strength. By comparing bond strength to tensile strength of the adhesives films in Table 3, it appeared that the bond strengths of Tenure and Universal Bond-2 were limited by the tensile strength of the adhesive film. The bond strength of Scotchbond-2 was 80% of the tensile strength of the film. The static and dynamic elastic modulus of Universal Bond-2 was definitely less than the other dentin adhesives. Therefore, it should be more effective if used as a thick adhesive film to relieve the bond stress from composite resin restoration polymerization shrinkage by elastic strain of the thick film. There was not a wide variation in glass transition temperature of the adhesives as demonstrated by the loss tangent peak temperatures. Scotchbond-2 appeared to present a more loss damping molecular structure as indicated by its higher loss modulus and loss tangent maximum.

Results of Computer Finite Element Analysis for Two-Dimensional Class 5 Composite Resin Restoration Polymerization Shrinkage Bond Stress to Dentin

Figures 2 through 4 show the interfacial bond stress acting perpendicular to the preparation wall for different curing conditions with the adhesive film thickness assumed to be zero. Tensile stress values are positive and compressive stress values are negative. The interfacial bond will fail in tension when the tensile shrinkage stress exceeds the bond strength. For all curing conditions that the bond stress exceeded the bond strength, a gap will be formed at the interface between the restoration and tooth which can cause staining, secondary decay, and pulp sensitivity from microleakage. For autocuring in Fig. 2, high tensile stresses were found at the margin and at the wall nodes near the preparation floor. Figure 5 demonstrated the effect of

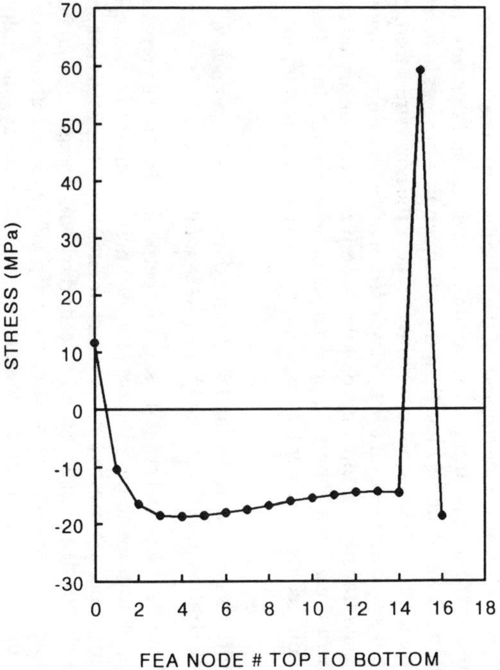

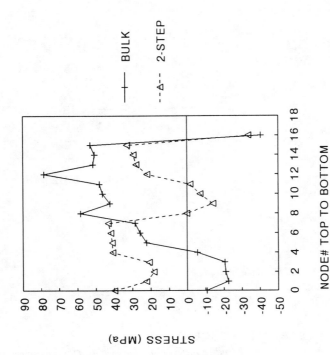

FIG. 3—*The wall interfacial stress for bulk cure and two-step VLC Class 5 composite restoration FEA model cured top down. The zero node represented the surface margin of the restoration. Each succeeding node was 125 μm apart measured down the interfacial wall of the preparation and composite restoration to the bottom corner of the preparation. Node 16 was the bottom corner of the wall at a depth of 2 mm from the zero node at the margin. The adhesive bond film thickness was zero in these models.*

FIG. 2—*The wall interfacial stress for autocured Class 5 composite restoration FEA model. The zero node represented the surface margin of the restoration. Each succeeding node was 125 μm apart measured down the interfacial wall of the preparation and composite restoration to the bottom corner of the preparation. Node 16 was the bottom corner of the wall at a depth of 2 mm from the zero node at the margin. The adhesive bond film thickness was zero in this model.*

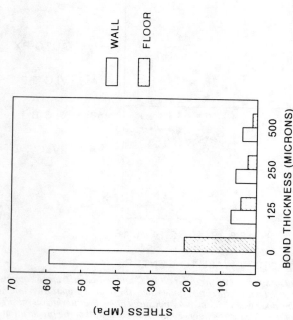

FIG. 5—A bar graph showing how the maximum interfacial wall and floor stress of an autocured Class 5 composite restoration was decreased by thick adhesive bond layers as calculated by FEA models of increasing resin bond layer thickness (0, 125, 250, and 500 µm, respectively).

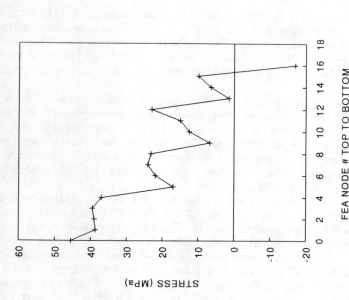

FIG. 4—The wall interfacial stress for bulk VLC Class 5 composite restoration FEA model cured bottom up through the tooth. The zero node represented the surface margin of the restoration. Each succeeding node was 125 µm apart measured down the interfacial wall of the preparation and composite restoration to the bottom corner of the preparation. Node 16 was the bottom corner of the wall at a depth of 2 mm from the zero node at the margin. The adhesive bond film thickness was zero in this model.

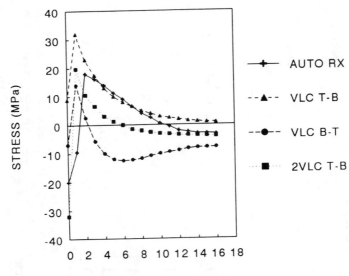

FIG. 6—*The floor interfacial stress for all the different VLC and self-cured Class 5 composite restoration FEA models. The zero node represented the corner node where the floor of preparation intersected the preparation wall. Each succeeding node was 125 µm apart measured along the interface at the preparation floor. Node 16 was at the center of the preparation floor, 2 mm from each wall of the preparation. By symmetry the stress across the remaining floor nodes would be the mirror image of the first 16 nodes. The adhesive bond film thickness was zero in these models. Auto RX = self-cured; VLC T-B = light-cured bulk top to bottom; VLC B-T = light-cured bulk bottom to top; 2VLC T-B = light-cured top to bottom in two steps.*

increasing bonding resin thickness on lowering these high tensile stress observed in the auto-cured composite with no bonding resin in Figs. 2 and 6. This analysis demonstrated that the use of a 125-µm or thicker bond layer of UB-2 was sufficient to lower the peak tensile stress below the bond strength of this adhesive. Therefore, the use of a thick bond layer is expected to be an effective way of lowering the shrinkage bond stress by using elastic strain relaxation of the thick film.

A comparison of the wall stress values for the different curing conditions in Figs. 2 through 4, indicated that bulk VLC top to bottom of the restoration produced the greatest peak tensile stress. However, the two-step VLC top to bottom and bulk VLC bottom to top through the tooth produced much greater stress at the margins. However, when the bond stresses perpendicular to the floor of the prep were compared in Fig. 6, it was evident that curing through the tooth was the most effective way to lower the floor's peak tensile stress for these models that assumed a minimum bond resin layer thickness.

The bond stresses that were calculated using finite element methods are based on total volume shrinkage measurements which vary between 1.2% to about 4% for different composite resins [9]. The value used for the composite resin, P 50, of 2.5% was provided by the manufacturer. Recent measurements with strain gages of composite resin shrinkage have recorded linear shrinkage [10,11]. These strain measurements are "post-gelation" shrinkages that occur after the elastic modulus has developed to the degree that bond stresses can be generated. For these reasons, the post-gelation volume shrinkage may be on the order of only 0.8% and bond stress reported for finite element analysis may be a factor of three high [12]. However, polymerization may produce uneven and localized areas of reaction where stresses are raised due to inhomogeneous reaction.

Conclusions

1. Universal Bond-2 with its lower elastic modulus and higher ductility was the most effective material to use for a thick dentin bond layer to relax shrinkage stress of bonded composite resins.
2. The tensile strength of adhesive films limited the bond strength of adhesive bonds to dentin.
3. Finite element analysis showed that polymerization shrinkage produced tensile bond stress that exceed the bond strength of adhesive resins to dentin if no mode of stress relaxation was present.
4. Finite element analysis showed that thick adhesive film of 125 μm or more reduced the peak shrinkage bond stress to below the bond strength of the adhesive films to dentin.
5. Finite element analysis showed that two-step visible light curing (VLC) from the top down and bulk VLC from the bottom up greatly increases the tensile stresses at the margins of restorations.
6. Finite element analysis showed that VLC from the bottom up through the tooth was the most effective way to reduce the tensile stress on the floor of the restoration.

References

[1] Tsai, Y. H., Swartz, M. L., Phillips, R. W., and Moore, B. K., "Bond Strength and Microleakage with Dentin Bond Systems," *Operative Dentistry*, Vol. 15, March 4, April 1990, pp. 53–60.
[2] Barkmeier, W. W. and Haang, C. T., "Bond Strength and Microleakage of New Dentin Adhesive Systems," *Journal of Dental Research*, IADR Abstract #1098, Vol. 65, March 1990, p. 128.
[3] Venz, S. and Dickens, B., "Effect of Primers and Adhesives on Micromorphology and Strength of Adhesives/Dentin Bonds," *Journal of Dental Research*, IADR Abstract #786, Vol. 70, March 1991, p. 363.
[4] Erickson, R. L., "Mechanism and Clinical Implications of Bond Formation for Two Dentin Bonding Agents," *American Journal of Dentistry*, Vol. 2, July 1989, pp. 117–123.
[5] Ruyter, I. E., "Monomer Systems and Polymerization," *International Symposium on Posterior Composite Resin Dental Restorative Materials*, G. Vanherle and D.C. Smith, Eds., Peter Szulc Publishing Co., The Netherlands, 1985, pp. 109–138.
[6] Park, J. B., *Biomaterials Science and Engineering*, Plenum Press, New York, 1990.
[7] "Directions for XR Bond," Kerr Manufacturing Co., Romulus, MI 1990.
[8] Van Noort, R., Cardew, G. E., Howard, I. C., and Norwozi, S., "The Effect of Local Interfacial Geometry on Measurement of Tensile Bond Strength to Dentin," *Journal of Dental Research*, Vol. 70, 1991, pp. 889–893.
[9] Byerly, T. J., Eick, J. D., Chen, G. P., et al., "Synthesis and Polymerization of New Expanding Dental Monomers," *Dental Materials*, Vol. 8, November 1992, pp. 345–350.
[10] Sakaguchi, R. L., Sasik, C. T., Bunczak, M. A., and Douglas, W. H., "Strain Gauge Method for Measuring Polymerization Contraction of Composite Resins," *Journal of Dentistry*, Vol. 19, 1991, pp. 312–316.
[11] Sakaguchi, R. L., Peters, M. C. R. B., Nelson, S. R., et al., "Effects of Polymerization Contraction in Composite Resins," *Journal of Dentistry*, Vol. 20, 1992, pp. 178–182.
[12] Moon, P. C. and Carter, R. H., "3D Measurement of Gelation Shrinkage of VLC Resins," *Journal of Dental Research*, V74, abstract to be published March 1994.

Robert R. Peterson[1]

Taguchi Experiment on Strength Correlation Between a Customer and Supplier of Porous Coatings

REFERENCE: Peterson, R. R., **"Taguchi Experiment on Strength Correlation Between a Customer and Supplier of Porous Coatings,"** *Biomaterials' Mechanical Properties, ASTM STP 1173,* H. E. Kambic and A. T. Yokobori, Jr., Eds., American Society for Testing and Materials, Philadelphia, 1994, pp. 96–108.

ABSTRACT: Problems in correlating porous coating pull-off strength test results through the use of test coupons led to the use of Taguchi methods to isolate the variables that contribute to test result differences between the customer and supplier of these coatings.

In the past, the supplier would test the coupons representative of the parts and ship the parts believing the pull-off strength requirements were met. The customer then tested additional coupons and usually found a lower strength (sometimes below specification) which resulted in rejection of the material. This, of course, led to problems. If both testing sources had correlated at a particular strength level, whether it be high or low, there would be no question as to the disposition of the material. Therefore, the major concern was that the numbers from both testing sources agree.

Since there are scores of variables that could affect the pull-off test, general categories were selected to determine major sources of variation that could be further analyzed at a later date if necessary. The four sources of variation (factors) that were selected included: (1) who performed the gluing operation on the coupons (the supplier or the customer); (2) at which facility the pull-off test was performed (the supplier's or the customer's); (3) what testing fixture configuration was used (two different types); and (4) at what speed was the tensile machine run (two different speeds).

Two analysis methods were used which concluded that the difference in fixturing was probably the most important source of variation. While the other factors were significant, it was discovered that the highest pull-off strength values were obtained by having the customer glue the sample and the supplier run the test. This would mean that neither the customer nor the supplier had an overall better technique, further verifying the main source of variation was in the fixturing.

KEYWORDS: Taguchi, porous coating tensile strength, pull-off orthogonal array, analysis of variance (ANOVA), experiment, titanium, beads

Quality Control methods fall into two categories: on-line and off-line. On-line Quality Control refers to the monitoring of current manufacturing processes to verify the quality levels produced. The on-line method uses tools such as statistical process control (SPC). The off-line portion of the Quality Control methods are valuable as they impact the cost that is obtained by improving quality at the earliest times in a product's life cycle [1]. One of the newly used methods for off-line quality improvement is the Taguchi method. Taguchi stresses the need to control both the mean (centering) of a process as well as its variation. Experiments are set up to determine what factors are significant in controlling the necessary output. Taguchi techniques allow these factors to be checked simultaneously so that both money and time are

---

[1] Quality control metallurgist, Smith and Nephew-Richards, Memphis, TN 38116.

saved. Designs are carefully chosen with the triangular table to minimize false results due to mixing of interactions or confounding. While criticized for not being as accurate as a full factorial experiment, many times it supplies the needed information at a lower cost. The Taguchi method does not need very high powered statistics to work; only elementary statistics are used. The Taguchi method has been taught in Japan since the mid-1960s and has allowed Japanese companies to become world economic competitors [1].

Purpose

The purpose of this experiment was to determine what factor or factors were responsible for creating the most discrepancy between the results of a porous coating supplier and those obtained by the customer of these coatings in coupon pull-off tests.

Background

To verify the strength of the porous coating on implants, round coupons which are porous coated at the same time the implants are coated are produced. These coupons are placed in the furnace alongside the parts and are subjected to the same sintering/heat treatment cycles as the parts are. This is to ensure that the coupon, which is of a simpler geometry, will have a strength level similar to the actual parts. Upon completion of the thermal cycles, the coupons are glued in a fixture and pulled in an axial tension test to failure. Acceptance or rejection of the implants is determined in part by meeting the minimum strength requirement of the pull-off test.

Problems in the past have arisen when there is a difference between the porous coating supplier's results and those obtained by the customer. Such differences can mean rejecting good parts and accepting bad ones. In either case, unnecessary delays, cost, and debating are the result of these differences.

Experimental Setup

As there are literally scores of different variables that can affect the results of the pull-off test, it was decided that large general categories would be selected first, and if the study would need to be continued at a later date with additional variables, it could. Four variables (factors) were initially selected. They are the following:

(A) Who glues the coupon fixtures to the coupon?
(B) Who performs the tension test?
(C) What tensile machine fixtures are used to pull the coupons?
(D) At what speed is the test run?

All the factors had two levels assigned to them. Factors A and B were both assigned the following two levels:

(1) The porous coating supplier, and
(2) The porous coating customer.

While these two factors were uncontrollable as both the supplier and the customer will continue testing, it was felt that they should be included, as it would be helpful to know if they were the sources of variation. The main difference in the test fixturing is the number of U-joints in the setup. One U-joint had been historically used by the customer in the past (Fig. 1),

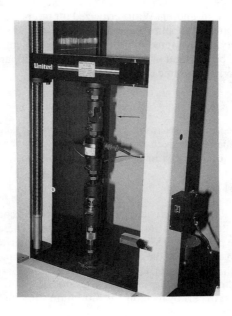

FIG. 1—*Tensile machine showing 1 U-joint setup (or, Table 6).*

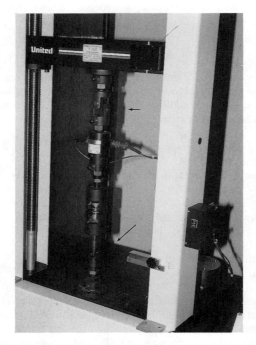

FIG. 2—*Tensile machine showing 2 U-joint setup (or, Table 7).*

while two U-joints had been used by the porous coating supplier (Fig. 2). No reason was given to why each used a particular design. Both were thought to have been acceptable for the application. Hence, the two levels set up here for Factor C were one and two U-joints. Finally, it was thought that the speed of the test might make a difference. The speeds selected for Factor D were .04 in./min (1 mm/min) and 0.1 in./min (2.54 mm/min) as these were the speeds the supplier and the customer ran, respectively.

Methods

The titanium 6Al-4V coupons, which were round slugs, were all made from the same diameter and lot of barstock and cut approximately ⅜ in. (9.5 mm) high. All coupons were porous-coated at the same time, using beads from the same lot (C.P. grade titanium) and were all placed in the same location in the furnace to minimize the effect of hot and cold spots in the oven. Next, all specimens were subjected to the same thermal cycles. While the exact thermal process is proprietary, the parts were heated to extremely high temperatures for a long period of time. This allows the atoms to diffuse between the beads and the coupon substrate and form a bond. The coupons were then submitted to the customer where they were physically mixed up and randomly separated into one of the eight trials. Twenty-four coupons allowed for three repetitions of the eight trials. The experiment up to this point was fully randomized. After the coupons were placed in the various groups and shipped to the supplier (if necessary), the experiment took more of a block design. This is because coupons of a particular group were glued together. While this was not fully randomized, it did have some advantages. First of all, this practice is the way it is done in production, thereby simulating day-to-day standard setups. In addition, there was thought to be more variation from the individual gluing operations as compared to "bulk" gluing a whole group. Gluing was done by placing heat-cured sheets of glue between both sides of the coupon and the fixture and heating the coupons/fixtures for 2½ h at 350°F (177°C) while under spring tension to aid in the bonding. Both the supplier and customer used basically the same bonding process. While both shared many variables in this process (i.e., the same glue), many minor variables were similar, but not controlled (i.e., different curing ovens, cooling rates, spring tension). This was intentional as both the customer and supplier were to bond their coupons following their own similar but not identical procedure. Again, the intent of this experiment was to verify which of the four selected factor(s), if any, was causing significant variation in the tensile strength results. Effects of specific variables that were not controlled in the gluing process would be combined and their results would be seen in Factor A—who glues the coupon fixtures to the coupon? If this factor was found to be significant, additional Taguchi experimentation would be required if it was deemed necessary to determine which variable(s) within this factor was causing the variation. The specimen was then placed in a standard tensile machine and subjected to an axial load until the specimen broke. When this occurred, the maximum load was recorded. Three trials of each test group were performed.

Data

The tables (data sheets) containing the information obtained in setting up and running the experiment are outlined below:

Table 1–Selected variables, interactions, and levels for experiment
Table 2–Linear graph
Table 3–Triangular table
Table 4–Orthogonal array

TABLE 1—*Selected variables, interactions, and levels for experiment.*

Factor	Col. #	Description	Level 1	Level 2
A	1	Glued by	supplier	customer
B	2	Test performed by	supplier	customer
A × B	3	Interaction	n/a	
C	4	Fixture	1 U-joint	2 U-joints
A × C	5	Interaction	n/a	
B × C	6	Interaction	n/a	
D	7	Speed of test	0.1 in./min	0.04 in./min
			(2.54 mm/min)	1 mm/min)

Table 5–Test specimen (Fig. 3)
Table 6–Tensile machine showing 1 U-joint setup (Fig. 1)
Table 7–Tensile machine showing 2 U-joint setup (Fig. 2)
Table 8–Test results
Table 9–Observations of results
Table 10–First and second level calculations
Table 11–Auxiliary calculations
Table 12–Graph of auxiliary interactions
Table 13–ANOVA table
Table 14–Pooled calculations
Table 15–Calculated S/N ratios
Table 16–S/N ANOVA table
Table 17–S/N ANOVA (pooled) table
Table 18–S/N ANOVA (pooled) nominal is best table

TABLE 2—*Linear graph.*

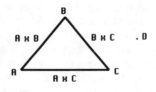

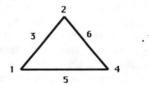

Experimental Graph   **Standard Graph**

Match corresponding points:

1 - A
2 - B
3 - A × B
4 - C
5 - A × C
6 - B × C
7 - D

TABLE 3—*L8 Triangular table (for determination of interaction locations).*

	Column No.					
	2	3	4	5	6	7
Column No. 1	3	2	5	4	7	6
2	—	1	6	7	4	5
3	—	—	7	6	5	4
4	—	—	—	1	2	3
5	—	—	—	—	3	2
6	—	—	—	—	—	1

Results

Table 1 shows the variables, interactions, and levels that were selected which were thought to affect the differences in the pull-off results. These factors were symbolized with dots and the interactions between them were symbolized by lines. This graph was then compared to a standard reference graph to determine what columns to assign the factors and interactions (see Table 2) [1]. An L8 design suited the experiment's needs and was also selected for simplicity. Effort was focused on the factors; interactions were of secondary concern. However, since the array allowed the group to test for these, they were included as this information was basically free. The triangular table (see Table 3)[1] was used as a way of verifying the factor and interaction setup. Whenever possible, factors should not be placed in columns where major interactions are to occur. For example, Column 3 will contain the interaction of Columns 1 and 2, and therefore this location should be reserved for the 1 × 2 interaction. The experiment was then ready to be set up. As can be seen in Table 4, the eight trials which were repeated three times each show the various levels of the factors set in this orthogonal array. For example, in Trial 1, all of the factors were set to level one. Interactions were not set, they were merely evaluated.

The experiment was then followed using the method previously described, with each of the factors set to the proper level for each trial. Table 5 (shown as Fig. 3) shows what this specimen looks like right before axial loading in a standard tensile machine. Table 6 (shown as Fig. 1) displays the single U-joint setup, while Table 7 (shown as Fig. 2) shows the two U-joint setup. Test results can be seen in Table 8.

TABLE 4—*Orthogonal array.*

	Factor							
	A	B	A × B	C	A × C	B × C	D	Specimen
Trials # \Cols.	1	2	3	4	5	6	7	#
1	1	1	1	1	1	1	1	1, 9, 17
2	1	1	1	2	2	2	2	2, 10, 18
3	1	2	2	1	1	2	2	3, 11, 19
4	1	2	2	2	2	1	1	4, 12, 20
5	2	1	2	1	2	1	2	5, 13, 21
6	2	1	2	2	1	2	1	6, 14, 22
7	2	2	1	1	2	2	1	7, 15, 23
8	2	2	1	2	1	1	2	8, 16, 24

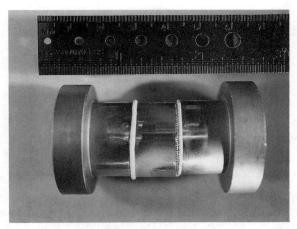

FIG. 3—*Test specimen (or, Table 5).*

In reviewing the results, obvious conclusions were found first. It was initially assumed that everyone was using methods and techniques to obtain the highest pull-off values. Therefore, by looking at Trials 5 and 6 in Table 9 (which had the highest average) and checking the level of factors they had in common (A and B), the first conclusion that could be drawn was that these factors were the most significant in determining maximum pull-off strength.

Next, first level and second level summaries were performed on each factor column (see Table 10). First level totals were subtracted from second level totals and the greater the difference, the more significant the factor. It can be seen here that in addition to Factors A and B, Factor C also appeared considerably different. Additional computations can be seen in Table 11 which were used to produce the graphs in Table 12 of three other interactions which could not be tested for in the original array. These interactions were A × D, B × D, and C × D. As all three of these graphs had lines that crossed each other, all displayed significant interactions.

The significance of the factors were then verified mathematically. Table 13 shows the sum

TABLE 8—*Tensile strength test results.*

Trial #	Specimen Numbers	Tensile Strength psi × 1000 (ksi)			Trial Average	
					(ksi)	(MPa)
1	1, 9, 17	9.822	9.728	9.024	9.52	65.6
2	2, 10, 18	9.592	11.393	10.594	10.52	72.6
3	3, 11, 19	7.235	8.410	9.223	8.28	57.1
4	4, 12, 20	9.947	11.066	9.537	10.18	70.2
5	5, 13, 21	11.828	11.338	10.285	11.15	76.9
6	6, 14, 22	10.717	11.068	12.002	11.26	77.6
7	7, 15, 23	10.332	8.028	11.165	9.84	67.9
8	8, 16, 24	11.005	9.701	11.164	10.62	73.2

NOTE: 1 ksi = 6.894 MPa.

TABLE 9—*Observations of results.*

Trial #	Factor							Avg.	
	A	B	A × B	C	A × C	B × C	D	ksi	MPa
1	1	1	1	1	1	1	1	9.52	65.6
2	1	1	1	2	2	2	2	10.52	72.6
3	1	2	2	1	1	2	2	8.28	57.1
4	1	2	2	2	2	1	1	10.18	70.2
5	2	1	2	1	2	1	2	11.15	76.9
6	2	1	2	2	1	2	1	11.26	77.6
7	2	2	1	1	2	2	1	9.84	67.9
8	2	2	1	2	1	1	2	10.62	73.2

Note: 1 ksi = 6.894 MPa.

TABLE 10—*First and second level calculations.*

Factor	Level		ksi	MPa
A	L_1	9.52 + 10.52 + 8.28 + 10.18 = 38.5 /4 =	9.625	(66.4)
	L_2	11.15 + 11.26 + 9.84 + 10.62 = 42.87/4 =	10.718	(73.9)
		Difference =	1.093	(7.5)
B	L_1	9.52 + 10.52 + 11.15 + 11.26 = 42.45/4 =	10.612	(73.2)
	L_2	8.28 + 10.18 + 9.84 + 10.62 = 38.92/4 =	9.730	(67.1)
		Difference =	.882	(6.1)
A × B	L_1	9.52 + 10.52 + 9.84 + 10.62 = 40.5 /4 =	10.125	(69.8)
	L_2	8.28 + 10.18 + 11.15 + 11.26 = 40.87/4 =	10.218	(70.5)
		Difference =	.093	(.7)
C	L_1	9.52 + 8.28 + 11.15 + 9.84 = 38.79/4 =	9.698	(66.9)
	L_2	10.52 + 10.18 + 11.26 + 10.62 = 42.58/4 =	10.645	(73.4)
		Difference =	.947	(6.5)
A × C	L_1	9.52 + 8.28 + 11.26 + 10.62 = 39.68/4 =	9.920	(68.4)
	L_2	10.52 + 10.18 + 11.15 + 9.84 = 41.69/4 =	10.423	(71.9)
		Difference =	.503	(3.5)
B × C	L_1	9.52 + 10.18 + 11.15 + 10.62 = 41.47/4 =	10.368	(71.5)
	L_2	10.52 + 8.28 + 11.26 + 9.84 = 39.9 /4 =	9.975	(68.8)
		Difference =	.393	(2.7)
D	L_1	9.52 + 10.18 + 11.26 + 9.84 = 40.8 /4 =	10.2	(70.3)
	L_2	10.52 + 8.28 + 11.15 + 10.62 = 40.57/4 =	10.142	(69.9)
		Difference =	.058	(.4)

TABLE 11—*Auxiliary calculations.*

Interaction	ksi	MPa
A $\times$ D		
$A_1 D_1 = (9.52 + 10.18)/2 =$	9.85	(67.9)
$A_1 D_2 = (10.52 + 8.28)/2 =$	9.40	(64.8)
$A_2 D_1 = (11.26 + 9.84)/2 =$	10.55	(72.8)
$A_2 D_2 = (11.15 + 10.62)/2 =$	10.89	(75.1)
B $\times$ D		
$B_1 D_1 = (9.52 + 11.26)/2 =$	10.39	(71.6)
$B_1 D_2 = (10.52 + 11.15)/2 =$	10.84	(74.8)
$B_2 D_1 = (10.18 + 9.84)/2 =$	10.01	(69.0)
$B_2 D_2 = (8.28 + 10.62)/2 =$	9.45	(65.2)
C $\times$ D		
$C_1 D_1 = (9.52 + 9.84)/2 =$	9.68	(66.8)
$C_1 D_2 = (8.28 + 11.15)/2 =$	9.72	(67.0)
$C_2 D_1 = (10.18 + 11.26)/2 =$	10.72	(73.9)
$C_2 D_2 = (10.52 + 10.62)/2 =$	10.57	(72.9)

of squares, degrees of freedom, variance, and the resulting F ratios which were compared to standard critical values to determine significance. This resulting analysis of variance (ANOVA) table verifies that Factors A, B, and C were significant to the 0.10 level. An additional technique called "pooling" was used to combine insignificant factors and recalculate the F values. Table 14 displays the pooling calculations. It can be seen that the values are not significantly changed and the conclusions that were drawn remain the same.

TABLE 12—*Graph of auxiliary interactions.*

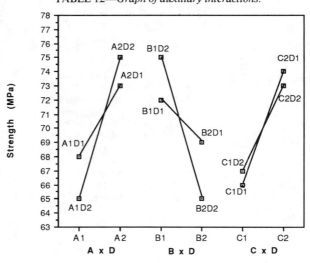

TABLE 13—*ANOVA table.*

	SS			V	F	(V Factor)
	Psi	MPa	DF	Psi	MPa	(V Error)
$SS_A = \dfrac{[12(1.093)]^2}{24} =$	7.16	337.3	1	7.16	337.3	8.63[a]
$SS_B = \dfrac{[12(.882)]^2}{24} =$	4.67	222.0	1	4.67	222.0	5.63[a]
$SS_{AXB} = \dfrac{[12(.093)]^2}{24} =$	.051	2.4	1	.051	2.4	.06
$SS_C = \dfrac{[12(.947)]^2}{24} =$	5.38	257.6	1	5.38	257.6	6.49[a]
$SS_{AXC} = \dfrac{[12(.503)]^2}{24} =$	1.51	72.1	1	1.51	72.1	1.83
$SS_{BXC} = \dfrac{[12(.393)]^2}{24} =$	.92	43.2	1	.92	43.2	1.11
$SS_D = \dfrac{[12(.058)]^2}{24} =$	.02	0.8	1	.02	0.8	.02
$SS_E = SS_T \Sigma_{remainder} =$	13.27	669.8	16	.83	41.9	
$SS_{Total} = \Sigma y^2 - \dfrac{T^2}{N} =$	33.0	1605.2	23			

[a] Significant F.90, 1, 16 = 3.05.

Next, an ANOVA table was created using signal-to-noise ratios (S/N). This is a more accurate way of determining significance when there are several repetitions of the trials such as in this experiment. Table 15 shows the calculation of the S/N ratio. The S/N ANOVA table can be seen in Table 16. Pooling must be done on this table as an error term which is needed to calculate the F values is not produced in the S/N analysis. A pooled table with the corresponding F values can be seen in Table 17. As seen in this table, the significant factors again calculated to be A, B, and C.

As a final analysis, it was thought that instead of viewing the problem as the higher the better, it was suggested that if all of the data were averaged together and analyzed as a nominal is best, it was thought that factors causing large amounts of variability could be isolated. This was done by computer and the results can be seen in Table 18. This analysis picked Factor C as significant, as well as the interaction B × C. This additional analysis would tend to reinforce a conclusion that the fixture type (Factor C) is one of the most important factors. The interactions the computer picked out in both the "nominal is best" and the "higher is better" scenarios are not easily explained. However, with all but one of the factors showing some significance in either analysis, several interactions in this experiment would not be surprising.

Summary

Four factors were tested for significance in determining if they contributed to test result variation. In the first analysis, assuming higher is better, it was discovered that three of the factors were significant. These factors were: (1) who glued the coupons, (2) who pulled the coupons, and (3) what fixture was used. Three interactions were also deemed significant. The speed of

TABLE 14—*Pooled calculations.*

psi Calculations

$$V_{e1} = \frac{13.27 + .02 + .051 + .92}{16 + 1 + 1 + 1} = \frac{14.26}{19} = .75$$

$$F_1 = \frac{1.51}{.75} = 2.01 \ \text{F.90.1, 19} = 2.99 \ (\text{Not significant } 2.01 < 2.99)$$

$$V_{e2} = \frac{13.27 + .02 + .051 + .92 + 1.51}{16 + 1 + 1 + 1 + 1} = \frac{15.78}{20} = .789$$

$$F_2 = \frac{4.67}{.788} = 5.92 \ \text{F.90, 1, 20} = 2.97 \ (\text{Significant } 5.92 > 2.97)$$

MPa Calculations

$$V_{e1} = \frac{669.8 + 0.82 + 2.4 + 43.2}{16 + 1 + 1 + 1} = \frac{716.2}{19} = 37.7$$

$$F_1 = \frac{72.1}{37.7} = 1.91 \ \text{F.90, 1, 19} = 2.99 \ (\text{Not significant } 1.91 < 2.99)$$

$$V_{e2} = \frac{669.8 + 0.82 + 2.4 + 43.2}{16 + 1 + 1 + 1 + 1} + 72.1 = \frac{788.3}{20} = 39.4$$

$$F_2 = \frac{222.0}{39.4} = 5.63 \ \text{f.90, 1, 20} = 2.97 \ (\text{Significant } 5.63 > 2.97)$$

Therefore, pool everything up to and including 1.51 (7.21).

Factor	f	SS		V		F
		Psi	MPa	Psi	MPa	
A	1	7.16	(337.3)	7.16	(337.3)	9.07[a]
B	1	4.67	(222.0)	4.67	(222.0)	5.92[a]
A × B		(pooled)	(pooled)	(pooled)	(pooled)	
C	1	5.38	(257.6)	5.38	(257.6)	6.82[a]
A × C		(pooled)	(pooled)	(pooled)	(pooled)	
B × C		(pooled)	(pooled)	(pooled)	(pooled)	
D		(pooled)	(pooled)	(pooled)	(pooled)	
error	20	15.783	(788.3)	0.789	(39.4)	
Total	23	33.003	(1605.2)			

[a] Significant F.90, 1, 20 = 2.97

TABLE 15—*Calculated signal to noise ratios.*

For higher is better: $S/N_{HB} = -10 \log (1/r \ \Sigma \ 1/y^2)$

Psi	$\Sigma 1/y^2$	$1/r$	$-10 \log (1/r \ \Sigma \ 1/y^2)$
1	0.0332	0.33	19.55
2	0.0275	0.33	20.38
3	0.0451	0.33	18.23
4	0.0293	0.33	20.10
5	0.0244	0.33	20.90
6	0.0238	0.33	21.00
7	0.0329	0.33	19.59
8	0.0269	0.33	20.47
MPa			
1	0.000699	0.33	36.32
2	0.000577	0.33	37.15
3	0.000946	0.33	35.01
4	0.000615	0.33	36.88
5	0.000513	0.33	37.67
6	0.000501	0.33	37.77
7	0.000692	0.33	36.37
8	0.000566	0.33	37.24

TABLE 16—*S/N ANOVA table (computations use signal to noise ratio from the test results).*

Col.		Factors	f	S	V	F
1	A	Glued by	1	1.7112	1.7112	—
2	B	Test performed by	1	1.4792	1.4792	—
3	A × B	Interaction	1	0.0071	0.0071	—
4	C	Fixture	1	1.6926	1.6926	—
5	A × C	Interaction	1	0.3696	0.3696	—
6	B × C	Interaction	1	0.4141	0.4141	—
7	D	Speed of test	1	0.0088	0.0088	—
All other/error			0			
Total:			7	5.682		

TABLE 17—*S/N ANOVA pooled table (computations use signal to noise ratio from the test results).*

Col.		Factors	f	S	V	F
1	A	Glued by	1	1.711	1.711	8.561
2	B	Test performed by	1	1.479	1.479	7.400
3	A × B	Interaction	(1)	(0.01)	Pooled	
4	C	Fixture	1	1.693	1.693	8.468
5	A × C	Interaction	(1)	(0.37)	Pooled	
6	B × C	Interaction	(1)	(0.41)	Pooled	
7	D	Speed of test	(1)	(0.01)	Pooled	
All other/error			4	0.800	0.200	
Total:			7	5.682		

NOTE: Insignificant factorial effects are pooled as shown ( ).

TABLE 18—*S/N (pooled) ANOVA viewing nominal is best (computations use signal to noise ratio from the test results).*

Col.		Factors	f	S	V	F
1	A	Glued by	(1)	(4.02)	Pooled	
2	B	Test performed by	(1)	(2.52)	Pooled	
3	A × B	Interaction	1	10.465	10.465	3.061
4	C	Fixture	1	23.154	23.154	6.773[a]
5	A × C	Interaction	(1)	(2.92)	Pooled	
6	B × C	Interaction	1	31.800	31.800	9.302[a]
7	D	Speed of test	(1)	(4.22)	Pooled	
All other/error			4	13.674	3.419	
Total:			7	79.094		

NOTE: Insignificant factorial effects are pooled as shown ( ).
[a] Significant F.90, 1, 4 = 4.54.

the test did not show to be a significant factor in the selected ranges. In the second analysis, setting nominal is best, it was determined that the fixture used was a significant factor, as well as one interaction. None of the interactions in either of the analyses were found to have any assignable causes.

Conclusions

In reviewing both methods of analysis, it was the author's opinion that the fixture was the most important factor and if the customer switches to two U-joints, this significant factor will be eliminated by duplication by both parties. A better correlation of tensile strength values between both groups will be the result.

The factors of who glued the specimen and who pulled the specimen were also significant. However, since the optimum strength was achieved by having the customer glue the specimen and the supplier pull it, there appeared to be no clear overall technique which gives either the customer or the supplier the ability to produce a superior strength coupon. The significant interactions have no positively assignable causes at this time.

Recommendations

The two U-joint fixtures should be used in testing all coupons. Additional data may then be collected as this process appears to be somewhat sensitive and variable. If correlation problems still exist, then a repeat of this experiment would probably be in order with the known factors optimized. Additional analysis of the subvariables in Factors A and B may then need to be performed.

Acknowledgment

I would like to acknowledge the following people who helped me make this project possible: Susan Bell, Mari Crosslin, Rolf Klein, Nelda Peterson, Henry Pleasants, Dave Walker, and Shawn Wood.

Reference

[1] Ross, P. J., "Taguchi Techniques for Quality Engineering," McGraw-Hill, 1988.

Evaluation of Metallic Materials

Sushil K. Bhambri[1] and Leslie N. Gilbertson[1]

Characterization and Quantification of Fretting Particulates Generated in Ceramic/Metal and Metal/Metal Modular Head/Taper Systems

REFERENCE: Bhambri, S. K. and Gilbertson, L. N., **"Characterization and Quantification of Fretting Particulates Generated in Ceramic/Metal and Metal/Metal Modular Head/Taper Systems,"** *Biomaterials' Mechanical Properties, ASTM STP 1173*, H. E. Kambic and A. T. Tokobori, Jr., Eds., American Society for Testing and Materials, Philadelphia, 1994, pp. 111–126.

ABSTRACT: The use of modular head/Morse taper joints in total hip replacements has become a preferred surgical practice in consideration of the flexibility in surgical procedures and reduced inventory. The modular joints also offer an advantage in selection of appropriate material for components of a prosthesis depending upon the performance requirements. These modular joints have performed successfully *in vivo* for well over a decade. Recently, however, the release of fretting wear particulates from prosthetic implants in total hip arthroplasty has received greater attention, and a concern has been expressed for the modular head/taper joint to be a source of metal debris.

In this paper, an experimental setup is described for conducting fretting/corrosion fatigue testing of modular head/taper assemblies in simulated body environments. The test setup consisted of a special cell designed to contain simulated body environment and to retain all particles greater than 0.20 μm, generated due to fretting fatigue. For this purpose, in-line filters were used and the environmental chamber was made of acrylic material to avoid any contamination. The test environment was aerated Ringer's solution circulated in a closed loop at 37°C. The fatigue load was applied on the head in 15° mediolateral anatomic orientation. The functional capabilities of this setup was demonstrated by testing alumina ceramic and cobalt-chromium-molybdenum femoral heads fitted on titanium alloy tapers, at a fatigue load of 5.34 kN and a stress ratio of 0.1. The results are summarized in terms of characterization and quantification of any particulates generated, and surface topographical changes on both head and taper contact surfaces.

KEYWORDS: fatigue, fretting, Ringer's solution, wear, alumina, surface roughness, scanning electron microscope

Total Hip Replacements are indispensable in successful treatment of many medical disorders such as rheumatoid arthritis, osteoarthrosis, congenital hip dysplasia, and accidental fractures. These artificial joints facilitate most of the functional capabilities of the natural bone joint, with a few restrictions depending on the activity level of the recipient. Since the first hip replacement surgeries three decades ago, considerable research effort has been expended in the development of modern hip joints. Today, the use of modular head/Morse taper joints in total hip replacements has become a preferred surgical practice and the manufacturers of prosthetic implant devices the world over offer modular hip prostheses. The modular joints offer a great flexibility in surgical procedures in terms of component interchangeability for head size, neck

[1] Senior research engineer and group manager, respectively, Engineering Test Laboratory, Zimmer, Inc., A Division of Bristol-Myers Squibb Company, Warsaw, IN 46580-0708.

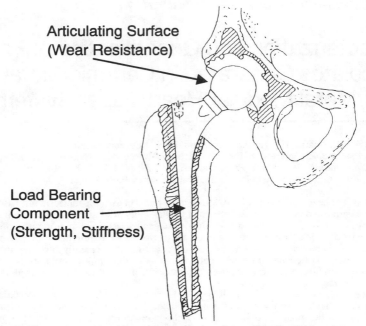

Articulating Surface
(Wear Resistance)

Load Bearing
Component
(Strength, Stiffness)

FIG. 1—*Articulating and load bearing components of a modular head/hip stem taper joint.*

length, and head material and the benefit of a reduced inventory accompanied with a reduced cost of arthroplasty. The modular joints also offer an advantage in selection of appropriate materials for articulating surfaces and load-bearing components of the prosthesis. While the biocompatibility or bioinert nature of implant materials is of prime importance, the wear resistance of the head articulating against the acetabular cup and load-bearing capability and stiffness of the stem are major considerations in material selection (Fig. 1). Different material combinations can be employed to meet these specific requirements of the head and the stem in total hip replacements. The modular joint, however, has some inherent disadvantages in creating a crevice and causing fretting due to micromovement of two components under cyclic loading. This is further aggravated by the hostile environment of the body which is fluid and oxygenated, conducive to corrosion induced phenomena such as crevice corrosion and corrosion enhanced fretting/fatigue. Crevice corrosion is a form of intense local attack that occurs in shielded areas or annular spaces formed at the contact surfaces of the metallic components. Fretting is a mechanical process whereby contact stresses between two surfaces under cyclic micromovements cause removal of material from one or both surfaces.

A number of studies has been carried out to understand various aspects of modular joint for application in total hip replacements [1–3]. These studies have addressed issues such as locking force, fatigue loading, fretting, and corrosion. The modular hip joints have now been successfully employed in service for nearly a decade and some of the retrievals at varying length of service are available for evaluation of their *in vivo* performance [4–6]. The appearance of the contact surfaces of head and stem tapers have indicated some topographical changes, the cause for which has not been understood conclusively. However, none of the reported retrievals was due to any improper function or failure of the implant device. The release of metal to body tissues by the metal prostheses has been recognized by many authors

7–10], the sources of which were identified as head articulating against acetabular socket, wear at metal/bone cement interface and, in case of cementless total hip replacements, the wear at metal/bone interface. In this respect modular joints have not been studied in isolation, and their contribution to metal particulates released into the body is not known with certainty. Recently, Mathiesen et al. [4] reported to have observed black deposits at the junction of modular head and stem tapers in four out of nine retrieved cobalt-chromium prostheses. McKellop et al. [5] have expressed a concern for the modular head/taper joint as an additional source of metal debris.

In this study an experimental setup is described to determine the fretting fatigue behavior of modular head/taper joint in Ringer's solution. The experimental setup was developed to retain any fretting debris generated during fatigue loading and to prevent external contamination from entering into the test environment. The test setup was used in characterizing the fretting behavior of cobalt-chromium-molybdenum alloy and alumina ceramic heads tested with Ti-6Al-4V alloy tapers, with and without surface nitriding treatment. The results are presented in terms of surface topographical changes on the contact surfaces and characterization of any debris generated during fatigue loading to 10 million cycles.

Experimental Procedures

Test Setup

The test setup was comprised of four basic components: (1) the test environment, (2) a container for aqueous environment and test sample, (3) a circulation system for continuous flow of the environment at 37°C, and (4) filters for entrapping any wear debris. The test environment was Ringer's solution prepared to a pH of 7.8. The container for Ringer's solution was machined out of ultra high molecular weight polyethylene. The container had a dimple (spherical cavity) 25 mm in diameter and 3 mm in depth at its base for centering and seating the femoral head during fatigue testing. Two nozzles were provided for inlet and outlet of the fluid. Polypropylene tubing was used for circulation of Ringer's solution at 37°C. The temperature of the Ringer's solution was maintained at 37°C by immersing a major length of the tubing in a heated water bath. At both inlet and outlet, 0.45-μm and 0.20-μm pore size filters were used to retain all the particulates larger than 0.20 μm in the test container. The filters used were 47-mm vericel membrane filters held by nalgene polycarbonate in-line filter holders. A schematic of the experimental test arrangement is shown in Fig. 2a. A closeup view of the modular head/taper joint is shown in Fig. 2b.

Material and Specimens

Cobalt-chromium-molybdenum alloy heads are commonly used with both cobalt-chromium-molybdenum and Ti-6Al-4V alloy hip stems. Ceramic heads are increasingly finding applications in total hip replacements. In this investigation both cobalt-chromium-molybdenum alloy and alumina ceramic heads were selected for fretting fatigue testing with Ti-6Al-4V alloy tapers. A part of the tapers were thermal nitrided to form a ceramic layer of TiN on the surface. The heads used in testing were the actual production parts used in total arthroplasty, but the tapers were simulated hip stem taper cones. The metal heads were 32-mm-long neck heads to simulate the worst fretting fatigue condition due to (1) lower stiffness, resulting from the thin section of the skirt (Fig. 2b) and (2) a larger offset. The ceramic heads used for fatigue testing were 28-mm alumina heads. The tapers tested with ceramic heads had a rougher surface finish and a larger diameter in comparison to the tapers used with metal heads. This variation in surface finish and diameter of the taper was made to match the taper with the ceramic

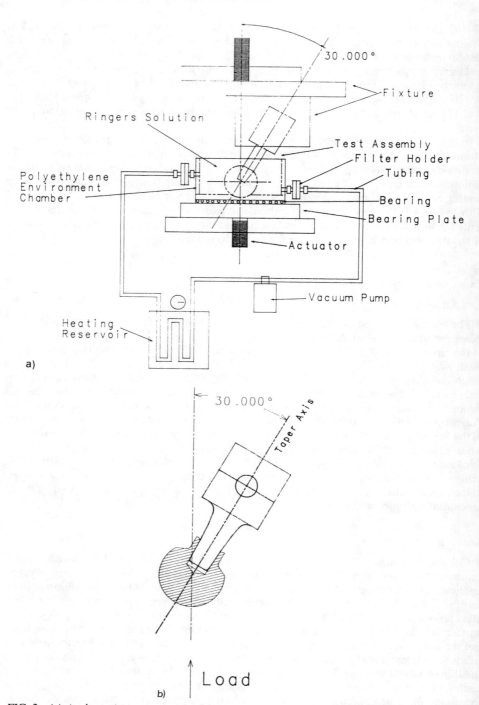

FIG. 2—(a) *A schematic representation of the experimental arrangement for fretting/corrosion fatigue testing of simulated modular head/taper joints in Ringer's solution.* (b) *Schematic of a modular head/taper joint showing section through a long neck head and method of loading.*

head taper and to comply with the recommended surface finish of tapers for use with the ceramic heads. No attempt was made to study the effect of these variables on the fretting behavior. Likewise, different head materials and surface treatments were selected to determine the efficacy of the experimental setup and not to compare materials or surface treatments. Three assemblies in each combination of head/taper system were tested.

Test Method

The heads were assembled on the tapers by hand impaction simulating the surgical technique. The taper cone base was held in a specially made fixture such that load on the head was applied at 30° simulating a 15° mediolateral anatomic orientation. The material of the test block was Ti-6Al-4V titanium alloy. The specimen was loaded axially on the head with the head resting in the dimple at the bottom of the environmental chamber. The environmental chamber was filled with Ringer's solution above the head neck/taper contact, and the circulation system was made operational prior to cyclic loading. The fatigue tests were run to 10 million cycles at a frequency of 5 Hz. A fatigue load of 5.34 kN (1200 lb), six times the body weight of a 0.89 kN (200 lb) person, was applied at a stress ratio of 0.1. The fatigue tests were carried out on MTS testing machines and a test setup is shown in Fig. 3. It should be noted that only the head and taper of the test specimen are immersed in Ringer's solution, and no other metal part of the test fixtures or test machine came in contact with the test environment.

At the completion of fatigue testing to 10 million cycles, Ringer's solution in the closed circuit was filtered using a 0.20 μm filter and a Milipore filtering apparatus. The filter was dried in a desiccator and weighed to determine weight gain due to any entrapped wear particulates. The filtered Ringer's solution was analyzed by inductively coupled plasma spectrometry for metal ion release during fatigue testing.

Evaluation of Surface Topography

The head and taper of each assembly was identified for medial and lateral orientations prior to removal of the head from the taper. The head and taper were left in distilled water for 24 h

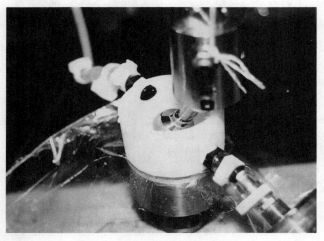

FIG. 3—*Test setup for a fretting fatigue test in Ringer's solution.*

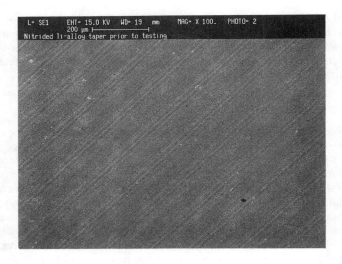

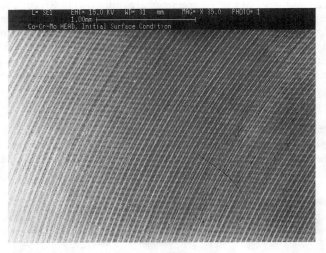

FIG. 4—*Typical surface morphology of a Ti-6Al-4V titanium alloy taper and a cobalt-chrome alloy head-taper surfaces, prior to fatigue testing.*

and then ultrasonically cleaned for 30 min. Surface morphology of head-taper and taper over the contact length was photodocumented. The metal heads were sectioned along the antero-posterior plane for scanning electron microscopic examination.

Method of Analysis

The evaluation of fretting fatigue behavior was carried out based on the following evaluations: (1) surface color changes, (2) changes in surface roughness, (3) amount of fretting debris generated, and (4) area fraction showing surface damage. In addition, attempts were made to characterize any corrosion induced damage. The changes in surface topography and color were recorded by visual observations. Further surface topographical changes were documented by optical and scanning electron microscopic examination. The changes in surface roughness were measured by using a Perthometer. The Perthometer is a surface roughness measurement device using a noncontact optical sensor. Characterization of fretting debris and any corrosion induced damage was carried out by using the scanning electron microscope and the energy dispersive X-ray analyzer (EDXA).

Results and Discussion

Surface Topography

A typical surface morphology of a nitrided titanium alloy taper surface and a cobalt-chromium-molybdenum head-taper prior to fatigue testing is shown by the scanning electron micrographs in Fig. 4. Representative surface roughness profiles obtained by the Perthometer for taper and head surfaces are shown in Fig. 5. The surface roughness was measured in terms of the average roughness parameter, R_a, which is the arithmetic average of all departures of the roughness profile from the center line within the evaluation length. Representative R_a values

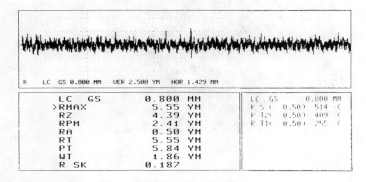

taper

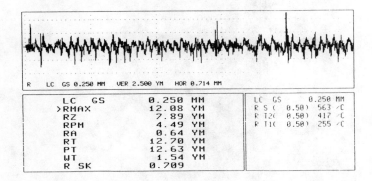

head-taper

FIG. 5—*Representative surface roughness profiles for titanium alloy taper and Co-Cr-Mo alloy head-taper surfaces.*

obtained were 0.50 and 0.70 μm for non-nitrided and nitrided taper surfaces, 0.64 μm for the Co-Cr-Mo head-taper surface and 2.0 μm for the alumina head-tapers. The rougher surface condition of the tapers for tests with ceramic heads had typical R_a values of 2.94 and 3.69 μm for non-nitrided and nitrided tapers. In each case, three surface roughness measurements were taken on the medial surface. The mean R_a values were in the range 0.50 to 0.56 and 0.68 to 0.78 μm for the non-nitrided and nitrided tapers, 0.62 to 0.67 μm for the Co-Cr-Mo head-tapers, and 1.98 to 2.12 μm for the alumina head-tapers. The mean R_a values for rough tapers ranged 2.0 to 2.19 and 2.94 to 3.11 μm for non-nitrided and nitrided conditions.

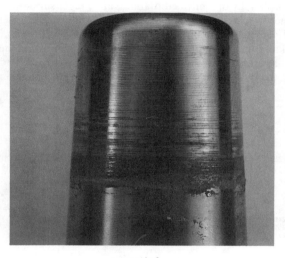

medial

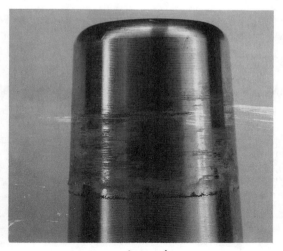

lateral

FIG. 6—*The morphology of medial and lateral surfaces of Ti-6Al-4V titanium alloy taper fatigue tested with a cobalt-chromium-molybdenum alloy head in Ringer's solution at 37°C.*

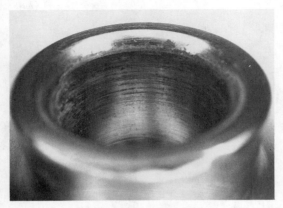

FIG. 7—*The surface morphology of cobalt-chromium-molybdenum alloy head-tested with Ti-6Al-4V titanium alloy taper.*

The morphology of medial and lateral surfaces of the non-nitrided titanium alloy taper fatigue tested with a cobalt-chrome head is shown in Fig. 6. In this *in vitro* study, the surface of head and taper on the side of the applied load is the lateral surface while the opposite side in compression is the medial surface. Figure 7 shows the medial contact surface of the cobalt-chrome head. The taper surface showed a dark band at its junction with the head, covering almost the entire medial circumference. The lateral side was least affected with almost no changes in color or surface morphology. The surface morphology showing fretting induced changes on the medial side of a non-nitrided taper are observed at high magnifications in Fig. 8. The discolored band at high magnifications showed particulates on the taper surface. EDXA

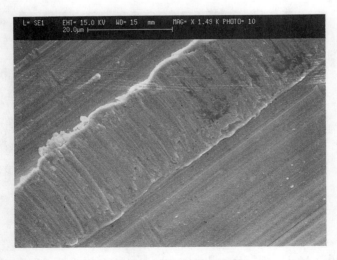

FIG. 8—*Scanning electron micrograph showing fretting induced changes in surface morphology of Ti-6Al-4V taper tested with cobalt-chrome head.*

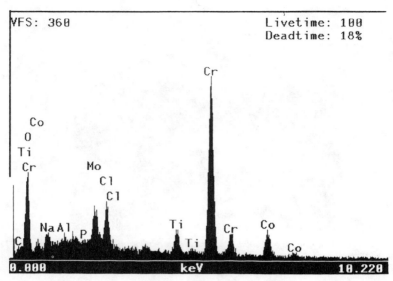

FIG. 9—*Chemical analysis of taper surface showing elemental peaks characteristic of head material.*

analysis in this region indicated cobalt, chromium, and molybdenum peaks in the spectrum (Fig. 9), suggesting transfer of head material onto the taper surface. At the dark band, the surface deposits at higher magnification showed "mud cracks" (Fig. 10). The mud cracks have been observed on retrieved implant devices like a stainless steel jewett nail and are formed due to drying of the body fluids [11]. In the present study, dried up saline solution, rich in chromium ions, may have resulted in the formation of mud cracks. At this location on the taper, machining marks were not observed, indicating a severe change in surface morphology. Away

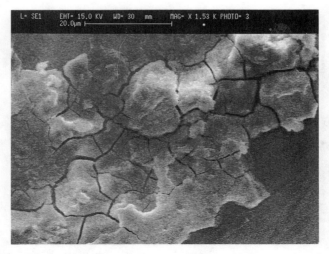

FIG. 10—*"Mud cracks" observed on taper surface tested with Co-Cr-Mo alloy head.*

from this location (the head/taper junction) towards the taper-end, the machining marks were clearly observed with occasional smearing of the peaks due to fretting. The head surface also showed changes in color on the medial side when observed visually. The head-taper contact surface, when examined by scanning electron microscope, revealed a small area on the medial side that showed fretting damage accompanied by discoloration (Fig. 11). Backscattered electron imaging clearly distinguished between the base cobalt-chrome alloy of the femoral head and titanium alloy transferred from the taper onto the head-taper. The transferred titanium alloy appeared as a dark region over the gray areas of the cobalt-chrome alloy. The EDXA spectrum obtained at the dark region indicated elements characteristic of titanium alloy (Fig. 12). In addition, a high chromium peak was observed in this spectrum. The head surface showed no evidence of pitting on the surface.

The nitrided titanium alloy taper fatigue tested with cobalt-chromium alloy head showed minor changes in surface topography (Fig. 13). The discoloration observed on the taper surface was in the form of a narrow dark band at the head opening, covering the entire medial surface. The extent of these topographical changes was much less in comparison to the non-nitrided titanium alloy taper. The EDXA spectrum obtained from the discolored site indicated transfer of head material onto the taper. In this spectrum, the chromium peak was very high and out of proportion in comparison to the head material. The surface topographical changes observed on the head-taper contact surface are also shown in Fig. 13. The EDXA spectrum obtained from the medial surface of the head-taper at various locations did not indicate elemental peaks characteristic of titanium alloy, suggesting no material transfer occurred from taper onto the head. A disproportionally higher chromium peak was obtained in the EDXA spectrum, as with the stem taper. Similar to the non-nitrided titanium alloy, there was no evidence of pitting on either of the contact surfaces. The absence of pitting on titanium alloy taper surfaces is in agreement with previously reported studies [12,13]. Levine and Staehle [12] in their study of crevice corrosion in various orthopedic implant materials observed no pitting or visible changes in the surface condition of titanium alloy, other than slight discoloration. Solar et al. [13] reported that even at low pH levels no significant effect on passivation behavior of tita-

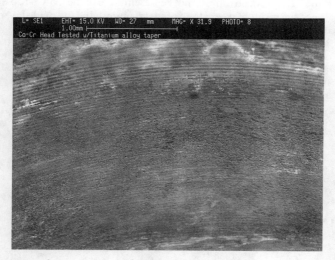

FIG. 11—*Scanning electron micrograph of the medial head-taper surface showing topographical changes due to fretting fatigue.*

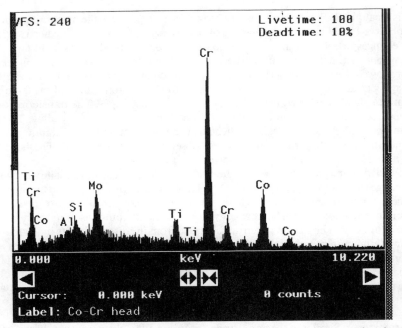

FIG. 12—*Chemical analysis of the Co-Cr-Mo head-taper surface showing elemental peaks characteristic of taper material.*

nium alloy was observed. An extensive distribution of chromium and, to a smaller extent, of molybdenum on the titanium alloy taper and Co-Cr-Mo head contact surfaces, is perhaps due to the shredding of the oxide film from the Co-Cr-Mo head. However, since the elemental peak ratio observed in the EDXA spectrum was not representative of the Co-Cr-Mo head alloy, the observed debris is not the result of wear alone of metal underlying the oxide layer. In this spec-

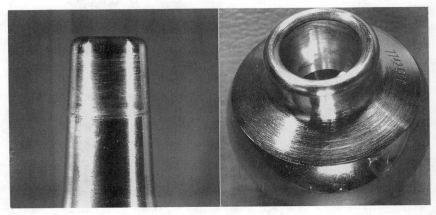

FIG. 13—*The medial surface morphology of a nitrided titanium alloy taper and a Co-Cr-Mo head after fatigue testing in Ringer's solution.*

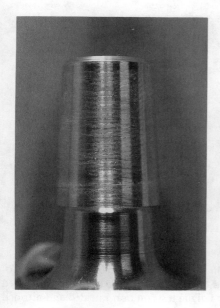 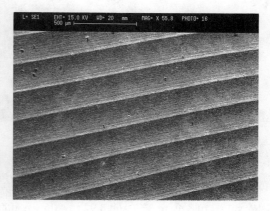

FIG. 14—*The medial surface of a Ti-6Al-4V alloy taper showing machining marks after fatigue test with an alumina head*: (a) *photomicrograph*, (b) *scanning electron micrograph.*

trum, the chromium peak was much higher than the cobalt peak whereas in a typical spectrum for a Co-Cr-Mo alloy used in this study, the cobalt peak is higher than the chromium peak. The preferential dissolution of chromium from the head material and a disturbance in its stoichiometry indicates a chemical induced phenomenon.

The titanium alloy tapers tested with alumina ceramic did not show discoloration over the entire contact area with the head, except for a light-colored ring on the medial side at the socket opening (Fig. 14a). The scanning electron microscopic examination revealed that machining marks were undeformed (Fig. 14b), suggesting no significant fretting damage occurred on the taper surface. The nitrided titanium alloy taper also showed no discoloration or damage to machining marks and the taper contact surface was free from any particulates. The ceramic heads also showed no debris but a small area of discoloration was observed on the contact surface (Fig. 15). Scanning electron microscopic examination and EDXA analysis indicated the presence of titanium, transferred from the non-nitrided taper. Such discoloration is generally observed when metal and ceramic come in contact even while driving the head on to the taper following surgical practice. The machining marks on the taper surface of the ceramic head were not deformed, suggesting that the contact surface did not experience fretting damage.

Surface Roughness

The surface roughness profiles were obtained from the contact surfaces of taper and head, and R_a values were recorded for various combinations of head/taper modular joints after each test. Typical R_a values for one set in each combination are given in Table 1. The other two sets in each condition showed similar changes in surface topography, indicating consistency in results. The R_a values were in the range 0.94 to 1.17 and 0.75 to 0.83 μm for the titanium alloy

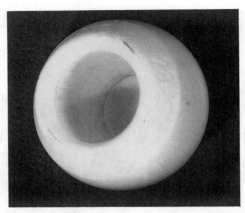

FIG. 15—*Post-fatigue condition of an alumina head tested on a Ti-6Al-4V titanium alloy taper.*

tapers in non-nitrided and nitrided conditions, 0.46 to 0.53 and 0.50 to 0.54 μm for the Co-Cr-Mo heads tested with non-nitrided and nitrided tapers. The ceramic head-tapers showed R_a values of 3.49 to 3.67 and 3.92 to 4.06 μm after fatigue tests on non-nitrided and nitrided tapers, respectively. A slight change in R_a values due to surface disturbances on both the mating surfaces is apparent from Table 1. These changes are not significant since some magnitude of fretting damage is inevitable between any two surfaces undergoing micromovement with respect to one another. The influence of change in the reflectivity of the surfaces on the peak-sensitive R_a values is negligible in these measurements, since for R_a values greater than 50 μm the geometric factor is dominant and the optical profile component is negligible. Further, utmost care was taken to align the pickup with respect to the test surface such that the stylus moved downward square to the measuring surface.

Filter Weights and Fretting Particulates

Representative filters, after the completion of 10 million cycles and after drying in a desiccator, are shown in Fig. 16. A few particulates were captured on filters during the testing of cobalt-chrome heads with titanium alloy tapers. Filters from the nitrided titanium alloy/cobalt-chrome alloy head had fewer particles in comparison to the non-nitrided. All the particulates entrapped were on the 0.45-μm filters, and the 0.20 μm filters neither showed any particulates nor any weight gain. These results conform to the findings of Willert and Sem-

TABLE 1—*Surface disturbances due to fretting fatigue in terms of R_a value measured by perthometer.*

Head	Taper	Initial R_a Value (μm)		Post-Fatigue R_a Value (μm)	
		Head	Taper	Head	Taper
Co-Cr-Mo	Ti-6Al-4V	0.64 ± 0.08	0.50 ± 0.04	0.50 ± 0.11	1.11 ± 0.16
Co-Cr-Mo	Nitrided Ti-6Al-4V	0.64 ± 0.07	0.70 ± 0.09	0.56 ± 0.10	0.75 ± 0.12
Alumina	Ti-6Al-4V	2.03 ± 0.12	2.94 ± 0.19	1.95 ± 0.17	3.56 ± 0.07
Alumina	Nitrided Ti-6Al-4V	2.00 ± 0.16	3.69 ± 0.21	1.77 ± 0.19	3.92 ± 0.09

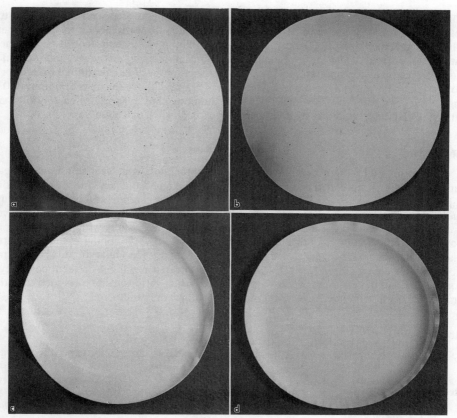

FIG. 16—*Representative filters at completion of 10 million cycles and drying in desiccator for 24 h, for various head/taper combinations fatigue tested in Ringer's solution: (a) Ti-6Al-4V taper/Co-Cr-Mo head, (b) nitrided Ti-6Al-4V taper/Co-Cr-Mo head, (c) Ti-6Al-4V taper/ alumina head, and (d) nitrided Ti-6Al-4V taper/alumina head.*

litsch [14]. These authors observed metallic wear particles in tissues adjoining endoprostheses predominantly in the range of 0.50 to 5.0 μm, with occasional occurrence of larger pieces of debris up to 100 μm. The particulates on the filter paper of this study were identified to be titanium alloy by EDXA. The filters used with ceramic heads had no particulates entrapped on them and were practically clean. Table 2 shows the weights of filters both before and after the fatigue test in dry condition. Drying of filters under identical conditions in a desiccator

TABLE 2—*Representative values of weight gain by filters.*

Material Taper/Head	Initial Weight of Filter (g)	Post-Fatigue Weight of Filter (g)	Weight Gained by Filter (g)
Ti-6Al-4V/Co-Cr-Mo	0.10491	0.12296	0.01805
Nitrided Ti-6Al-4V/Co-Cr-Mo	0.13670	0.13725	0.00055
Ti-6Al-4V/Alumina	0.14685	0.14689	0.00004
Nitrided Ti-6Al-4V/Alumina	0.14490	0.14484	—

eliminated any possibility of error being introduced in these measurements due to moisture retained from the test environment or pickup of humidity from the laboratory environment. The filtered Ringer's solution from the Ti-6Al-4V titanium alloy taper/cobalt-chrome head fatigue test indicated 0.94 mg/L of aluminum. Aluminum is very pervasive, and it could be easily picked up as contamination. However, the exact source of its contamination cannot be pointed out with certainty. No other element was detected above the detection limit of 0.02 mg/L. Ringer's solution from the Ti-6Al-4V titanium alloy taper/alumina ceramic head fatigue tests did not show any metallic elements exceeding the detection limit.

Conclusions

An experimental setup for conducting fretting/corrosion fatigue testing of modular head/taper assemblies in simulated body environments was designed and fabricated. The functional capability of this setup was illustrated by testing alumina ceramic and cobalt-chromium-molybdenum alloy femoral heads on Ti-6Al-4V titanium alloy tapers. The experimental arrangement permitted the use of 0.20 μm in-line filters successfully without impairing the flow of Ringer's solution used as a test environment and, thus, entrapping all the wear particulates greater than 0.20 μm generated during fretting fatigue of modular joints. The wear particulates were characterized by EDXA, and the effect of fretting fatigue on the topography of contact surfaces of heads and tapers were examined using various techniques such as optical and scanning electron microscopy and surface roughness measurement.

Acknowledgment

The authors would like to thank Jennifer Price for her assistance in the experimental work.

References

[1] Asgian, C., Gilbertson, L., and Hori, R., "Fatigue of Tapered Joints," *Biomaterials '84 Transactions*, Vol. 7, 1984, p. 145.
[2] Fessler, H. and Fricker, D. C., *Proceedings, Institution of Mechanical Engineers, Journal of Engineering in Medicine*, Vol. 203, 1989, p. 1.
[3] Fricker, D. C. and Shivnath, R., *Biomaterials*, Vol. 11, 1990, p. 495.
[4] Mathiesen, E. B., Lindgren, J. U., Blomgren, G. G. A., and Reinholt, F. P., *Journal of Bone Joint Surgery* (Br), Vol. 73- B, 1991, p. 569.
[5] McKellop, H., Gogan, W., Ebramzadeh, E., et al., "Metal-Metal Wear in Metal-Plastic Prosthetic Joints," *Transactions of the Society for Biomaterials*, 1990, p. 144.
[6] Collier, J. P., Surprenant, V. A., Jensen, R. E., and Mayor, M. B., *Transactions of the Society for Biomaterials*, 1991, p. 292.
[7] Michel, R., Hofmann, J., Loer, F., and Zilkens, J., *Arch Orthopedic Trauma Surgery*, Vol. 103, 1904, p. 85.
[8] Jacobs, J. J., Skipor, A. K., Black, J., et al., *The Journal of Bone and Joint Surgery*, Vol. 73-A, 1991, p. 1475.
[9] Pazzaglia, U. E., Minola, U., Gualtieri, G., et al., *Acta Orthopedic Scandinavia*, Vol. 57, 1986, p. 415.
[10] Agins, H. J., Alcock, N. W., Bansal, M., et al., *The Journal of Bone and Joint Surgery*, Vol. 70-A, 1988, p. 347.
[11] *Fractography, Metals Handbook,* Ninth ed., Vol. 12, ASM Publication, 1989, p. 364.
[12] Levine, D. L. and Staehle, R. W., *Journal Biomedical Materials Research*, Vol. 11, 1977, p. 553.
[13] Solar, R. J., "Corrosion Resistance of Titanium Surgical Implant Alloys: A Review," in *Corrosion and Degradation of Implant Materials, ASTM STP 684*, B. C. Syrett and A. Acharya, Eds., American Society for Testing and Materials, Philadelphia, 1979, p. 259.
[14] Willert, H. G. and Semlitsch, M., "Tissue Reactions to Plastic and Metallic Wear Particles of Joint Endoprosthesis," in *Total Hip Prosthesis*, N. Gschwerd and H. U. Debrunner, Eds., The Williams & Wilkins Company, Baltimore, 1976, p. 205.

Yuji Tanabe,[1] Koichi Kobayashi,[1] Makoto Sakamoto,[2] Toshiaki Hara,[1] and Hideaki Takahashi[1]

Identification of the Dynamic Properties of Bone Using the Split-Hopkinson Pressure-Bar Technique

REFERENCE: Tanabe, Y., Kobayashi, K., Sakamoto, M., Hara, T., and Takahashi, H., **"Identification of the Dynamic Properties of Bone Using the Split-Hopkinson Pressure-Bar Technique,"** *Biomaterials' Mechanical Properties, ASTM STP 1173,* H. E. Kambic and A. T. Yokobori, Jr., Eds., American Society for Testing and Materials, Philadelphia, 1994, pp. 127–141.

ABSTRACT: A method has been developed for the identification of the viscoelastic characteristics of compact bone using transient response information obtained from the split-Hopkinson pressure-bar (SHPB) test. The method combines the solution procedures of two problems. One is the identification (or inverse) problem and the other is the associated problem, i.e., the prediction (or direct) problem of stress wave propagation in the SHPB. The solutions are accomplished by means of the method of Laplace transformation and Gauss-Newton iterative scheme for nonlinear least squares problems. Numerical experiments are performed to demonstrate the validity of the method established. The method is also applied to the SHPB experiments on bovine femoral compact bone (plexiform bone), assuming that the mechanical behavior of the bone can be represented by the three-element standard linear solid model. The applicability of the model to the bone is also discussed and the orientational dependence of the viscoelastic characteristics of the bone is determined.

KEYWORDS: biomechanics, compact bone, viscoelasticity, split-Hopkinson pressure-bar (SHPB) technique, stress wave propagation, inverse problem

Compact bone in the support bones of the human skeleton continuously remodels its microstructure in response to physiological loading. Therefore, in order to develop a stable interface between compact bone and an implanted material, it is necessary to ensure a biomechanical matching at the tissue-implant interface so as to maintain the tissue within its normal physiological strain range [1]. In other words, the development of bone-analogue materials which combine suitable mechanical compatibility with a favorable bioactive response requires the evaluation of mechanical properties of the bone.

Many investigations concerning the mechanical properties of compact bone have been reported in the field of biomechanics [2] but only a limited amount of work has been done on its dynamic response under high strain rates. These studies have used the split-Hopkinson pressure-bar (SHPB) technique to investigate the dynamic constitutive relations [3,4], the dependence of the fracture stress on strain rate [3], variation of the viscoelastic response with

[1] Associate professor, Department of Mechanical Engineering; graduate student, Graduate School of Engineering; professor, Department of Mechanical Engineering; and professor, Department of Orthopaedic Surgery, respectively, Niigata University, Niigata, Japan.
[2] Associate professor, Niigata College of Technology, Niigata, Japan.

post mortem age [5], and the dependence of stiffness on orientation under impact compression [6]. SHPB technique is an impact test on a reasonable consideration of wave propagation [7] and can be used as a concise method to determine the unknown parameters in the dynamic constitutive relations of various kinds of viscoelastic materials [8]. However, application of such a method is very scarce in the field of biomechanics. This study deals with the inverse problem of determining the unknown parameters in the constitutive equation for compact bone from experimental data obtained in the SHPB test and also evaluates the orientational dependence of the viscoelastic characteristics of bovine femoral compact bone.

Hence, the objectives of this study can be explicitly stated as:

1. To develop a method for the identification of the dynamic properties of bone using the transient response information obtained from the SHPB test, and
2. To apply this method to bovine femoral compact bone and to determine the orientational dependence of its viscoelastic characteristics such as the compressive elastic modulus and damping loss.

In this paper, assuming that the linear viscoelastic model can be applied to the bone, we consider the identification (or inverse) problem and the associated wave propagation problem in the SHPB, i.e., the prediction (or direct) problem. The solutions are performed by means of the method of Laplace transformation and Gauss-Newton iterative scheme for nonlinear least squares problems and are shown to be coupled. The SHPB tests on bovine femoral compact bone are conducted and its viscoelastic properties are estimated from the records of transmitted stress by using the identification method developed. The applicability of the viscoelastic model to the bone is also discussed.

Theory

Formulation of the Problem

According to the theory of poroelasticity [9], it has been shown that the mechanical behavior of compact bone agrees well with the three-element standard linear solid model. The model can be represented by a parallel spring and dashpot in series with another spring (Fig. 1). Now consider the longitudinal stress wave propagation in SHPB which comprises two long elastic bars, input and output bars, with a small viscoelastic cylindrical specimen (Fig. 2). The mechanical behavior of the specimen is represented by the model as shown in Fig. 1. If each bar length is much larger than its diameter and the lateral contraction (or the Poisson's ratio effect) is negligible, we can analyze the dynamic stress state in each bar based on the one-dimensional wave propagation theory. It is further assumed that the lengths of the input and output bars are such as to guarantee that the reflected waves from their free-ends would not arrive at the observation points during the time interval of interest [0,T].

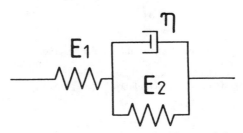

FIG. 1—*Three-element standard linear solid.*

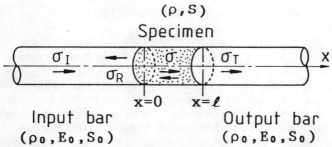

FIG. 2—*Wave propagation in the split-Hopkinson pressure-bar with a viscoelastic specimen.*

From the well known solutions of the elastic wave equation [10], Eqs 1 and 2 and Eqs 3 and 4 are established for the input and output bars, respectively.

$$v = v_I + v_R = \frac{c_0}{E_0} (\sigma_R - \sigma_I) \ , x \leq 0 \tag{1}$$

$$\sigma = \sigma_I + \sigma_R \qquad\qquad , x \leq 0 \tag{2}$$

$$v = v_T = \frac{c_0}{E_0} (-\sigma_T) \qquad , x \geq l \tag{3}$$

$$\sigma = \sigma_T \qquad\qquad , x \geq l \tag{4}$$

where subscripts I, R, and T refer to the incident, reflected and transmitted waves, respectively, and

x = longitudinal spatial coordinate, m,
v = particle velocity, m/s,
σ = longitudinal stress, Pa,
$c_0 = (E_0/\rho_0)^{1/2}$ = elastic wave velocity in the input and output bars, m/s,
E_0 = Young's modulus of the input and output bars, Pa,
ρ_0 = density of the input and output bars, kg/m³, and
l = length of specimen, m.

Equations 1 to 4 are used as boundary conditions for the specimen input and output bars interfaces.

For the specimen, the wave equation and the constitutive equation are given as follows

$$\frac{\partial \sigma}{\partial x} = \rho \frac{\partial v}{\partial t} \tag{5}$$

$$\sigma + \frac{\eta}{E_1 + E_2} \frac{\partial \sigma}{\partial t} = \frac{E_1 E_2}{E_1 + E_2} \epsilon + \frac{E_1 \eta}{E_1 + E_2} \frac{\partial \epsilon}{\partial t} \tag{6}$$

where

ϵ = longitudinal strain, m/m,
ρ = density of the specimen, kg/m³,
t = time, s,
E_1, E_2 = stiffness of the springs in the model shown in Fig. 1, Pa, and
η = viscosity coefficient of the dashpot in the model shown in Fig. 1, Pa·s.

Differentiating Eq 6 with respect to time t and combining the result with Eq 5, Eq 7 is obtained.

$$\frac{\partial^2 \sigma}{\partial t^2} + \frac{\eta}{E_1 + E_2} \frac{\partial^3 \sigma}{\partial t^3} = \frac{E_1 E_2}{\rho(E_1 + E_2)} \frac{\partial^2 \sigma}{\partial x^2} + \frac{E_1 \rho}{\eta(E_1 + E_2)} \frac{\partial^3 \sigma}{\partial x^2 \partial t} \tag{7}$$

Equation 7 is a linear differential equation that governs the longitudinal stress wave propagation phenomenon in the specimen. Once we get the stress produced at the specimen-output bar interface ($x = l$) from the solution of Eq 7, the stress history at any point on the output bar, or the transmitted stress history can be easily obtained by using Eq 4.

Now suppose that the transmitted stress pulse profile is measured at a point on the output bar, designated $\sigma_m(t)$. The problem is to identify the parameters $P = (E_1, E_2, \eta)$ in Eq 6 and to predict stress history at the same point based on this stress measurement.

The Solution of a Wave Equation

In order to solve the problem of wave propagation in the specimen, let us first consider solving Eq 7 for time interval $0 \le t \le T$ subject to the initial conditions

$$\sigma(x,0) = \frac{\partial \sigma(x,0)}{\partial t} = 0, \, 0 \le x \le l \tag{8}$$

and the boundary conditions

$$v = \frac{c_0}{E_0} (\sigma_R - \sigma_I) \,, x = 0 \tag{9}$$

$$\sigma = \frac{S_0}{S} (\sigma_R + \sigma_I) \,, x = 0 \tag{10}$$

$$v = -\frac{c_0}{E_0} \sigma_T \quad\quad ,x = l \tag{11}$$

$$\sigma = \frac{S_0}{S} \sigma_T \quad\quad ,x = l \tag{12}$$

where

S, S_0 = cross-sectional area of the specimen and of the input-output bars, respectively, m².

The origin of time ($t = 0$) is selected to be the time when the incident stress pulse arrives at the specimen-input bar interface ($x = 0$). Applying the Laplace transformation with respect to time t to Eq 5 and Eqs 7 to 12 yields

$$\frac{d^2 \bar{\sigma}}{dx^2} - \phi(p)\bar{\sigma} = 0 \tag{13}$$

$$\frac{d\bar{\sigma}}{dx} = \rho p \bar{v} \tag{14}$$

$$\bar{v} = \alpha(\bar{\sigma}_R - \bar{\sigma}_I) \,, x = 0 \tag{15}$$

$$\bar{\sigma} = \frac{1}{\beta} (\bar{\sigma}_R + \bar{\sigma}_I) \,, x = 0 \tag{16}$$

$$\bar{v} = -\alpha \bar{\sigma}_T \qquad , x = l \tag{17}$$

$$\bar{\sigma} = \frac{1}{\beta} \bar{\sigma}_T \qquad , x = l \tag{18}$$

where a bar over its symbol "-" denotes the Laplace transformation, i.e.,

$$\bar{f}(p) = \int_0^\infty f(t) e^{-pt} dt$$

where p = subsidiary variable and

$$\alpha = \frac{c_0}{E_0}, \beta = \frac{S}{S_0}, \phi(p) = \frac{\rho p^2 (\eta p + E_1 + E_2)}{\eta E_1 p + E_1 E_2} .$$

Equation 13 has a solution

$$\bar{\sigma} = C_1 \exp\{-\sqrt{\phi(p)}\, x\} + C_2 \exp\{\sqrt{\phi(p)}\, x\} \tag{19}$$

Evaluating the constants C_1 and C_2 from the boundary conditions given by Eqs 15 to 18, we obtain

$$C_1 = \bar{\sigma}_I \frac{2\alpha}{\{\delta + \Psi(p)\}} \cdot \frac{1}{G(p)} \tag{20}$$

$$C_2 = -\bar{\sigma}_I \frac{2\alpha\{\delta - \Psi(p)\}}{\{\delta + \Psi(p)\}^2} \cdot \frac{\exp\{-2\sqrt{\phi(p)}\, l\}}{G(p)} \tag{21}$$

where

$$\delta = \alpha\beta, \Psi(p) = \phi(p)/(\rho p), G(p) = 1 - \left\{\frac{\delta - \Psi(p)}{\delta + \Psi(p)}\right\}^2 \exp\{-2\sqrt{\phi(p)}\, l\} \tag{22}$$

Once we have the Laplace transformation of the arbitrarily prescribed incident stress pulse $\bar{\sigma}_I$, we can get that of the stress $\bar{\sigma}$. The actual solution of the stress in the specimen is the inverse of Eq 19 and it can be evaluated by means of the method of numerical inverse Laplace transformation (see Appendix). For the sake of simplifying the computation, profile of the incident stress pulse measured is reduced to a certain specific function as shown in the Appendix.

The Solution of the Identification and Prediction Problem

Recall that $\sigma_m(t)$ is the measured stress history at an arbitrary point on the output bar. The solution of the direct problem, i.e., the solution of the initial-boundary value problem represented by Eqs 8 to 12 is given by Eq 19 and the actual numerical solution of stress in the specimen, i.e., $\sigma(x,t)$ for $0 \leq x \leq l$ and $0 \leq t \leq T$ can be obtained accurately by the aforementioned method. According to the theory of one-dimensional wave propagation in elastic bar [10], the stress histories to be observed at arbitrary points on the output bar, designated transmitted stress $\sigma_T(t)$, should be the same and they can be readily evaluated from the stress at the specimen-output bar interface by using Eq 12, i.e., $\sigma_T(t) \equiv \sigma_T(x,t) \equiv \beta\sigma\left(l, t - \dfrac{x - l}{c_0}\right)$ for $x \geq l$ and $0 \leq t \leq T$. Obviously if the parameters P were given the correct values, we would expect $\sigma_T(t)$ to be in good agreement with $\sigma_m(t)$. Accordingly, we may state that the identification problem is to find the best P so as to bring $\sigma_T(t)$ as close to $\sigma_m(t)$ as possible. Since both $\sigma_m(t)$ (experimental data) and $\sigma_T(t)$ (calculated by the computer) are given by their values at discrete time points, we introduce the least squares distance function

$$F = \sum_{k=1}^{N} [\sigma_T(t_k;P) - \sigma_m(t_k)]^2 \tag{23}$$

where

t_k = discrete time point ($k = 1, 2, \ldots, N$), s, and
N = number of data

and then the problem can be reduced to finding the best P so that Eq 23 attains its minimum value. Since $\sigma_T(t_k)$ depends on the parameters P, the problem can be explicitly stated as

$$\min_P F = \min_P \left\{ \sum_{k=1}^{N} [\sigma_T(t_k;P) - \sigma_m(t_k)]^2 \right\} \tag{24}$$

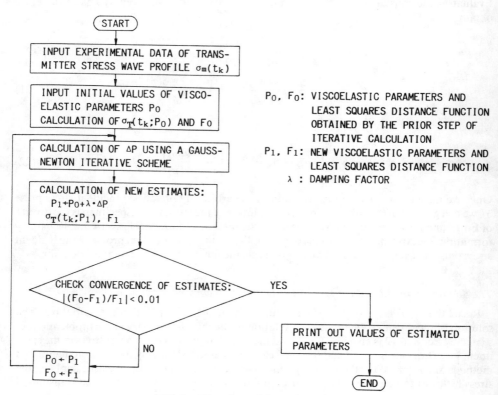

FIG. 3—*Flow chart of the methodology.*

TABLE 1—*Results of parameter identification.*

Iteration	Parameter Value		
	E_1, GPa	E_2, GPa	η, MPa·s
0 (Initial Guess)	4.00	10.0	1.50
5 (Converged)	5.24	8.38	1.91
Exact Value	5.00	8.00	2.00

Using the Gauss-Newton iterative scheme with a damping factor [*11*], the minimization problem (Eq 24) can be successfully carried out. Convergence is achieved if the function F changes by less than 1% of its value. A detailed description of this iterative scheme can be found in Ref *11*. The flow chart of the methodology previously described is shown in Fig. 3.

Numerical Experimentation

In order to demonstrate the feasibility and accuracy of the solution procedure in the preceding section, numerical simulations were performed. To generate numerical data, the transmitted stress was computed using Eqs 19 to 22 with the exact values of the parameters E_1, E_2 and η given in Table 1. Values of the other variables necessary for the computation, such as dimensions and material constants of the specimen, input, and output bars were taken from the experimental setup used in this study. For the incident stress in Eqs 20 and 21, an approximate expression given in the Appendix was used. Solution for the transmitted stress at $x = l$ was recorded, which constituted the numerical data $\sigma_m(t)$. For identification, the procedure previously described was used. Values of the parameters were assumed to be unknown and the data $\sigma_m(t)$ were used for their determination. The parameter values at different stages of iteration are given in Table 1 and the corresponding predictions of the stress history are shown in Fig. 4. It is clear from Table 1 that the final identified values agree well with their exact values (maximum relative error < 5%) implying that the identification procedure is correct and reli-

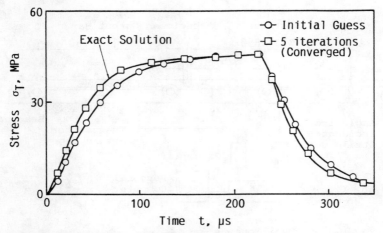

FIG. 4—*Results of numerical simulation. Numerically generated stress history (exact solution) and pulse prediction at various stages of identification.*

able. It is also shown in Fig. 4 that the stress prediction is hardly distinguished from the data designated as "exact solution."

Characterization of the Dynamic Properties of Bovine Femoral Compact Bone

A series of SHPB experiments on bovine femoral compact bone was conducted to obtain data for the purpose of identifying its viscoelastic properties by means of the method previously described. The experimental procedure and results are presented.

Experimental Setup

The conventional SHPB apparatus was used (Fig. 5). The apparatus is composed of input and output steel cylindrical rods containing a specimen sandwiched between them. The diameter of both the bars was 11 mm. The input and output bars, 1850- and 1960-mm-long, respectively, were supported by ball bearings mounted on a long angle-iron; eccentric bushings were used so that the vertical position of each bearing could be easily adjusted to align the bars. Using a compact air compressor, a striker bar (diameter = 13 mm, length = 600 mm) was fired through an air gun tube. The striker bar impacted on the input bar as a result. The impact velocity of the striker was selected to be about 1.3 m/s by regulating the pressure of air so that the maximum strain rate of about 100 s^{-1} was obtained.

The incident and transmitted stress pulse profiles were detected by the surface-bonded foil electrical-resistance strain gages (gage length = 1 mm) mounted on the input and output bars. The strain gage on the input bar was located at the center of the bar while the gage on the output bar was at a distance of 440 mm from the specimen interface. Profile of the stress pulses was recorded and stored in a digital storage oscilloscope. Subsequent operations of the recorded data were performed with the help of a personal computer. During testing a lubricant was placed on the contact surfaces to reduce the frictional constraint and all tests were done at room temperature (20°C).

Specimen Preparation

All specimens were fabricated from batches of fresh frozen bovine femurs of an average age of seven or eight months. Bone samples were machined from the dense cortical material of the

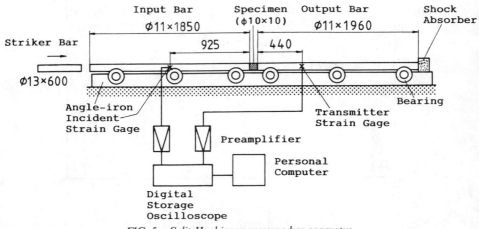

FIG. 5—*Split-Hopkinson pressure-bar apparatus.*

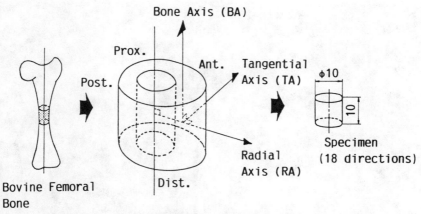

FIG. 6—*Cartesian coordinate system chosen for compact bone specimens.*

anterior part of the femoral mid-diaphysis into cylinders (diameter = 10 mm, length = 10 mm). Since mechanical properties were determined as a function of direction, a reference system had to be chosen for the orientation of the specimens in the cortical bone. A Cartesian coordinate system as shown in Fig. 6 was assumed. The bone axis was parallel to the long axis of the bone. The tangential axis was in the circumferential direction while the radial axis was in the endosteal-periosteal direction. These axes were specified by eye and denoted BA, TA, and RA, respectively. Specimens were cut with their long axis in the BA-, TA-, and RA-directions. Off-axis specimens were also prepared with their long axis in the BA-TA plane, BA-RA plane, and TA-RA plane at angles of 15°, 30°, 45°, 60°, and 75° to the BA, TA, and RA, respectively. After sectioning, specimens were stored in saline solution at 5°C till testing and were tested within 12 hours. Figures 7a to 7c show the typical optical micrographs of bone surfaces. Samples were taken perpendicular to the BA-, TA- and RA-directions, respectively. Specimens tested in this study consisted of primary bone (plexiform bone) devoid of any secondary Haversian system. In this study, only one specimen was taken from one individual bovine and five specimens were tested for each orientation.

Results and Discussion

The results are shown in Figs. 8 and 9. Figure 8 shows the record of the transmitted stress for a specimen oriented parallel to the BA-direction and the corresponding predictions of the stress history. The parameter values at different stages of iteration are also given. To speed up the process of identification, initial parameter values of E_1, E_2, and η were guessed as follows: E_1 was taken as the slope of the dynamic stress-strain curve obtained from conventional analysis of the SHPB technique (see Appendix); E_2 was estimated using the relation

$$E_s = \frac{E_1 E_2}{E_1 + E_2} \tag{25}$$

where E_s is the slope of the static stress-strain curve obtained from a quasi-static compression test, and this equation is derived from Eq 6 when $\partial\sigma/\partial t \rightarrow 0$ and $\partial\epsilon/\partial t \rightarrow 0$; the viscosity coefficient η was obtained by trial and error. As can be seen from Fig. 8, the final parameter values yielded fairly good prediction for the transmitted stress pulse profile. Thus, Fig. 8 emphasizes

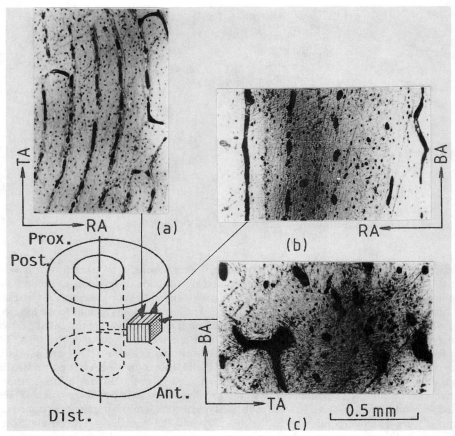

FIG. 7—*Microstructures of bone specimens observed at* (a) *BA-,* (b) *TA-, and* (c) *RA-surfaces.*

that bovine femoral compact bone (plexiform bone) can be well represented by the three-element standard linear solid model. Since similar results were obtained for other specimen directions, we examined the variation in the viscoelastic characteristics for the bone with respect to the orientation of the specimen axis. Figure 9 shows the mean value (with minimum and maximum values) of identified viscoelastic parameters plotted against the orientation of specimen axes. The stiffness E_1 is constant throughout the RA-TA plane and increases to a maximum in the BA-direction. The scatter in the stiffness E_2 is less than that in the other two parameters (E_1 and η) and the value of E_2 is approximately 7 GPa in all directions. The viscosity coefficient η varies with orientation similar to the stiffness E_1. In other words, Fig. 9 means that at higher strain rates Young's modulus increases and its orientational dependence becomes more significant (E_1 gives the upper bound for the elastic modulus of the bone). This has been ascertained through the experiments conducted on the same bone samples using the ultrasonic technique and quasi-static compression tests [12]. Hence, it is concluded that the rigidity and the internal frictional loss of the bone under impact compression are greatest in the BA-direction.

Our previous work has revealed that plexiform bone used here has linear stress-strain characteristics both under quasi-static and impact loading [13]. Hence, the application of the

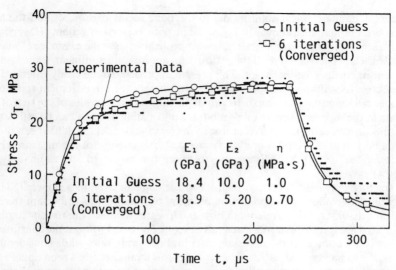

FIG. 8—*Transmitted pulse prediction at various stages of identification. Measured and predicted stress histories for bovine compact bone specimen (Specimen axis: BA-direction).*

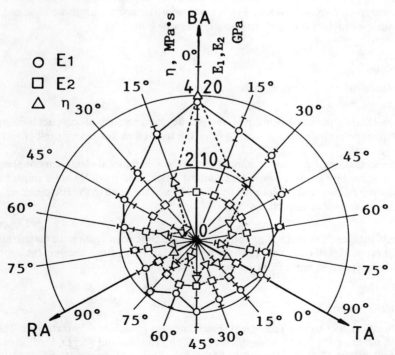

FIG. 9—*Viscoelastic characteristics as a function of orientation. Each datum point represents the mean (with maximum and minimum) of five specimens.*

three-element standard linear solid model to the bone seems reasonable and the adequate result has been obtained as shown in Fig. 8. Bone with Haversian system (Haversian bone) obviously shows nonlinear stress-strain relations probably due to the existence of many small pores such as Haversian canals and this requires an appropriate nonlinear viscoelastic model to represent its mechanical behavior. The present approach can be easily extended to such nonlinear case. In addition, though it is uncertain whether the three-element standard linear solid model can represent the creep behavior of plexiform bone because of the lack of the necessary data at the moment, the Young's modulus under static loading can be estimated from the identified model using Eq 25. According to the previous work [13], it has been shown that the estimated values of Young's modulus agree approximately with the measured results at strain rate of $1.67 \times 10^{-4} \mathrm{s}^{-1}$ (discrepancy between the measured and estimated values is within 10%).

Bone fracture may easily occur in high-speed accidents or even in a slow fall. Therefore, from a clinical viewpoint of the prediction of injury or fracture, it is important to reveal the mechanical behavior of bone under both high and low strain rates. The stress or strain state in bone subjected to arbitrary external loads can never be evaluated without the constitutive relation. There is not enough of the necessary data for high strain rates while considerable work on studies of mechanical properties of bone under low strain rates has been done. Hence, in order to establish the constitutive relation applicable to bone over a wide range of strain rates, impact mechanical tests such as the present study are still more significant.

Furthermore, only compressive loading was considered in this study. Bending, torsion, and various combined loading modes (such as compression-bending, compression-torsion, etc.) are also important as actual loading conditions or *in vivo* stress state. It has been confirmed that the parameter values given in Fig. 8 agree approximately with those obtained from the impact three-point bending experiments on the same bone [14].

Conclusions

The results obtained are summarized as follows:

1. A method for the identification of viscoelastic characteristics of compact bone using transient response information arising from the split-Hopkinson pressure-bar test has been developed.
2. The mechanical behavior of compact bone (bovine femoral plexiform bone) can be well represented by the three-element standard linear solid model. Under impact compression, the rigidity and the internal frictional loss of the bone in the BA-direction are larger than those in other directions.

The advantage of the method presented is that the time required for characterization of the dynamic properties of bone can be sharply reduced. Furthermore, the present approach can be readily extended to nonlinear materials.

Acknowledgments

Financial support by the Yamaguchi Foundation is gratefully acknowledged. The authors also wish to thank Professor W. Bonfield, Dr. K. E. Tanner, and Mr. D. Vashishth (Interdisciplinary Research Centre in Biomedical Materials, Queen Mary and Westfield College, London, U.K.) for their helpful suggestions.

APPENDIX

Numerical Inverse of the Laplace Transformation by the Use of the Fast Fourier Transformation (FFT) Algorithm

Rewriting the equations defining the inverse Laplace transformation in the form of discrete Fourier transformation, we have

$$f(h \cdot \Delta t) = \frac{\exp(\gamma h \cdot \Delta t)}{T} \sum_{n=0}^{N-1} \overline{f_n} \exp(i2\pi nh/N), (h = 0, \ldots, N-1)$$

$$\overline{f_n} = f(\gamma + in \cdot \Delta\omega), \gamma = \text{const.}, i = \sqrt{-1},$$ (26)

$$\Delta t = T/N, \Delta\omega = 2\pi/T$$

where

$T = $ finite time interval of interest, s, and
$N = $ number of data points and has to be of the form 2^m ($m = 1, 2, \ldots$).

Applying the algorithm of the FFT to Eq 26, we can reduce the amount of computation to find the final solution [15]. In this study, we set $\gamma = 6/T$ and $N = 2^{13}$. A check on the accuracy of the numerical solution obtained by this method has been done in Ref 16 by comparing it with the known exact solution of the elastodynamic problem, and it has confirmed that the first three significant digits in the numerical solution agree with those in the exact solution.

Approximate Expression for the Incident Stress Wave Profile

The wave form of the incident stress measured by the SHPB apparatus used here (Fig. 10) can be expressed as

$$\sigma_I = H(t) \left[1 - \exp\left(\frac{t}{t_R}\right) \right] - H(t - t_H) \left\{ 1 - \exp\left[\frac{-(t - t_H)}{t_D} \right] \right\}$$ (27)

where

$H(t) = $ Heaviside's step function, and
$t_R, t_H, t_D = $ rise, hold, and decrease time characterizing the pulse profile measured, s.

The Laplace transformation of Eq 27 then becomes

$$\overline{\sigma_I} = \frac{1 - \exp(-pt_H)}{p} - \frac{t_R}{t_R p + 1} + \frac{t_D\exp(-pt_H)}{t_D p + 1}$$ (28)

Evaluation of the Dynamic Stress-Strain Characteristics Using SHPB Technique

If the relation $\sigma_I + \sigma_R = \sigma_T$ is established, the strain rate ($\dot{\epsilon}$), strain (ϵ), and stress (σ) in the specimen at any time t can be estimated by the following equations [7]

$$\dot{\epsilon} = \frac{2}{\rho_0 c_0 l}(\sigma_I - \sigma_T)$$ (29)

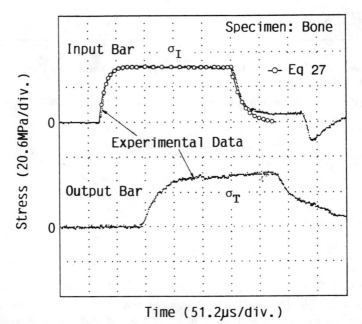

FIG. 10—*Typical oscilloscope records for SHPB test on bovine femoral compact bone. Top trace: incident stress pulse in input bar along with its approximate expression (upward is compression); Bottom trace: transmitted stress pulse in output bar (upward is compression).*

$$\epsilon = \frac{2}{\rho_0 c_0 l} \int_0^t (\sigma_I - \sigma_T) dt \qquad (30)$$

$$\sigma = \frac{S_0}{S} \sigma_T \qquad (31)$$

The dynamic stress-strain curve on the specimen can be readily derived from experimental data (Fig. 10) using Eqs 30 and 31. A check on the accuracy of the strain estimated by Eq 30 could be done by comparing it with the strain measured directly from the strain gage pasted on the specimen. It has been confirmed that discrepancy between estimated and measured strain was within 5%.

References

[1] Bonfield, W., "Bioactive Materials for Bone Replacement," *Digest of the World Congress on Medical Physics and Biomedical Engineering, Part 1,* Kyoto, Japan, July 1991, p. 47.
[2] Natali, A. N. and Meroi, E. A., "A Review of the Biomechanical Properties of Bone as a Material," *Journal of Biomedical Engineering,* Vol. 11, July 1989, pp. 266–276.
[3] Lewis, J. L. and Goldsmith, W., "The Dynamic Fracture and Prefracture Response of Compact Bone by Split Hopkinson Bar Methods," *Journal of Biomechanics,* Vol. 8, 1975, pp. 27–40.
[4] Yang, G., Wu, W., and Fan, X., "Dynamic Properties of Bone Under High Rate of Strain," *Progress and New Directions of Biomechanics,* Mita Press, Osaka, 1989, pp. 343–347.
[5] Tennyson, R. C., Ewert, R., and Niranjan, V., "Dynamic Viscoelastic Response of Bone," *Experimental Mechanics,* Vol. 12, November 1972, pp. 502–507.
[6] Tateishi, T., Shirasaki, Y., Kinoshita, Y., and Tateishi, K., *Transactions of the Japan Society of Mechanical Engineers,* Vol. 46A, No. 404, April 1980, pp. 438–448 (in Japanese).

[7] Lindholm, U. S., "Some Experiments with the Split Hopkinson Pressure Bar," *Journal of Mechanical and Physics of Solids,* Vol. 12, 1964, pp. 317–335.

[8] Lin, I. H. and Sackman, J. L., "Identification of the Dynamic Properties of Nonlinear Viscoelastic Materials and Associated Wave Propagation Problem," *International Journal of Solids and Structures,* Vol. 11, 1975, pp. 1145–1149.

[9] Nowinski, J. L., "Bone Articulations as Systems of Poroelastic Bodies in Contact," *AIAA Journal,* Vol. 9, No. 1, 1971, pp. 62–67.

[10] Akao, M. and Nakagawa, N., *Preprint of the Japan Society of Mechanical Engineers,* No. 754-1, March 1975, pp. 65–67 (in Japanese).

[11] Levenberg, K., "A Method for the Solution of Certain Nonlinear Problems in Least Squares," *Quarterly of Applied Mathematics,* Vol. 2, No. 4, 1944, pp. 164–168.

[12] Tanabe, Y., Tanaka, S., Sakamoto, M., and Hara, T., "The Evaluation of Mechanical Properties of Bone under Compressive Impact Loading,"*Proceedings of the Thirty-fourth Japan Congress on Materials Research,* 1991, pp. 233–237.

[13] Tanabe, Y., Sakamoto, M., Hara, T., Koga, Y., and Takahashi, H., "Influence of Loading Rate on Anisotropy of Compact Bone," *Journal de Physique IV: Proceedings of the Third International Conference on Mechanical and Physical Behaviour of Materials under Dynamic Loading,* Strasbourg, France, October 1991, pp. 305–310.

[14] Tanabe, Y., Kobayashi, K., Shinohara, A., and Koga, Y., "The Determination of Viscoelastic Properties of Compact Bone by Using Impact Three-Point Bending Test," *Proceedings of the Seventh International Conference on Biomedical Engineering,* Singapore, December 1992, pp. 422–424.

[15] Krings, W. and Waller, H., "Contribution to Numerical Treatment of Partial Differential Equations with the Laplace Transformation—An Application of the Algorithm of the Fast Fourier Transformation,"*International Journal for Numerical Methods in Engineering,* Vol. 14, 1979, pp. 1183–1196.

[16] Tanabe, Y., Maekawa, I., Handa, S., and Hara, T., "The Propagation of Shear Wave in a Viscoelastic Rod," *Transactions of the Japan Society of Mechanical Engineers,* Vol. 55A, No. 520, December 1989, pp. 2452–2457 (in Japanese).

Yoshinori Miyasaka,[1] *Masamizu Ohyama,*[1] *Minoru Sakurai,*[1]
A. Toshimitsu Yokobori,[2] *and Shigeru Sasaki*[2]

Mechanical Properties of Immature Callus in Long Bones

REFERENCE: Miyasaka, Y., Ohyama, M., Sakurai, M., Yokobori, A. T., and Sasaki, S., **"Mechanical Properties of Immature Callus in Long Bones,"** *Biomaterials' Mechanical Properties, ASTM STP 1173,* H. E. Kambic and A. T. Yokobori, Jr., Eds., American Society for Testing and Materials, Philadelphia, 1994, pp. 142–147.

ABSTRACT: Callus distraction had long been believed to be harmful to fracture healing until the development of a new method named callotasis, which gave the green light to the field of long bone lengthening. This revolutionary method showed that the distraction does not disturb bone formation, which was confirmed by our results of clinical cases. One of our callotasis cases was presented to show its characteristic X-ray features in the course of callotasis.

We made experimental callotasis in rabbit femurs and performed mechanical tests for callus of the bones in order to investigate its mechanical behavior when tensile loads were applied. Femurs of eight rabbits were osteotomized at the level of the midshaft with a bone saw and fixed with a mini-model external fixator. Gradual callus distraction was performed at the rate of about 0.7 mm per day. The femurs were removed after sacrifice and served as bone specimens for the mechanical tests. Control long bones were twelve osteotomized femurs fixed with the same external fixator without callotasis and ten osteotomized tibiae fixed with an intramedullary Kirschner wire.

This immature callus showed the characteristics of hysteresis in the load-deformation curves and also those of stress relaxation in stress relaxation test. We conclude that the callus in callotasis has the property of viscoelasticity, and infer that this property is one of the mechanical bases making callotasis possible.

KEYWORDS: callotasis, callus, mechanical test

Orthopaedic surgeons have given much attention to callus formation in fracture healing [1,2]. Fracture healing of a long bone proceeds as the following [2,3]. At first, hematoma and fibrous tissues appear around the fracture site, and then cartilaginous tissues also appear. They are called callus, which is composed of many tissues. This callus gradually becomes harder with its mineralization process and finally develops into mature bone. In an initial stage of fracture healing, immobilization of the callus site is believed to be essential. In a later stage, it had long been considered that local distraction force exerted an inhibiting factor and was harmful for fracture healing. However, a new method named callotasis, in which gradual callus distraction produces new bone formation, was introduced to orthopaedic practice. Callotasis became highlighted as a revolutionary method in long bone lengthening because its clinical results are excellent compared to ordinary methods.

[1] Assistant professor, lecturer, and professor, respectively, Department of Orthopaedic Surgery; [2]associate professor and postgraduate student, respectively, Department of Mechatronics and Precision Engineering; Tohoku University, Sendai, Japan.

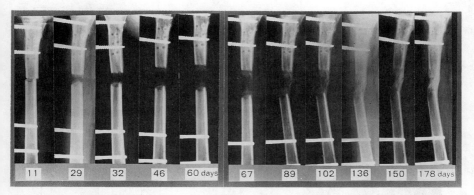

FIG. 1—*A case of a twelve-year-old boy. Radiographic change of the osteotomized femur during the course of callotasis. Numbers show the days after osteotomy.*

Clinical Case of Callotasis

A representative case, a twelve-year-old boy, had shortening of the left femur due to the dysfunctional growth plate associated with the residual femoral head deformity after the treatment of congenital hip dislocation. He underwent osteotomy of the left femur and its site was fixed with an external fixator (Orthofix type) under general anesthesia. After a two-week waiting period, callus distraction was started. His leg length discrepancy was corrected by final lengthening 40 mm after 47 days of intermittent distraction of about 0.5 mm twice a day. Radiographic change of osteotomized long bone during the course of callotasis is shown in Fig. 1. Callus formed in the osteotomized site not only increased in volume, but gradually mineralized as callotasis proceeded. This mineralization started in the peripheral zones of the callus which showed relatively sclerotic (white) in the radiograph. Its central zone remained black while being distracted and was thought to be immature callus (Fig. 1).

Experimental Materials and Methods

Japanese white rabbits were used. Femurs of eight rabbits were osteotomized at the midshaft with a bone saw and fixed with a mini-model external fixator. Callotasis was started at the rate of about 0.35 mm twice a day one week after the osteotomy. The femurs were removed after sacrifice during callotasis. Materials were the femurs from which the external fixator was detached. Controls were twelve osteotomized femurs fixed with the same external fixator without callotasis and ten osteotomized tibiae fixed with an intramedullary Kirschner wire. Tibiae were also removed after sacrifice one, two, or three weeks after osteotomy. The tibiae were also used as materials after the Kirschner wire was removed.

Mechanical tests were performed on the removed long bones with intact callus by using a Multi-applicable-micro-strength testing machine (YSGS type) which was developed by the authors (Fig. 2) [7]. Two ends of the whole bone specimens were firmly fixed with the chucks. Applied tensile loads were monitored by load cell, and deformation was also monitored. The container was filled with saline water to keep the specimens wet. Load-deformation hysteresis and stress relaxation tests were performed with the deformation rate of 11 mm per minute [4]. In the former test, the curve was obtained by applying a distractive load first, and then by decreasing the load before callus breakage and to zero level.

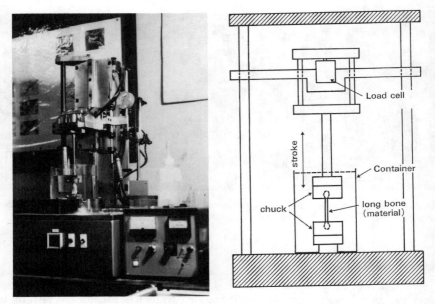

FIG. 2—*The system of the testing machine. Multi-applicable micro-strength testing machine (YSGS type).*

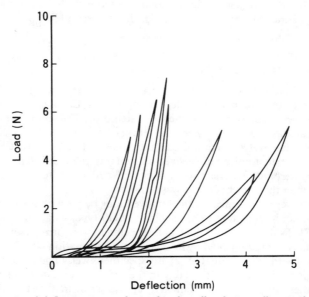

Fig. 3—*Load-deflection curves obtained in the callus during callotasis (femurs).*

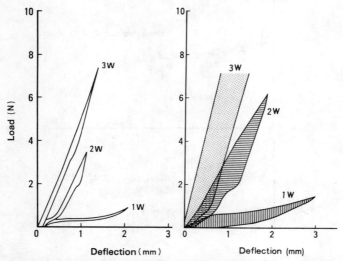

FIG. 4—*Load-deflection curves in the callus obtained one week, two weeks, and three weeks after oste-otomy. The left half of the figure shows a representative example of the curve (femur controls) in each group. The right half illustrates the range of each group of the curve (femurs and tibia controls).*

Results

Load-Deformation Hysteresis Test

Load-deflection curves (loading-unloading curve) obtained in the callus during callotasis (femurs) are shown in Fig. 3. It was found that the curves had a loop, or a characteristic of hysteresis. The slope of the curve was very small under smaller deflection, and then became larger under larger deflection; in short, the curves have two phases. Under the smaller deflection, the slope is similar to that of control long bones one week after osteotomy (Figs. 3 and 4).

All three types of load-deflection curves of control long bones also have a characteristic of hysteresis (Fig. 4). The order of slope degree of the curves is as follows: that of three weeks, two weeks, and one week after osteotomy (Fig. 4). In other words, younger and more immature callus had larger compliance and were more easily distracted.

These results in controls had, of course, differences between individual bone which were not smaller than bone differences between femurs and tibiae.

Stress Relaxation Test

Stress relaxation curves are shown in Fig. 5. All the curves of one, two, and three weeks after osteotomy demonstrated to have the stress relaxation characteristic, which was time-dependent. The curves of elongated callus (during callotasis) also demonstrated the stress relaxation characteristic.

Discussion

Many investigators have reported the mechanical properties of mature callus and its strength in the process of fracture healing [1,6]. But few reports have been presented on the mechanical behavior of callus when distractive force is applied. In this paper, we studied the

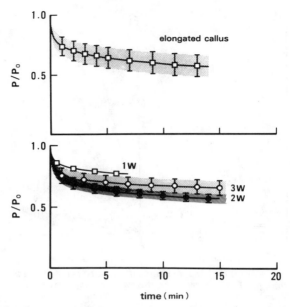

FIG. 5—*Stress relaxation curves are shown respectively, during callotasis (elongated callus of femur, upper graph) one week, two weeks, and three weeks after osteotomy (femurs controls, lower graph). The width in each time represents the range of the curve.*

behavior of immature callus in long bones from two viewpoints: stress relaxation and hysteresis in load-deformation curve. The obtained results revealed that callus has viscoelasticity because of its characteristics of both hysteresis and stress relaxation. It was also revealed that viscous deformity was produced when a minimal displacement of distraction was applied and maintained for a certain time. These observations led us to infer that this viscoelasticity of immature callus is one of the mechanical bases for callotasis.

A theoretical viscoelastic model for the callus was introduced (Fig. 6) and was used for a computer simulation study. This model contains both Maxwell and Kelvin units as its elements (Fig. 6). The details of the mechanical properties in callus were discussed in the computer simulation study [5], which made possible the more precise interpretation of the results in this study. Its conclusion is that the viscoelasticity of the callus in experimental callotasis can be related to the radiographic zonal structure of the callus, which is often observed in

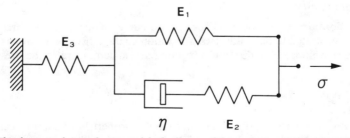

FIG. 6—*The theoretical viscoelastic model of callus used for computer simulation study. E1, E2, and E3 represent stiffness in each spring model, and η represents viscous coefficient in the dash-pot.*

radiographs also in clinical cases. Furthermore, the viscoelasticity is not simple enough to be explained by a single Kelvin model or a single Maxwell model. This is the reason we introduced the more complicated viscoelastic model.

References

[1] Albright, J. A. and Brand, R. A., *Scientific Basis of Orthopaedics,* Norwalk, CT, Appleton & Lange, 1987.
[2] Rockwood, C. A. Jr. and Green, D. P., *Basic Fracture Healing in Fractures in Adults,* J. B. Lippincott Co., Philadelphia, 1984, pp. 147–152.
[3] American Academy of Orthopaedic Surgeons, "Bone Repairs in Orthopaedic Science Syllabus," Chicago, 1986.
[4] Miyasaka, Y., Sakurai, M., and Yokobori, A. T. Jr., "Mechanical Test Method for Immature Callus Formed After the Experimental Osteotomy of Long Bones," *Journal of the Japan Orthopaedics Association,* Vol. 64, No. 8, 1990, S1152 (in Japanese).
[5] Miyasaka, Y., Sakurai, M., Ohyama, M., Yokobori, A. T. Jr., et al., "Analysis of Visco-elastic Behaviors in the Callus of Rabbit Femurs by Computer Simulation," *Japan Society for Orthopaedic Biomechanics,* Vol. 13, 1992, (in Japanese) pp. 321–325.
[6] White, A. A., Panjabi, M. M., and Southwick, W. O., "The Four Bio-Mechanical Stages of Fracture Repair," *Journal of Bone Joint Surgery,* Vol. 59A, 1977, pp. 188–193.
[7] Yokobori, A. T. Jr., Ohkuma, T., Yoshinari, H., et al., "Mechanical Test Method of Micro Blood Vessel," *Proceedings of the First Biomechanical Symposium, Journal of the Society for Mechanical Engineers,* 1990, pp. 21–22 (in Japanese).

Y. Higo[1] and Y. Tomita[2]

Evaluation of Mechanical Properties of Metallic Biomaterials

REFERENCE: Higo, Y. and Tomita, Y., **"Evaluation of Mechanical Properties of Metallic Biomaterials,"** *Biomaterials' Mechanical Properties, ASTM STP 1173,* H. E. Kambic and A. T. Yokobori, Jr., Eds., American Society for Testing and Materials, Philadelphia, 1994, pp. 148–155.

ABSTRACT: In this paper, some methods for evaluating the properties of metallic biomaterials are proposed and discussed, with special interest in the requirements of biomaterials which strongly relate to corrosive properties. A simple evaluation method for determining metallic elution was proposed, and the results are shown.

The most important mechanical property of a biomaterial is the fatigue life under consideration of actual usage and environment. The methods employed for the artificial joint were used as an example. The appropriate fatigue test for the biomaterial component is a four-point side notch bend specimen and the dimensions of the specimen are given. The notch tip radius of curvature should be the smallest radius of curvature of the implant design. The notch tip surface finishing condition should especially be examined, because not only notch radius (stress concentration) but also notch surface condition (scratch and structure sensitivity) affect the fatigue properties. The corrosion characteristics of biomaterials are also estimated by measuring the difference of the fatigue life in a laboratory air environment to that in a physiological saline solution environment. The details of the results on pure titanium, titanium alloy, and stainless steel are given.

KEYWORDS: titanium, titanium alloy, corrosion, galvanic corrosion, fatigue life

The difference between biomaterials and ordinary constructive materials is the requirement for long life of the component in the human body without any corrosion or fracture. A priority is also to minimize leaching of metal ions from the component. When we compare a door hinge subjected to sea water to an artificial joint, the door opens and closes more than 5000 times a day in the enrivonment for more than 20 years. During this period, the hinge should not corrode or wear. In addition to these characteristics, the fixation between the door and the hinge must not loosen throughout this period. Such a hinge has not yet been developed. Therefore, the mechanical properties of metallic biomaterials must be evaluated considering they will be subjected to severe environments analogous as in the hinge example.

The most important properties for metallic biomaterials are as follows:

1. minimal metal ion release reactions within human body, and
2. maintenance of mechanical strength with use.

These two requirements are closely related and affect each other. Corrosion and its effect on mechanical strength has been studied and discussed for a long time [1,2] and many kinds of

[1] Associate professor, Precision and Intelligence Laboratory, Tokyo Institute of Technology, Yokohama 227, Japan.
[2] Associate professor, Department of Orthopedic Surgery, The Jikei University, School of Medicine, Tokyo, Japan.

testing methods have been reported [1,3,4]. The methods for testing biomaterials are quite similar to methods for testing ordinary constructive materials. However, the test method to evaluate the elution of component atoms has not been clarified sufficiently.

In this paper, some methods for evaluating the properties of biomaterials are proposed and discussed.

Evaluation of the Component Atoms Elution—Corrosion

This property is the most important basic requirement for metallic biomaterials and is strongly related, not only to the mechanical properties, but also to the elution of component atoms of the material made by corrosion occurring in the human body. The corrosive properties are usually examined by measuring the anodic polarization curve [5,6]. However, the corrosive properties of biomaterials are rather different from the corrosion characteristics of other structural materials. The surfaces of biomaterials must be covered by a very strong and stable passive film that should not be damaged under static conditions. Therefore, the elution of component atoms is considered to occur when the material comes into contact with other materials (Galvanic corrosion), or when the surface is damaged by scratching or plastic deformation, or when both of these instances occur.

Galvanic corrosion is considered not to occur in pairs of materials, such as stainless steel, titanium, titanium alloys, and cobalt chromium alloys where the surface is covered by strong and stable passive films in a human body environment. However, very small amounts of the total metallic composition elute into the environment [7]. The elution is very important for the human body because the usage of biomaterials requires that an inserted implant can remain in the human body for more than 20 years. During this period, the eluted metallic ions are thought to be diffuse and to have little effect on the body as the amount is very small. However, even if the corrosion is incredibly slow, the corrosion is thought to be cumulative and may damage the strength of the biomaterial component over time. The corrosion is named Galvanic pico-corrosion because of the very small amount of elution. Therefore, it is important that the corrosive properties of the materials are known thoroughly.

The simple evaluation method of determining elution has been proposed by Roppongi et al. [7]. The specimen for evaluating the pico-corrosion properties consists of two pieces as shown in Fig. 1. Specimen A inserts into the hole of Specimen B. The specimen component pairs are immobilized and immersed in 250 mL of a physiological saline solution at 30°C for

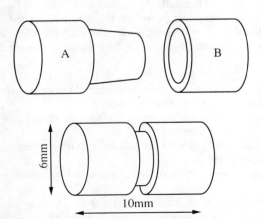

FIG. 1—*Specimen dimensions for examining elution (Galvanic pico-corrosion and crevice corrosion).*

TABLE 1—*Results of atomic absorption analysis.*

| | (Al, Ni, Cr, Mo, V, Ti, Co, Zr, Fe) (μg/100mL) | | | | |
A-B Pair	Co-Cr	316L	Ti	Ti-6Al-4V	Ti-5Al-2.5Mo-4Zr
Co-Cr	N				
316L	Fe; 3	Fe; 4			
		Ni; 2			
Ti	Co; 4	Fe; 7	N		
Ti-6Al-4V	N	Fe; 4	N	N	
Ti-5Al-2.5Mo-4Zr	N	N	Fe; 1	N	N

six months. The chemical composition of the solution is precisely analyzed by atomic absorption spectrochemical analysis (Jarell-Ash analyzer was used). When both materials A and B are the same, crevice corrosion may also be examined. When each material is different, the specimen may be used not only to examine galvanic pico-corrosion but also crevice corrosion. Therefore, the environment should be motionless because the occurrence of crevice corrosion is a function of diffusion [5] and is sometimes delayed by shaking or stirring. The Galvanic pico-corrosion test was performed between a Co-Cr alloy (supplied by Tainaka Mining Co.), 316L stainless steel (supplied by Nippon Stainless Co.), pure titanium (Ti), Ti-6Al-4VELI (supplied by Sumitomo Metal Industry), and Ti-5Al-2.5Mo-4Zr alloy (supplied by NKK Corporation). As shown in the results in Table 1 [8], the pair of pure titanium and Co-Cr alloy elute 4 μg/100mL of cobalt atoms show that all pairs except for Ti-5Al-2.5-Mo-4Zr alloy with stainless steel elute 4 to 7 μg/100mL of iron or nickel, or both.

The corrosion characteristics of biomaterials are also possible to estimate by measuring the difference of the fatigue life in a laboratory air environment and in a physiological saline solution environment as discussed in the next section.

Evaluation of Mechanical Properties

The mechanical properties required are not only a higher tensile strength and fracture toughness, but also good fatigue properties and wear resistance. The methods of evaluating these mechanical properties are essentially the same as those adopted for ordinary constructive materials, except for the environment. However, the method adopted for biomaterials must also consider the eventual usage of the materials. For example, the method to evaluate the mechanical properties of materials employed for the artificial joint must consider the following conditions:

1. stress concentrations that are caused by the design of the joint, namely the groove on the surface and the radius of curvature at the corners.
2. the effect of scratching and surface damage that are introduced during surgical operation and handling by scalpel or hammer.
3. the effect of surface finishing such as polishing, porous coating, atom implantation, ceramic coatings, and others.
4. the effect of Galvanic pico-corrosion which is caused by different component materials.

The monotomic test methods, such as the tensile and fracture toughness test for ordinary constructive materials, have been well established and there is no difference between these methods used for biomaterials or constructive materials. However, the fatigue test method is rather different and must be considered under these conditions. The implant cannot be repaired once it is inserted into the human body. Therefore, the implant must not crack or fracture while in the human body. Thus the most important fatigue property of biomaterials is the fatigue life.

Fatigue Tests and Specimen

The components for implants are usually used under bending stress conditions, where the maximum stress is loaded at the corner or at the groove on the surface. Therefore, the appropriate fatigue test specimen for the biomaterial component is a four-point side notch bend specimen. Effects of stress concentration on fatigue life of stainless steel (S316) and titanium alloy (T130 and T318) in NaCl solution is not the same as in laboratory air environment. High cycle fatigue life decreases $\frac{1}{10}$ or shorter in NaCl solution than in air. Therefore, the notch tip radius of curvature is the smallest radius of curvature of the implant design. This allows the finishing condition of notch surface to be the same condition as the actual implant surface, because not only the notch radius but also the surface flow and metallurgical structure effect fatigue life. This surface layer is very important on fatigue behavior of Ti-6Al-4V. Only a small amount of pre-cyclic deformation decreases more than $\frac{1}{10}$ of the fatigue life without pre-cyclic deformation [9]. Figure 2 shows an example of a four-point side notch bend specimen

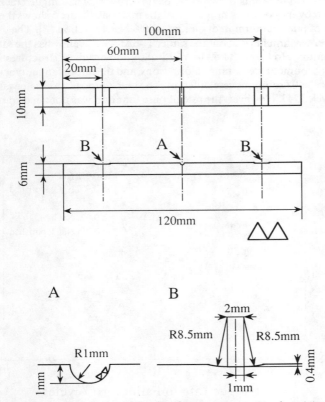

FIG. 2—*The dimensions of the four-point bending fatigue specimen. Notch tip (A) and loading point of notch side (B) are also precisely shown in A and B, respectively.*

employed to evaluate materials used for an artificial hip joint. The notch tip radius of curvature is 1 mm due to the design of the artificial hip joints. The effect of surface finishing is also examined by changing the finished condition of the notch tip. To examine the effect of galvanic pico-corrosion on the fatigue life, other materials may be fixed on the end surface of the specimen or the loading pin may be used. It must be noted that the specimen should be insulated electrically from other materials (loading pins or jig) to avoid the effect of galvanic corrosion. Therefore, ceramic loading pins are recommended for use.

Results

Effect of Environment—Figure 3 shows the typical results of fatigue life (S-N curve) of Ti-5Al-3Mo-4Zr (open symbols) and Ti-6Al-4VELI (solid symbols) alloys in air (square symbols) and in 0.9% NaCl solution (triangle symbols) using the four-point bending specimens shown in Fig. 2. There is only a small difference between the test environments on both materials. The results suggest that these titanium alloys have a good corrosion resistance. On the contrary, the results of fatigue life of 316L stainless steel are different. The fatigue life in air is comparable to that of titanium alloys in a high cycle fatigue range. However, the life of stainless steel in 0.9% NaCl solution is shorter than that in air (Fig. 4) because the passive films on the stainless steel are not stable in the environment containing chloride ions. These results are in the same tendency as the results of Galvanic pico-corrosion. The fatigue crack propagation rate is also affected by the corrosive properties of the material. Figure 5 shows the fatigue crack propagation rate of pure titanium in dry air and 0.9% NaCl solution [8]. The crack propagation rate in both environments is about the same. Ti-6Al-4VELI alloy has the same properties as the pure titanium. However, Ti-6Al-4VELI alloy for ordinary structures is very much affected by the environment containing chloride ions, and the rate of fatigue crack propagation in air and in 3.5% NaCl solution were different. The crack propagation rate was also affected by the loading cycle [11]. However, the rate of pure titanium was not affected by the loading

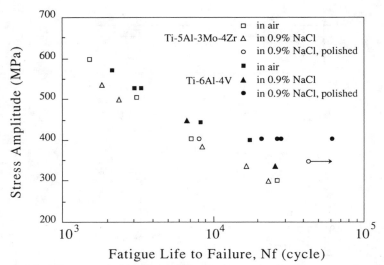

FIG. 3—*Results of four-point bending fatigue life, N_f, of titanium alloys in air and in 0.9% NaCl solution. The notch tip surface conditions of specimens were as-machined and polished.*

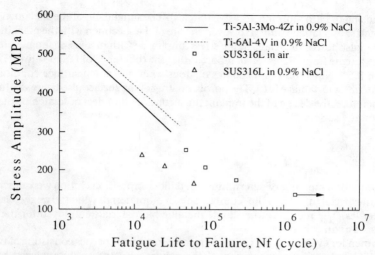

FIG. 4—*Comparison of the fatigue life, N_f, of 316L stainless steel, and titanium alloys in air and 0.9% NaCl solution.*

cycle [8]. Thus, the fatigue life (also fatigue crack propagation rate) clearly reflects the effect of environment and suggests the corrosion resistivity of the materials. Therefore, comparing the fatigue life in air and in 0.9% NaCl solution or a physiological saline solution is a very good evaluation method of biomaterials, not only for examining mechanical properties but also for resistivity of corrosion in the human body.

Effects of Surface Finishing—Figure 3 also demonstrates the effect of surface finishing on fatigue life in 0.9% NaCl solution. The finishing of the notch tip of specimens was machined

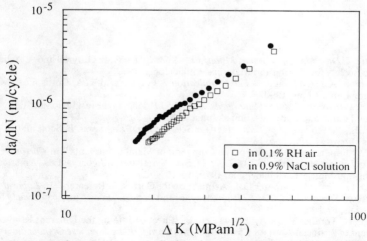

FIG. 5—*Fatigue crack propagation rate, da/dN, of titanium in air and in 0.9% NaCl as a function of stress intensity range, ΔK.*

or polished using 0.3 μm alumina abrasive (circles). The fatigue life of the specimen with the polished notch shows fatigue limit. However, the life of the specimen with the machined notch of both materials showed decreases in the stress amplitude with increasing fatigue life and did not show the fatigue limit. Peters et al. reported that the difference of fatigue life of Ti-6Al-4V in air and in 3.5% NaCl solution becomes obvious when the notch surface condition is not appropriate to fatigue damage [10]. The porous coating of the surface also decreases the fatigue life [12]. Therefore, the design of the implant must consider the effect of scratching or finishing conditions on the surface.

Conclusions

Simple evaluation methods of determining metallic composition elution were described and proposed with special interest in the requirements of biomaterials which strongly relate to corrosive properties. The methods to evaluate metallic biomaterials employed for the artificial joint were used as an example.

The specimen for evaluating the Galvanic pico-corrosion properties consisting of two pieces was shown. The chemical composition of the solution was precisely analyzed by atomic absorption spectrochemical analysis. When both materials A and B are the same, crevice corrosion may be examined also. The test was performed between a Co-Cr alloy, 316L stainless steel, pure titanium, Ti-6Al-4VELI, and Ti-5Al-2.5Mo-4Zr alloy. The pairs of pure titanium and Co-Cr alloy elute 4 μg/100mL of cobalt atoms and all pairs except for Ti-5Al-2.5Mo-4Zr alloy with stainless steel elute 4 to 7 μg/100mL of iron or nickel, or both.

The appropriate fatigue test specimen for the biomaterial component is a four-point side notch bend specimen and the dimensions of the specimen are given. The notch tip radius of curvature should be the smallest radius of curvature of the implant design. The notch tip surface finishing condition should be examined, not only for the notch radius (e.g., stress concentration), but also for the fine scratch and metallic fine structure of the notch tip surface effect on the fatigue properties. The corrosion characteristics of biomaterials are also estimated by measuring the difference of the fatigue life in a laboratory air environment to that in a physiological saline solution environment.

References

[1] *Corrosion and Degradation of Impact Materials, ASTM STP 684*, B. C. Syrett and A. Acharya, Eds., American Society for Testing and Materials, Philadelphia, 1979.

[2] "Environment Assisted Fatigue," *EGF Publication 7*, P. Scott and R. A. Cottis, Eds., Mechanical Engineering Publications, 1990.

[3] *Laboratory Corrosion Tests and Standards, ASTM STP 866*, Haynes and Baboian, Eds., American Society for Testing and Materials, Philadelphia, 1983.

[4] Mattsson, E., *Basic Corrosion Technology for Scientists and Engineers*, P. Scott and R. A. Cottis, Eds., Ellis Horwood, 1989, pp. 15–28.

[5] Kruger, J., "Fundamental Aspects of the Corrosion of Metallic Implants," in *Corrosion and Degradation of Impact Materials, ASTM STP 684*, B. C. Syrett and A. Acharya, Eds., American Society for Testing and Materials, Philadelphia, 1979, pp. 107–127.

[6] Tipton, D. G., "Micro-computer Data Acquisition for Corrosion Research," in *Laboratory Corrosion Tests and Standards, ASTM STP 866*, Haynes and Baboian, Eds., American Society for Testing and Materials, Philadelphia, 1983, pp. 24–35.

[7] Roppongi, T., Tomita, Y., Sugiyama, H., et al., "Effect of Joining the Different Kind of Metallic Component of Artificial Joint on Corrosion," *The Journal of the Japanese Orthopedic Association*, Vol. 64, 1990, p. S1279 (in Japanese).

[8] Shimojo, M., Higo, Y., and Nunomura, S., "Relation Between the Amount of Fresh Bare Surface at the Crack Tip and the Fatigue Crack Propagation Rate," *ISIJ International,* Vol. 31, 1991, pp. 870–874.

[9] Takemoto, T., Jing, K., Sakalakos, T., et al., "The Importance of Surface Layer on Fatigue Behavior of Ti-6Al-4V Alloy," *Metallurgical Transactions A,* Vol. 14, 1983, pp. 127–132.

[10] Peters, M., Gysler, A., and Lutjering, G., "Influence of Texture on Fatigue Properties on Ti-6Al-4V." *Metallurgical Transactions,* Vol. 15, 1984, pp. 1597–1605.

[11] Ryder, J. T., Krupp, W. E., Pettit, D. E., and Hoeppner, D. W., "Corrosion-Fatigue Properties of Recrystallization Annealed Ti-6Al-4V," in *Corrosion-Fatigue Technology, ASTM STP 642,* American Society for Testing and Materials, Philadelphia, 1978, pp. 202–222.

[12] Cook, S. D., Georgette, F. S., Skinner, H. B. and Haddad, R. J. Jr., "Fatigue Properties of Carbon- and Porous-coated Ti-6Al-4V Alloy," *Journal of Biomedical Materials Research,* Vol. 18, 1984, pp. 497–512.

C. A. C. Flemming,[1] *S. A. Brown,*[1] *and J. H. Payer*[2]

Mechanical Testing for Fretting Corrosion of Modular Total Hip Tapers

REFERENCE: Flemming, C. A. C., Brown, S. A., and Payer, J. H., **"Mechanical Testing for Fretting Corrosion of Modular Total Hip Tapers,"** *Biomaterials' Mechanical Properties, ASTM STP 1173,* H. E. Kambic and A. T. Yokobori, Jr., Eds., American Society for Testing and Materials, Philadelphia, 1994, pp. 156–166.

ABSTRACT: A recent advancement in the design of the total artificial hip is the introduction of modularity. Within the last year clinical retrievals have shown that significant corrosion can occur at the cone-taper interface in some variations of the modular hip. The hypothesis of this study was that the stability of the cone-taper interface affects the amount of fretting corrosion that occurs. The development of a method that can study the taper corrosion and determine the most stable design is therefore necessary.

Design characteristics that may affect corrosion include the use of dissimilar metals, taper angle, taper diameter, percent coverage, machining tolerance, and head neck extension. The fretting that occurred at the interface was initially studied by measuring potential changes while cyclically loading hips in a universal testing machine. This method of measurement proved ineffective at isolating the fretting at the taper interface so current changes were monitored instead. The current was measured when the saline was below the crevice and when it was just above the crevice, and the two measurements were subtracted from each other to produce the taper fretting current.

When comparing two different designs, one showed a significant taper fretting current while the other's was minimal. In a second study, when comparing two different head neck extensions placed on identical stem designs, a significant taper fretting current was seen with the +10-mm head as compared to a +0-mm head. It is concluded that this method can be used in the evaluation of designs to optimize stability and reduce the resulting fretting corrosion.

KEYWORDS: corrosion, fretting, modular hip, orthopaedics, titanium, cobalt-chrome, taper current, neck extension

The modular hip is one of the most recent advancements in the design of the total artificial hip. The design allows a surgeon to choose from a variety of femoral heads and stems in order to provide a patient with the best fit, while reducing the hospital's inventory and thereby reducing costs. From a materials standpoint, the design allows the optimal material to be chosen for each part of the hip according to the function that part fulfills. Within the last year, however, clinical retrievals have shown that there are specific corrosion problems related to the design of the modular hip. Alloys that were thought to be unsusceptible to corrosion have shown severe damage, and the need for a better understanding of the cone-taper interface has become apparent. Several characteristics of the design may lead to the resulting corrosion such as dissimilar metal combinations, taper angle, taper diameter, percent coverage, tolerances, and the use of different head neck extensions.

[1] Department of Biomedical Engineering and [2]Department of Material Science and Engineering, Case Western Reserve University, Cleveland, OH 44106.

The design of the modular hip presents three possible corrosion problems: crevice corrosion, galvanic corrosion, and fretting corrosion. Crevice corrosion is defined by Fontana [1] as an intense localized corrosion that takes place in narrow interfaces where liquid is present. The corrosion takes place in four steps: (1) General uniform corrosion takes place over the entire surface; (2) Metal ions are released inside the crevice leading to a reduction of oxygen, and eventually the oxygen is depleted because the crevice restricts oxygen convection; (3) In order to balance the positive metal ions that are still being produced, chloride ions begin to migrate into the crevice. The formation of metal hydroxide also results in a decrease in pH which accelerates the corrosion of the metal; and (4) As the corrosion in the crevice increases, the rest of the surface becomes cathodically protected, and the corrosion is localized [1]. Examination of the clinical retrievals has shown that fluid is present between the cone and taper.

Galvanic corrosion occurs from the use of dissimilar metals with differences in electrochemical potentials. The materials used in the modular hip are cobalt-chrome F75 and F799 (CoCr) and titanium F136 (Ti64). There has been much research on the use of these materials in the body and on their use in mixed metal combinations. Most of the research indicates that there is no increase in corrosion, but some suggest caution when using CoCr and Ti64. A slight tarnish formed on Ti64 and there was an increased fibrous capsule thickness when combined with CoCr *in vivo,* suggesting some corrosive activity [2]. Levine and Staehle [3] saw that this mixed metal combination could lead to an increased corrosion rate. Finally, the failure of a vitallium nailplate in a clinical environment was attributed to the combination of dissimilar types of vitallium; the nail was cast vitallium and the plate was wrought [4].

One must also consider the many studies which conclude that using CoCr and Ti64 together is acceptable. Kummer and Rose [5] saw that CoCr and Ti64 led to a stable passive layer and a decreasing corrosion current. Other electrochemical analyses have also shown that the coupling of the two did not lead to increased corrosion behavior [6,7], and that the corrosion resistance of wrought and cast CoCr were similar [8]. All of these studies concluded that the problem of dissimilar metals needed to be approached with caution, and a blanket statement on the galvanic corrosion of CoCr and Ti64 may not necessarily be true.

The final type of corrosion that may be occurring in the modular hip is fretting corrosion. As defined in ASTM F 897, Practice for Measuring Fretting Corrosion of Osteosynthesis Plates and Screws, fretting corrosion results from relative micromotion between the two components, and the rate of corrosion depends on load, frequency, materials, surface treatments, and environmental factors. This mechanical motion breaks the passive oxide layer that protects these metals, and the repassivation which then occurs can lead to a depletion in the oxygen concentration, thus setting up a crevice cell. Brown and Simpson stated that, "If the oxygen in solution in the contact area is consumed in the attempts to repassivate after each mechanical disruption of the passive film by fretting, then the metal can no longer repassivate and can freely corrode in the area which is by nature a crevice" [9]. They also showed that fretting can be measured using potential monitoring. As the passive layer is broken the potential decreases, and once the motion stops the potential immediately begins to increase.

Instead of potential measurements, corrosion rates can also be measured by monitoring current changes. Current monitoring has been used in the area of crevice corrosion, but has not been used for measuring fretting corrosion. Yao et al. [10] showed that the currents measured would be very small until crevice corrosion began at which point the current would increase to a plateau. Changes in the environment also led to changes to in the currents measured.

Three studies have specifically examined the corrosion of the modular hip and suggested possible mechanisms. First, Mathiesen et al. [11,12] studied nine cast CoCr Lord prostheses. In four cases, there was severe corrosion at the interface of the two components, and major amounts of corrosion products were released into the body possibly triggering an inflammatory response. At removal, black deposits were seen at the interface between the head and neck, and in one case these deposits showed up as a radiopaque shadow in the X rays. They concluded that the crevice corrosion that occurred had been facilitated by structural imperfections rather than fretting since no marks or scratches were present, and all of the heads were firmly fixed on the tapers.

An implant retrieval study by Collier et al. [13] showed corrosion in 56.6% of the mixed-metal hips studied, but they reported no incidences of corrosion in cases where similar metals were used. Corrosion was defined as the loss of material or the elimination of machining marks, or both, on the taper. The mechanism of corrosion was thought to be crevice corrosion which had an important galvanic contribution, and fretting was not considered a factor. They also concluded that the use of fiber mesh pads for increased fixation may lead to an unfavorable area effect which would increase the galvanic corrosion.

Finally, Fricker and Shivanath [14] studied several material combinations to determine if they would be affected by long-term fretting damage. They cyclically compressed the cone and tapers for one-hour periods in deaerated Ringer's solution. Visual and SEM inspection showed no signs of the start of fretting corrosion during these short-term tests, so they concluded that there should be no occurrence of long-term *in vivo* fretting corrosion.

Based on the examination of clinical retrievals from a study with the University Hospitals of Cleveland and the Cleveland Clinic [15], the hypothesis of this study has been that the corrosion begins with a fretting component which then leads to accelerated crevice corrosion, as described by Brown and Simpson [9]. The retrievals from this study were evaluated and scored on a scale of 1 to 8, with 8 indicating severe corrosion. In an extreme case, severe dendrites were seen in the cone-taper crevice after being implanted for only 44 months. Although corrosion was seen more frequently in the case of dissimilar metals, there were some CoCr-CoCr combinations that showed corrosion.

The purpose of this project was to develop a mechanical test method to study the fretting corrosion at the interface of the cone and taper and to validate that method. The project used both potential and current measurements to study the taper interface and showed that current monitoring was the best technique for examining this corrosion problem. Several tests were done to better understand this method, and finally, the method was used to study the contribution of neck extensions to the resulting corrosion.

Methods

The first approach in this study was to measure the potentials with a calomel reference electrode while cyclically loading the hip. The modular hip was mounted in PMMA, inverted and immersed in 0.9% saline, and placed in a mechanical testing machine (SCOTT) to be cyclically loaded between 0 N and 2000 N at a frequency of about 0.60 Hz. While mounting the hips, the alignment of the hips was determined visually to produce an axis of loading that was approximately vertical. An UHMWPE acetabular cup was used as the bearing surface during these tests. In order to separate the fretting at the cone and taper from that at the bearing surface, two methods were used: (1) taking the water level below the crevice, and (2) sealing the crevice with a glue gun or silicone caulk. Two stems which had been previously implanted, but showed minimal damage, were used during these tests, X1 + 5 and Y1 − 5.

Throughout this project, each stem was identified by a three part alpha-numeric code. The first letter indicated the manufacturer of the stem; these letters were chosen arbitrarily. The next number told which hip by that manufacturer was used, and the final number indicated the size of the head-neck extension used. All of the hips studied had a Ti64 stem and a CoCr head, except for T1 + 10 which was a CoCr-CoCr combination.

Potential measurements, however, proved to be insufficient because the specimen was not completely immersed in the saline. When the water level was changed, the potentials measured were significantly affected. Sealing the crevice also did not work because the seal was unable to withstand repeated loading, and there was no way to tell if it was defective. These problems led the use of current monitoring in order to measure the fretting.

The setup used for the current measurements is seen in Fig. 1. A separate total hip, or a sheet of commercially pure titanium (CPTi) was placed in the saline to act as an external cathode. A zero-resistance ammeter (Keithley 617) was then connected between the external cathode and the hip which was being loaded. The water level was adjusted to just above or just below the crevice to determine differences in the spontaneous current that was produced. The area of the external cathode was kept the same at both water levels. Because of the large external cathode, the current measurements were not affected by the small change in surface area on the loaded hip caused by adjusting the water level. To determine the taper fretting current, the current-time graphs were digitized, and the current just below the crevice was subtracted from the current produced just above the crevice. In order to reduce the fretting occurring at the bearing surface, an O-ring was used instead of the UHMWPE acetabular cup. This change significantly reduced the current below the crevice, and allowed the fretting at the cone and taper to be isolated and differences between different hips or designs to be detected.

In order to better understand using current to measure fretting, a series of tests was done to determine the effects of the size of the external cathode on the measured currents. In these tests, five different cathode sizes made from sheet CPTi were used: 372, 320, 240, 160, and 80 cm^2. Stem X1 + 5 was used in these tests, and the water level was kept above the crevice the entire time, allowing both potential and current to be monitored. The surface area of the hip was also measured to compare this area with the surface areas used for the external cathode. The area

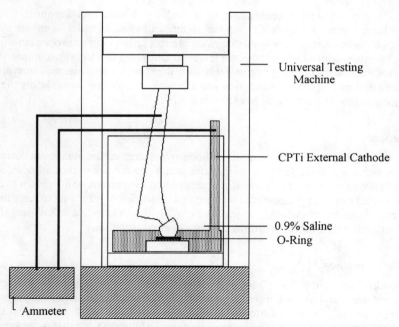

FIG. 1—*Setup for current measurements with a CPTi sheet as an external cathode and a zero-resistance ammeter. Instead of an UHMWPE cup, an O-ring was used as the bearing surface in order to reduce this fretting component. This setup allowed the cone and taper fretting to be isolated.*

of the porous pads was multiplied by 3 to take into account the increased surface area they provide.

After determining that current monitoring was a feasible method for studying fretting, the effect of head-neck extension was examined. Two identical stems, which had never been implanted or exposed to a corrosive environment, were used. Stem W1 was used to test the +0-mm (short) extension. The hip was repeatedly tested for 12-min periods at a frequency of 0.33 Hz, and the 372 cm^2 titanium sheet was used as the external cathode. The taper did not receive any special cleaning or preparation before testing was done which resulted in the hip requiring a period of time to adjust to the environment. Stem W2 was used to test the +10-mm (long) neck extension. Before testing, the crevice was passivated with 20% HNO$_3$ acid for 30 min, rinsed with water and ethanol, and dried. This pretreatment seemed to eliminate the adjustment period which had been seen with stem W1. Five 12-min tests were run above the crevice and below the crevice at a frequency of 0.5 Hz.

Results

Cone Taper Differences

Current monitoring produced a cyclic pattern which coincided with the loading. When testing stem X1 + 5, clear differences could be seen between the currents measured while the water level was above and below the crevice. The currents measured were in the μA range. The maximum current initially increased with time before reaching a plateau, and the minimum current did not return to zero between cycles when above the crevice. With stem Y1 − 5, the currents with the saline above and below the crevice were identical which would indicate less fretting. The above and below currents for both stem X1 + 5 and stem Y1 − 5 were then subtracted to produce a taper fretting current. Stem X1 + 5 had a very definite taper current, while the taper current for stem Y1 − 5 was significantly less. In order to ensure that these differences in taper current were from design differences rather than improper mounting, the fretting currents produced when the water level was below the crevice were compared. These showed that the fretting of the O-ring was relatively the same for both stems. Therefore, it was determined that using current monitoring was a feasible method for investigating the fretting of the modular hip, and needed to be explored further.

Cathode Size

In the cathode surface area tests, as the cathode area decreased the maximum current measured also decreased similarly to that of galvanic attack. As the size of the cathode decreased, the drop in potential increased. It was also observed that the current would return to a resting value in 5 to 30 min, but the potential took several hours before returning to a resting value. The estimated surface area of stem X1 was 88.2 cm^2 which would indicate that using the larger external cathode magnified the currents seen in a normal situation.

Head-Neck Extension

The results from stem W2 + 10 are seen in Figs. 2 and 3. Figure 2 shows the load cycle and the currents above and below the crevice, and Fig. 3 shows the taper current that is produced. The curves show a biphasic nature which indicates that there was a mechanical stick-slip behavior occurring at the taper. The currents increased whenever there was movement occurring which again supported fretting. In this test the taper current ranged from 3.49 to 10.22 μA.

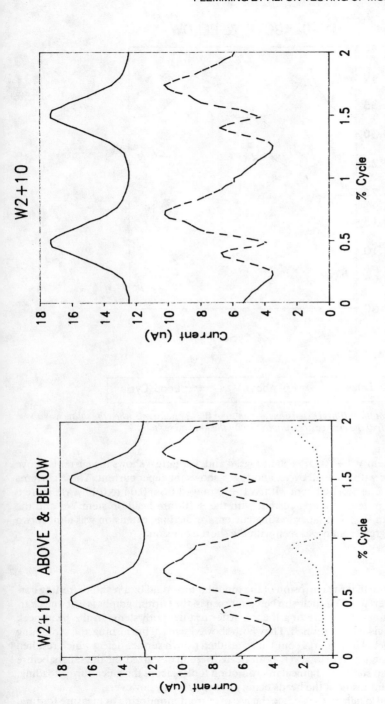

FIG. 3—*The taper fretting current (dashed) for the +10-mm extension tests on stem W2 is compared to the load cycle (solid). The currents range from 3.49 to 10.22 µA. The current is a biphasic wave which increases when there is movement occurring.*

FIG. 2—*The results for the +10-mm extension tests on stem W2. The currents when the saline was above (dashed) and below (dotted) the crevice are compared with the load cycle (solid).*

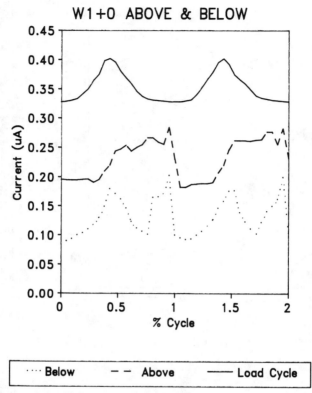

FIG. 4—*The results for the +0-mm extension tests on stem W1. The currents when the saline was above (dashed) and below (dotted) the crevice are compared with the load cycle (solid).*

The results from stem W1 + 0 are seen in Figs. 4 and 5. Figure 4 shows the currents above and below the crevice with the load cycle, and Fig. 5 shows the taper current. These currents are significantly less. The taper current with W1 + 0 ranged from 0.04 to 0.17 μA. Figure 6 shows the difference in taper fretting current with the +10-mm head on stem W2 and the +0-mm head on stem W1. The taper fretting current for the long extension was almost two orders of magnitude greater than was seen with the short extension.

Discussion

These results indicate that the corrosion of the modular hip could be a result of fretting corrosion at the taper interface. The stick-slip behavior seen in the current graphs is just one characteristic seen that supports the fretting theory. After testing, both stems in the head-neck extension study were visually examined. They both showed signs of burnishing and scratching halfway down the taper. These marks could have resulted from a surface defect which resulted in point loading of the tapers. However, both heads were firmly fixed on the tapers before removal indicating that some mechanical micromotion took place at the taper during loading. This movement did not result in the heads being physically loose, however.

Other results have also helped to validate the use of current monitoring to measure fretting.

First, fretting is dependent on the loading frequency, and tests showed that as the loading frequency was increased, the current measured also increased. The small difference in the frequencies used between stem W1 + 0 and stem W2 +10, however, would not account for the large difference in the currents measured. Second, the magnitude of the current has also been shown to be load dependent, another sign of fretting. In one case, while cyclically loading the hip between 0 and 100 N, the same cyclic patterns were observed, but they were at least one order of magnitude less than when loading the hip to 2000 N.

When considering design differences, some of the possible reasons for less fretting with stem Y1 − 5 as compared to X1 + 5 could be: (1) the head has a −5-mm neck extension compared to the +5-mm extension on stem X1; (2) the taper angle of stem Y1 − 5 is half that of stem X1 + 5; and (3) the taper diameter of X1 + 5 was smaller than that of Y1 − 5. Further tests on another stem, T1, with a +10-mm extension produced results similar to stem Y1 − 5, and T1 + 10 had a taper angle similar to Y1 − 5. This indicates that the taper angle could have more of an effect on the fretting corrosion than the head-neck extension. A smaller taper diam-

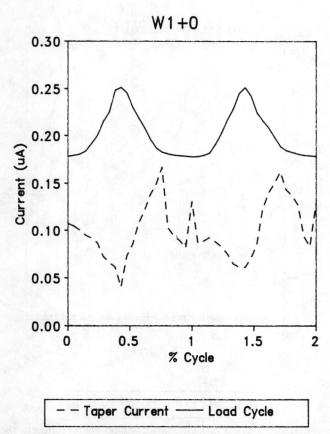

FIG. 5—*The taper fretting current (dashed) for the +0-mm extension on stem W1 is compared to the load cycle (solid). The currents range from 0.04 to 0.17 µA.*

eter could result in more bending of the taper during loading and more relative movement. Each of these variables needs to be studied further.

The current monitoring showed some interesting behavior in the measured currents when multiple tests were run in a single day. When the water level was above the crevice, the current at the very beginning of the first test in a day tended to rise slowly to a plateau, but in the second test the current began at a higher level and did not rise as much. This behavior was not seen when the water level was below the crevice. In this case, every test began at the low level and rose to the plateau. This result could suggest that the passive layer inside the crevice has not been completely restored between tests when the water level is above, but the fretting by the O-ring is less than the stem metal so the passive layer on the bearing surface is able to completely reform. The potential measurements from the surface area tests also suggested such a behavior.

Some of the problems encountered with using current monitoring in the head-neck extension study included "wicking" and alignment. After review it was discovered that when the below the crevice tests were done in some of the tests with W2 + 10, the area around the

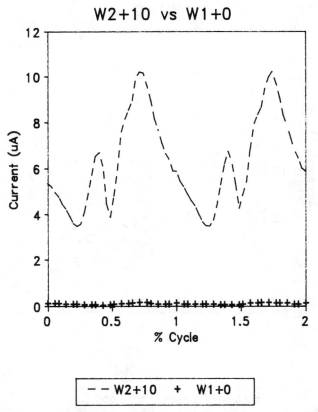

FIG. 6—*A comparison of the effects of neck extension. The taper fretting current for the +0-mm extension on stem W1 (cross-hatched) is compared with the taper fretting current for the +10-mm extension on stem W2 (dashed). The long extension's taper current is almost two orders of magnitude greater than the short extension's taper current.*

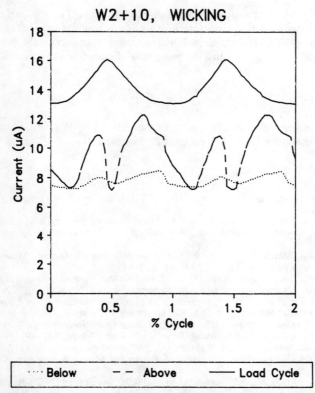

FIG. 7—*The results from stem W2 + 10 which showed "wicking." The currents when the saline was above (dashed) and below (dotted) the crevice are compared with the load cycle (solid). Because the crevice was not dry when the below the crevice test was run, an electrical pathway was present which caused the below the crevice current to be shifted higher.*

crevice had not completely dried. This allowed there to be an electrical pathway with the activity inside the crevice, and wicking occurred causing the below crevice curve to be shifted higher (Fig. 7). Therefore, the taper current would be lower than when the hip was handled carefully to ensure that no wicking occurred. Only those data in which no wicking occurred were included in the W2 + 10 results.

The alignment of the hip also was seen to have an effect on the currents measured. Some tests were done with the +0-mm extension on stem W2 which had been mounted for a +10-mm extension. This difference in alignment resulted in increased slipping, especially when the load had just been removed, which in turn resulted in spikes in the current. When compared with the results from W1 + 0, the currents were also much higher, and it was determined that using the same mounted stem to test two different extensions was not a valid option.

Conclusions

The results from this study show that there is a fretting component at the cone-taper interface which may be a factor in the corrosion that has been seen. This study also shows that current, rather than potential, is the most effective way of measuring the activity at the interface and is able to make distinctions between different designs. The study of the neck extensions showed that the +10-mm (long) neck extension is much more susceptible to fretting corrosion than the +0-mm (short) extension. The fretting currents for the two sizes were significantly different. This project is just the beginning of examining the corrosion of the modular hip.

Acknowledgments

This project was supported in part by NIH grant AR35590. We would also like to thank those companies that have given their support to this research.

References

[1] Fontana, M. G., *Corrosion Engineering: Third Edition,* McGraw-Hill Publishing Company, New York, 1986, pp. 51–9.

[2] Rostoker, W., Galante, J. O., and Lereim, P., "Evaluation of Couple/Crevice Corrosion by Prosthetic Alloys Under In Vivo Conditions,"*Journal of Biomedical Materials Research,* Vol. 12, 1978, pp. 823–29.

[3] Levine, D. L. and Staehl, R. W., "Crevice Corrosion in Orthopedic Implant Metals, *Journal of Biomedical Materials Research,* Vol. 11, 1977, pp. 553–61.

[4] Rose, R. M., Schiller, A. L., and Radin, E. L., "Corrosion-Accelerated Mechanical Failure of a Vitallium Nail-Plate," *Journal of Bone and Joint Surgery,* Vol. 54A, No. 4, June 1972, pp. 854–62.

[5] Kummer, F. J. and Rose, R. M., "Corrosion of Titanium/Cobalt-Chromium Alloy Couples," *Journal of Bone and Joint Surgery,* Vol. 65A, No. 8, October 1983, pp. 1125–6.

[6] Rostoker, W., Pretzel, C. W., and Galante, J. O., "Couple Corrosion Among Alloys for Skeletal Prostheses," *Journal of Biomedical Materials Research,* Vol. 8, 1974, pp. 407–19.

[7] Lucas, L. C., Buchanan, R. A., and Lemons, J. E., "Investigations on the Galvanic Corrosion of Multialloy Total Hip Prostheses," *Journal of Biomedical Materials Research,* Vol. 15, 1981, pp. 731–747.

[8] Sury, P. and Semlitsch, M., "Corrosion Behavior of Cast and Forged Cobalt-Based Alloys for Double-Alloy Joint Endoprostheses," *Journal of Biomedical Materials Research,* Vol. 12, 1978, pp. 723–41.

[9] Brown, S. A. and Simpson, J. P., "Crevice and Fretting Corrosion of Stainless-Steel Plates and Screws," *Journal of Biomedical Materials Research,* Vol. 15, 1981, pp. 867–78.

[10] Yao, L. A., Gan, F. X., Zhao, Y. X., et al., "Microelectrode Monitoring the Crevice Corrosion of Titanium," *Corrosion,* Vol. 47, No. 6, June 1991, pp. 420–3.

[11] Mathiesen, E. B., Lindgren, J. U., Blomgren, G. G. A., and Reinholt, F. P., "Corrosion of Modular Hip Prostheses," *Journal of Bone and Joint Surgery,* Vol. 73B, No. 4, July 1991, p. 569–75.

[12] Svensson, O., Mathiesen, E. B., Reinholt, F. P., and Blomgren, G., "Formation of a Fulminant Soft-Tissue Pseudotumor After Uncemented Hip Arthroplasty," *Journal of Bone and Joint Surgery,* Vol. 70A, No. 8, 1988, pp. 1238–42.

[13] Collier, J. P., Surprenant, V. A., Jensen, R. E., and Mayor, M. B., "Corrosion at the Interface of Cobalt-Alloy Heads on Titanium-Alloy Stems," *Clinical Orthopedics,* No. 271, October 1991, pp. 305–312.

[14] Fricker, D. C. and Shivanath, R., "Fretting Corrosion Studies of Universal Femoral Head Prostheses and Cone Taper Spigots,"*Biomaterials,* Vol. 11, September 1990, pp. 495–500.

[15] Bauer, T. W., Brown, S. A., Jiang, M., et al., "Corrosion in Modular Hip Stems," *Transactions of the Orthopaedic Research Society,* Vol. 17, 1992, p. 354.

Masaaki Nakamura,[1] *Shoji Takeda,*[1] *Koichi Imai,*[1] *Hiroshi Oshima,*[1]
Dai Kawahara,[1] *Hiroki Kosugi,*[1] *and Yoshiya Hashimoto*[1]

Cell-to-Materials Interaction—An Approach to Elucidate Biocompatibility of Biomaterials *In Vitro*

REFERENCE: Nakamura, M., Takeda, S., Imai, K., Oshima, H., Kawahara, D., Kosugi, H., and Hashimoto, Y., **"Cell-to-Materials Interaction—An Approach to Elucidate Biocompatibility of Biomaterials *In Vitro*,"** *Biomaterials' Mechanical Properties, ASTM STP 1173,* H. E. Kambic and A. T. Yokobori, Jr., Eds., American Society for Testing and Materials, Philadelphia, 1994, pp. 167–179.

ABSTRACT: The biomaterials used in the oro-maxillo-facial region, in particular the oral cavity, center of the region, require unique biocompatibility characteristics compared to those for other parts of the body. Cell-to-material interaction is a key approach in elucidating such aspects as biological, mechanical, and chemical compatibility of biomaterials *in vitro*. The results obtained by the *in vitro* tests under dynamic conditions mimicking the functions of this region are considered to better reflect the material's behavior *in vivo* than those obtained by the conventional, static testing methods. We have obtained data different from those obtained by the conventional methods. A simulation approach appears to be necessary to elucidate biocompatibility. Also, the measurement of the adhesive strength of cells on biomaterials is important in elucidating the cell-to-biomaterial interaction. Further refinement of methods is essential for standardization.

KEYWORDS: cell-to-material interaction, biocompatibility, biomaterials, biological safety, changes of biocompatibility, interface compatibility, dynamic extraction

Determining the interaction between cells and materials *in vitro* is a key approach in elucidating the biocompatibility of biomaterials. The present paper focuses on the study of biomaterials used in the oro-maxillo-facial region. The center of the region, the oral cavity, is a unique part of the body, the main biological functions of which are mastication, taste, respiration, speech, and emotional expression. Because it is exposed to the external environment when functioning, e.g., as in food intake, it is thereby subject to various influences, the most extreme of which is high-magnitude occlusal force, which is reported to be as great as 800 N [1]. Once the integrity of the oral cavity is damaged by disease, injury, congenital malformation, or developmental anomaly, restoration with various kinds of biomaterials is required, since the tissue restoring capacity of the region is extremely low. The biomaterials that are applied to the region must be biologically, physically, and chemically biocompatible in order to retain their functions. The investigation of cell-to-material interaction can contribute to the understanding of the biocompatibility of a biomaterial in terms of its biological safety, alteration due to its deterioration, and its interface compatibility.

---

[1] Professor, associate professor, lecturer, lecturer, instructor, graduate student, and instructor, respectively, Department of Biomaterials, Osaka Dental University, Osaka 540, Japan.

Materials and Methods

In vitro studies present advantages in terms of reproducibility, quantification, speed, simplicity, and cost over animal experiments, which have been challenged worldwide by animal rights groups and considerably restricted in recent years [2]. The three major elements in a cytotoxicity study in a tissue culture environment are the cells, medium, and material. The mode of contact between the cells and material can be direct, by extraction, or with the interposition of either dentin or agar (Fig. 1). Cytotoxicity is evaluated by assessing cell multiplication and cell function, as either cell metabolism or cell membrane permeability [3,4]. The purpose of an *in vitro* test is to detect possible biological inadequacy. First, the cells are tested after a material has been placed either directly on or within the same medium. The method is used to screen a given material for cytotoxicity. Second, cells are cultured with extracts obtained by extraction of a material in medium by static or gyrational action. This method is used to look beyond the purely localized effects of the material observed by the direct contact method, and allows us to test the material under conditions that simulate those of the region. Restorations in the oral cavity are constantly exposed to mechanical, chemical, and biological forces while fulfilling their biomechanical functions. This method is the most versatile way of examining contact between cells and material. Third, the interposition of either dentin or agar between the cells and material is a kind of *in vitro* reproduction of the conditions prevailing in tooth restoration, in which restorative materials are used to fill a cavity located above the tooth pulp. Tests under dynamic conditions, in which forceful motion is exerted upon a material during extraction, are considered interim simulation tests, while total simulation remains to be achieved. The alteration of biocompatibility due to its deterioration and its interface compatibility were examined hereunder.

The Approach to Alteration of Biocompatibility Due to Material Deterioration

As biomaterials change with time after application to the body, so does their biocompatibility, and the greater their resistance to mechanical, chemical, and biological wear, the longer will satisfactory restorations last. One way to investigate this question *in vitro* is to establish a model that totally simulates the condition of the oral environment both aseptic and septic.

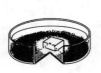
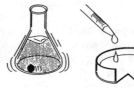

a: Direct contact method   b: Extraction method

c: Interposition of either dentin or agar method

FIG. 1—*The three methods of contact between cells and materials.*

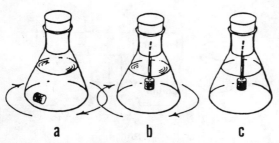

FIG. 2—*The three extraction methods:* (a) *Dynamic extraction with a freely moving specimen: To simulate the dynamic oral environment containing the inserted materials, the tightly sealed Erlenmeyer flask used to contain the specimens in minimum essential medium (MEM) is fixed in a gyrotory incubator, and dynamic extraction of the freely moving specimen is carried out at 200 r/min and 37°C. Gyration at 200 r/min exerts a dynamic load on the specimen that includes friction and collision with the vessel walls as well as extract flow.* (b) *Dynamic extraction with a suspended specimen; the specimen is suspended in the middle of the extract and gyrated at 200 r/min. Of the dynamic effects in* (a), *only the effect of the collision with the vessel walls is excluded.* (c) *Static extraction; no dynamic load is applied to a suspended specimen.*

Dynamic Extraction—Our tentative method is to extract the materials by dynamic extraction. Figure 2 shows three extraction methods of dynamic extraction with a freely moving specimen, dynamic extraction with a suspended specimen, and static extraction. In the first method, the cylindrically shaped specimen, 6.0 mm in diameter and 5.0 mm in height, is allowed to move freely; thus, the flow of extract can be expected, and the number of collisions, and the friction exerted on the specimen by the extraction vessel will also be increased. In the first dynamic extraction study, specimens of various dental amalgams, including a widely used restorative material constituted of metallic mercury and silver-tin-copper alloy at about a 1:1 ratio, were tested (Fig. 3) [6].

In our next step, we refined the method of dynamic extraction. In standard dynamic extraction, the effect on metal dissolution and cytotoxicity of specimen shape, i.e., a cylindrical, a spherical, and a square specimen, was examined. A cylindrical, a spherical, and a square specimen of Co-Cr alloy, Ni-Cr alloy, and titanium used in dental prostheses were subjected to 200 r/min gyration in an extract at 37°C for a unit period for a certain number of times [7,8]. The extracts obtained were then used for cell culture and atomic absorption spectroscopy.

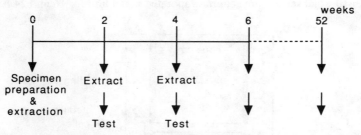

FIG. 3—*Test schedule. The specimen, 6.0 mm in diameter and 5.0 mm in height, was extracted in 15 mL of MEM in the tightly sealed 20 mL Erlenmeyer flask for a unit period of two weeks, after which the entire extract was obtained and used for cell culture. This condition, i.e., the relationship between surface area of a specimen and volume of extract, has been kept 1 cm² versus 10 mL throughout this series of experiments. The same specimen was used throughout the total testing period.*

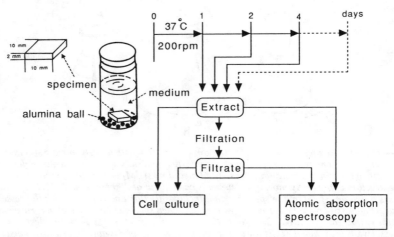

FIG. 4—*Accelerated dynamic extraction. A square specimen is placed on pure alumina balls and subsequently subjected to dynamic extraction.*

Accelerated Dynamic Extraction—In accelerated dynamic extraction, a square specimen is placed on pure alumina balls and subsequently subjected to dynamic extraction by the same method (Fig. 4) [9]. The filtrate was separated from the extract with a 0.22-μm filter. Metal dissolution in the extract and filtrate was measured by atomic absorption spectroscopy. Moreover, both noble and base alloys used for dental restorations were dissolved by the accelerated dynamic extraction method shown in Fig. 4 and the cytotoxicity of the wear debris of the alloy was examined. A definite concentration of wear debris was exposed to the L-929 cells for five days and then cell viability was measured by the neutral red method [10].

In another study, we examined the efficiency in extracting various biomaterials of three different extraction methods, i.e., static extraction at 37°C for 24 h, extraction by heating in an autoclave for 60 min, and dynamic extraction at 37°C for 24 h. Biomaterials included metals, plastics, and ceramics for medical and dental use [11,12].

The Approach to Interface Compatibility

Primary cultured cells of human dental pulp were cultivated with Medium 199 supplemented with 10% calf serum on vacuum evaporated metal film for 16 and 24 h in 5% CO_2-

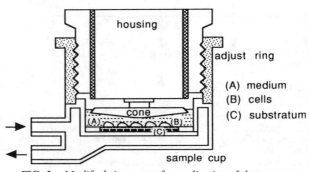

FIG. 5—*Modified viscometer for application of shear stress.*

95% air, humidified environment at 37°C, and the attachment of cells was investigated by scanning electron microscopy (SEM)[*13*].

In our next approach, we applied shear stress to cells. Production of shear stress was achieved by using a cone and disk type viscometer (Fig. 5). In this test, the cells were cultivated on a disk composed of biomaterials for a certain period and then the disk was placed at the bottom of the chamber of the apparatus while the cone was placed on top of it. After the apparatus was set up, the rotation of the cone caused the medium in the chamber to flow in one direction, thus exerting a force that detached the cells from the disk. The number of cells remaining on the disk was then measured with a photo pattern analyzer. Adhesive strength was expressed as the percent of the total number of cells on the disk remaining after application of the shear stress.

Results

The Approach to Alteration of Biocompatibility Due to Material Deterioration

Dynamic Extraction—Dental amalgams subjected to repeated dynamic extraction were found to show a wide fluctuation in cytotoxicity at various times up to 52 weeks (Fig. 6). Of five specimens tested, two showed marked wear after 52 weeks (Fig. 7) [*6*]. The results were in sharp contrast to our previous data obtained in a static environment, which had indicated diminution of cytotoxicity after 24 h following trituration [*14,15*]. Figures 8 and 9 showed the effects of specimen shape on cytotoxicity and element dissolved from Ni-Cr alloy. The cylin-

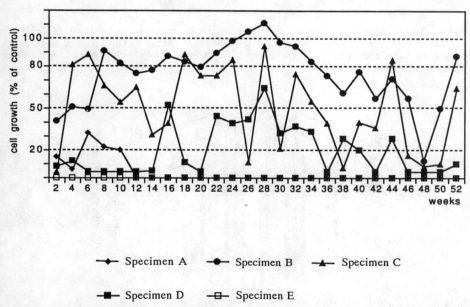

FIG. 6—*Cytotoxicity of the dental amalgams was tested. Cell growth is plotted on the ordinate and time on the abscissa. Five dental amalgams used were Specimen A (Spherical-D, 067690, non-zinc type, Shofu Co., Kyoto, Japan), Specimen B (Dispersalloy, 12 EF, Johnson & Johnson, NJ,), Specimen C (Dialloy, JW 2, non-zinc type, GC Dental Mgf. Co., Tokyo, Japan), Specimen D (Spherical, 037569, non-zinc type, Shofu Co., Kyoto, Japan), and Specimen E (Copper, OJ, Niimi Chemical Co., Kiryu, Japan) amalgams. Specimen E, copper amalgam (indicated by open squares), as a restorative has been prohibited.*

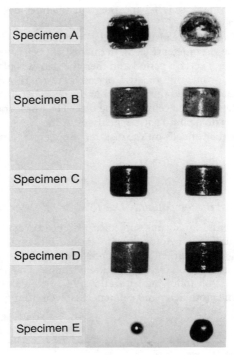

FIG. 7—*Two specimens to each kind of amalgams were shown. Wear occurred markedly in Specimens E and A during a 52-week period. Total weight loss amounted to average 86.4% of original weight of 1.5 g in Specimen E and average 11.2% loss in Specimen A. On the other hand, weight loss in others ranged only between average 1.7% to 4.4%.*

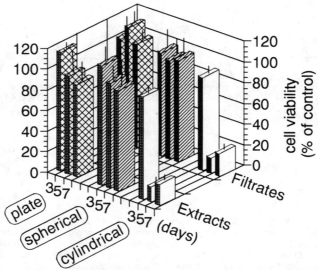

FIG. 8—*The effect on cytotoxicity of specimen shape. A cylindrical, a spherical, and a square specimen were subjected to 200 r/min gyration in an extract at 37°C for seven days.*

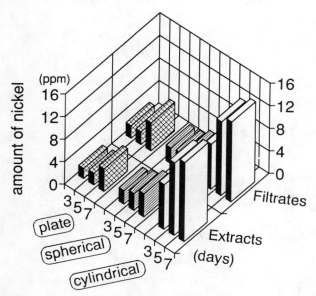

FIG. 9—*The effect of specimen shape on metal dissolution. Experimental methods were the same as in Fig. 8.*

drically shaped specimen of Ni-Cr alloy was more soluble and cytotoxic than the spherical or square specimen [7,8].

Accelerated Dynamic Extraction—Figure 10 shows the nickel dissolution from 316L stainless steel under accelerated dynamic extraction [16]. The dissolution of alloy components under an accelerated dynamic condition was greater than that under a static condition and the

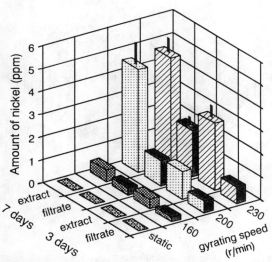

FIG. 10—*The effect of extraction condition on nickel dissolution from 316L stainless steel. The amount of nickel in the filtrate was less than that in the extract.*

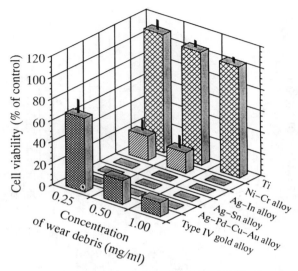

FIG. 11—*The effect of wear debris borne in MEM containing 0.4% albumin on cell viability.*

amount of nickel in the filtrate was less than that in the extract. Figure 11 shows the cytotoxicity of the wear debris borne under accelerated dynamic extraction. Wear debris of pure titanium was noncytotoxic, while that of an alloy including silver or nickel as a main component was cytotoxic [10]. As Fig. 12 shows, the dynamic extraction method surpassed the others in efficiency [11,12].

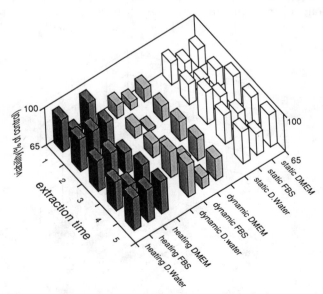

FIG. 12—*The effect on cytotoxicity of three different extraction methods, i.e., static extraction at 37°C for 24 h, extraction by heating in an autoclave for 60 min, and dynamic extraction at 37°C for 24 h.*

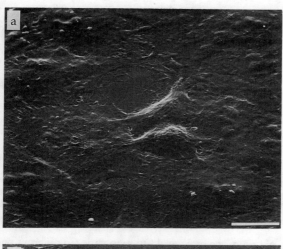

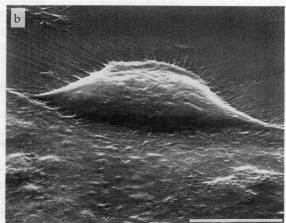

FIG. 13—*Primary cultured cells of human dental pulp were cultivated with Medium 199 supplemented with 10% calf serum on vacuum evaporated metal film for 16 to 24 h in 5% CO_2-95% air, humidified environment at 37°C. Bars: 50 μm for (a) gold and 30 μm for (b) platinum. Cells appear firmly attached to metal film. However, this observation did not provide data regarding cellular adhesive strength.*

The Approach to Interface Compatibility

Primary cultured cells of human dental pulp appeared firmly attached to metal film of gold and platinum (Fig. 13) [*13*].

The relative cell adhesion rate for the titanium alloy was identical to that for the control (Fig. 14). After application of shear stress, the number of cells remaining on the disk was reduced by 80 to 90% (Fig. 15).

Discussion

Biomaterials have been evaluated *in vitro* using conventional mechanical, chemical, and biological tests. Although a single, uniform method would be ideal, it would be difficult—if

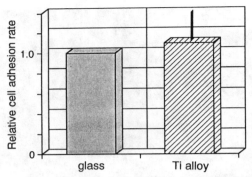

FIG. 14—*The attachment of L-929 cells to titanium alloy after a 4-h cultivation in Eagle's minimum essential medium supplemented with 5% newborn bovine serum. Relative cell adhesion rate was obtained by dividing the number of cells adhered to titanium alloy by those adhered to the glass surface.*

not impossible—to obtain, since biological function varies in different parts of the body. The study of cell-to-material interaction is considered to be valuable in the study of the combined effects of mechanical, chemical, and biological factors. This seems particularly true in regard to dental materials, the biomaterials used in the oro-maxillo-facial region which are stress bearing and subject to external influences. With respect to the topic of alteration of biocompatibility due to materials deterioration, our *in vitro* method with dynamic extraction could be a candidate for the simulation tests. However, the method has some shortcomings. First the uniformity of the surface finish may vary from one specimen shape to another, i.e., cylindrical, spherical, or plate. Second, the amount of mechanical stress is unknown. Although the load exerted on a specimen can be controlled by adjusting the speed of the gyrotory movement in the flask, i.e., revolutions per minute, it is hard to calculate the force per unit area. Third another difficulty is the differences of specific gravity among specimens composed of metal plastic, ceramic, or other substances. These differences may lead to a difference in the mechanical stress exerted on specimens during extraction. In order to offset the difference, lighter weight specimens were added with a glass tube and tissue embedding wax was added to the upper surface, both of which were not cytotoxic, and their weight was made 2.0 ± 0.1 g. The

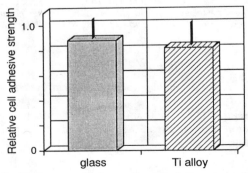

FIG. 15—*Relative cell adhesive strength after application of shear stress of 3.7 dyn/cm² for 5 min. Ce and culture condition were the same as in Fig. 14. Relative cell adhesive strength was obtained by dividing the number of cells adhered to biomaterials after application of shear stress by those before application of shear stress.*

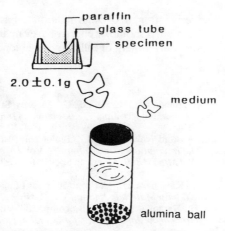

FIG. 16—*The weight of specimen, 10 × 10 mm, 1.5 mm in width, was adjusted to an even value of 2.0 ± 0.1 g by adding noncytotoxic glass tube and tissue embedding wax. Then it was put into a glass container, into which 20 mL of extract had been kept, and finally brought to dynamic extraction.*

treatment allowed the application of even stress to the specimen (Fig. 16) [*16*]. Finally, how well the load applied *in vitro* simulates real occlusal stress in the oral cavity is unknown, even though this is actually a key issue in being able to extrapolate from *in vitro* data to *in vivo* situations. Unfortunately, information is still lacking. Furthermore, it is important to standardize the methodology before the validity of the *in vitro* method can be tested.

The materials for comprehensive restorations must not only be safe with interface compatibility, i.e., adhesion, but must also be secure. This is particularly true in the case of dental restorations, since their longevity depends largely on good adhesion. Studies on cell adhesion to the substratum have been done by cell biologists and by material scientists in recent years [*17–28*].

Although the cells attached to the film appeared to differ from those in the medium, the results provided little information regarding adhesive strength, which is an important factor in the adherence of cells to biomaterials. However, our study was a preliminary step toward the quantification of adhesive strength. There have been some studies on this subject using mechanical principles such as micromanipulation [*22*], cell separation in a shear flow [*18*], and centrifugation [*14*]. The method reported in this paper is expected be effective in evaluating the relative cell adhesive strength necessary to prevent detachment of cells from the biomaterial surface. The effect of surface treatment and kinds of biomaterials in addition to the effects of shear stress and shear time all require further examination.

Conclusion

The interaction between the cell and biomaterials is important in determining the biocompatibility of materials. The present dynamic extraction approach was considered potentially useful in investigating the changes in the interaction between cells and materials over time and their relation to cytotoxicity. The method enabled the study of changes in biocompatibility due to material degradation, in particular of metallic materials, of medical devices. Degradation is an important factor in *in vitro* testing of dental materials, most of which are subject to mechanical forces such as occlusion and attrition in the oral cavity.

The measurement of the adhesive strength of cells on biomaterials is important in elucidating the cell-to-biomaterial interaction. It should be effective in evaluating the relative cell adhesive strength necessary to prevent detachment of cells from the biomaterial surface.

References

[1] *Restorative Dental Materials,* 7th ed., R. G. Craig, Ed., C.V. Mosby, St. Louis, 1985.
[2] Nakamura, M., "Dental Biocompatibility Testing," *Transactions of International Congress on Dental Materials,* 1989, pp. 180–189.
[3] Kawahara, H., Yamagami, A., and Nakamura, M., "Biological Testing of Dental Materials by Means of Tissue Culture," *The International Dental Journal,* Vol. 18, No. 2, 1968, pp. 443–467.
[4] *Cell-Culture Test Methods, ASTM STP 810,* American Society for Testing and Materials, Philadelphia, 1983.
[5] Nakamura, M., Koda, H., and Kawahara, H., "A Proposition for Long-term Biocompatibility Test of Dental Materials *in vitro,*" *Dental Materials Journal,* Vol. 2, No. 1, 1983, pp. 113–123.
[6] Nakamura, M., Kawahara, H., Kataoka, Y., et al., "Biocompatibility of Dental Amalgams *in vitro* During 52 Week Period," *Journal of the Japan Society for Dental Apparatus and Materials,* Vol. 21, No. 55, 1980, pp. 228–244.
[7] Kosugi, H., "*In vitro* Cytotoxicity Evaluation of Base Metals by Dynamic Extraction," *The Journal of the Japan Prosthodontic Society,* Vol. 36, No. 3, 1992, pp. 510–523.
[8] Takeda, S. and Nakamura, M., "The Effects of Dynamic Extractions on Cytotoxicity of Dental Alloys," *Abstracts of BIOMAT 91,* 1991, pp. 77–78.
[9] Nakamura, M., Takeda, S., Imai, K., et al., "V. A Proposal of Guideline on *in vitro* Cytotoxicity Tests of the Dental Materials," *Research Project on Biological Evaluation for Dental Materials,* A. Sato, Ed., Research Report for 1989 of the Scientific Research supported by the Ministry of Health and Welfare in Japan, 1990, pp. 48–63.
[10] Sano, Y. and Takeda, S., "Study of Cytotoxicity and Dissolution of Metallic Biomaterials Using Dynamic Extraction *(in vitro),*" *The Journal of the Osaka Odontological Society,* Vol. 55, No. 2, 1992, pp. 125–140.
[11] Oshima, H. and Nakamura, M., "Cytotoxicity Evaluation of Biomaterials by Extraction," *In Vitro,* Vol. 27, No. 3, 1991, p. 72A.
[12] Tsutsumi, N. and Oshima, H., "Cytotoxicity Evaluation of Crown and Bridge Materials by Extraction *(in vitro),*" *The Journal of the Japanese Society for Dental Materials and Devices,* Vol. 10, No. 5, 1991, pp. 555–565.
[13] Nakamura, M., Kawahara, H., Imai, K., and Kawamoto, Y., "Cell Contact to Metal Surface," *Journal of Japan Society for Dental Apparatus and Materials,* Vol. 19, No. 46, April 1978, pp. 98–111.
[14] Kawahara, H., Nakamura, M., Yamagami, A., and Nakanishi, T., "Cellular Responses to Dental Amalgam *in vitro,*" *Journal of Dental Research,* Vol. 54, No. 2, 1975, pp. 394–401.
[15] Nakamura, M. and Kawahara, H., "Cellular Responses to the Dispersion Amalgams *in vitro,*" *Journal of Dental Research,* Vol. 58, No. 8, 1979, pp. 1780–1790.
[16] Doi, H. and Takeda, S., "*In vitro* Metal Dissolution Under Various Extraction," *The Journal of the Japanese Society for Dental Materials and Devices,* Vol. 9, No. 3, 1990, pp. 375–386.
[17] Easty, G. C., Easty, D. M., and Ambrose, E. J., "Studies of Cell Adhesiveness," *Experimental Cell Research,* Vol. 19, No. 3, 1960, pp. 539–548.
[18] Weiss, L., "The Measurement of Cell Adhesion," *Experimental Cell Research Supplement,* Vol. 8, 1961, pp. 141–153.
[19] George, J. N., Weed, R. I., and Reed, C. F., "Adhesion of Human Erythrocytes to Glass: the Nature of the Interaction and the Effect of Serum and Plasma," *Journal of Cellular Physiology,* Vol. 77, No. 1, 1971, pp. 51–60.
[20] Milam, M., Grinnell, F., and Srere, P. A., "Effect of Centrifugation on Cell Adhesion," *Nature,* Vol. 244, No. 133, 1973, pp. 83–84.
[21] Mohandas, N., Hochmuth, R. M., and Spaeth, E. E., "Adhesion of Red Cells to Foreign Surfaces in the Presence of Flow," *Journal of Biomedical Materials Research,* Vol. 8, No. 2, 1974, pp. 119–136.
[22] McKeever, P. E., "Methods of Study Pulmonary Alveolar Macrophage Adherence Micromanipulation and Quantitation," *Journal of the Reticuloendothelial Society,* Vol. 16, No. 6, December 1974, pp. 313–317.
[23] Corry, W. D. and Defendi, V., "Centrifugal Assessment of Cell Adhesion," *Journal of Biochemical and Biophysical Methods,* Vol. 4, 1981, pp. 29–38.

[24] Forrester, J. V. and Lackie, J. M., "Adhesion of Neutrophil Leucocytes Under Conditions of Flow," *Journal of Cell Science*, Vol. 70, 1984, pp. 93–110.
[25] Hertl, W., Ramsey, W. S., and Nowlan, E. D., "Assessment of Cell-Substrate Adhesion by a Centrifugal Method," *In Vitro*, Vol. 20, No. 10, October 1984, pp. 796–801.
[26] Kawahara, H., Maeda, T., Iseki, T., and Sànchez, A., "Studies on Cell Adhesion to Biomaterials by Viscometric Method, *in vitro*, 2. Adhesive Strength of Cells to Glass Surface," *Journal of Japanese Society for Biomaterials*, Vol. 2, No. 3, August 1984, pp. 187–192.
[27] Shiga, T., Sekiya, M., Maeda, N., and Oka, S., "Statistical Determination of Red Cell Adhesion to Material Surface, by Varying Shear Force," *Journal of Colloid and Interface Science*, Vol. 107, No. 1, September 1985, pp. 194–198.
[28] Francis, G. W., Fisher, L. R., and Gamble, R. A., "Direct Measurement of Cell Detachment Force on Single Cells Using a New Electromechanical Method," *Journal of Cell Science*, Vol. 87, 1987, pp. 519–523.

Nathaniel J. Stewart,[1] Takeshi Muneta,[2] Jack Lewis,[1]* Conrad Lindquist,[1] and Elizabeth Arendt[1]

Mechanical Evaluation of Soft Tissue and Ligament Implant Fixation Devices

REFERENCE: Stewart, N. J., Muneta, T., Lewis, J., Lindquist, C., and Arendt, E., **"Mechanical Evaluation of Soft Tissue and Ligament Implant Fixation Devices,"** *Biomaterials' Mechanical Properties, ASTM STP 1173*, H. E. Kambic and A. T. Yokobori, Jr., Eds., American Society for Testing and Materials, Philadelphia, 1994, pp. 180–190.

ABSTRACT: The purpose of this study was to define a new mechanical measure of soft tissue fixation device performance and to use the method to assess the fixation performance of three fixation systems. The commonly used screw and spiked washer (SSW, Synthes) was tested as a method to fix both tendon and Ligament Augmentation Device (LAD, 3M Co.). Also tested was fixation of an LAD with a custom designed ligament implant fixation tab (LIFT). Specimens, goat tendons or LADs, were fixed under 44.5 N of tension to two flat segments of goat bone. Five specimens were tested for each group.

After specimen fixation, increasing loads were applied to the specimen. One bone block was cyclically moved an incrementally increasing distance away from the other, along the axis of the specimen. Between applied loads the bone blocks were returned to their original positions. Two measurements were made at each level of applied load. The first was the force remaining in the specimen with the bone segments in their original positions. The second was the elongation required to return the fixed specimen to its original tension. The second measure was termed slippage, and includes effects of viscoelastic and plastic deformation of the tendon/LAD at both fixation points and within the tendon/LAD. Cyclic loading was continued until failure.

The results are quantified in Table 1. This study demonstrates that soft tissue fixation devices may be characterized by loss of tension, and elongation required to regain original tension, as a function of applied loads. Such information may be useful to evaluate devices that are designed to reduce slippage.

KEYWORDS: soft tissue fixation, slippage, ligament reconstruction

The fixation of soft tissues, such as tendons and ligaments, to bone is a common aspect of many orthopaedic procedures. Which method of fixation is appropriate in a given procedure largely depends on the mechanical demands to be made on the tissue prior to its formation of a new insertion into the bone. Failure of soft tissue fixation can be primarily of two types: gross avulsion with loss of continuity between the tissue and the bone, and slippage of the fixation, either immediately or with gradual use. Slippage of the tissue increases its effective length. This may prevent the fixed tissue from performing its biomechanical task. Similar problems exist when fixing synthetic ligament implants.

Perhaps nowhere else is soft tissue fixation more critical than in the reconstruction of the anterior cruciate ligament (ACL) deficient knee, where both gross avulsion and slippage of the fixed tissue or ligament implant can result in failure of the procedure. In designing an ACL

[1] Department of Orthopaedic Surgery, University of Minnesota, Minneapolis, MN 55455.
[2] Department of Orthopaedic Surgery, Tokyo Medical and Dental University, Tokyo 113, Japan.
* To whom all correspondence should be addressed.

TABLE 1—*Test results.*

Fixation Measure	Applied Force (N, average ± SEM)		
	SSW with Tendon	SSW with LAD	LIFT with LAD
50% loss of set force	146.5 (± 23.9)	54.8 (± 7.14)	217.4 (± 28.5)
Slippage: 2-mm	293.8 (± 62.4)	118.3 (± 9.74)	539.1 (± 38.8)
5-mm	356.3 (± 82.8)	336.2 (± 10.8)	978.5 (± 67.3)
Maximum Force	486.8 (± 108)	776.4 (± 31.7)	1540.7 (± 139)

reconstructive procedure using soft tissue fixation, the method of soft tissue fixation should be characterized by both the maximal force it can support without avulsion and also by its ability to maintain the desired tension with the bones in their functional positions. The fixation should be maintained both immediately and with use until the graft material can be incorporated biologically.

Many of the modern methods of soft tissue fixation have been introduced relatively recently. Hurson and Sheehan [1] reported on the clinical use of screws and spiked washers for repair of avulsed ligaments. In an extensive cadaveric study, Robertson et al. [2] compared failure loads for methods of fixation using barbed staple, stone staple, suture techniques, screw with spiked washer, and screw with soft tissue plate for a variety of soft tissues. Their work identified the screw with spiked washer and soft tissue plate as superior methods in terms of maximal load to failure. While performing their investigation the authors were able to make qualitative observations on soft tissue slippage with the various methods of fixation, concluding that significant slippage took place before gross failure for both suture techniques and stone staples.

The purpose of this study was to examine not only the failure load obtained with common fixation devices but also the ability to fix tissue at a desired load, to maintain the stability of set tension and fixation length with cyclic unloading and reloading, and to resist loss of tension due to applied loads at the time of surgical fixation through the time of biological incorporation of the graft material. The methods developed allow evaluation of new and established fixation devices.

Materials and Methods

Tissue or Ligament Implant Fixation: General Procedure

The fixation devices tested in this study were the screw and spiked washer (SSW, Synthes U.S.A., Monument, CO) and screw with a custom designed ligament fixation tab (LIFT). The materials tested were goat tendons, similar in size to human semitendinosis tendons, and ligament augmentation devices (LAD, 3M Corporation, St. Paul, MN). Five repetitions were performed for each of the three groups tested: SSW with tendon, SSW with LAD, and LIFT with LAD.

The experimental setup is diagrammed in Fig. 1, using testing of the SSW fixation method as an example. In testing a particular method of soft tissue fixation, two portions of goat femoral or tibial diaphyseal bone were freed of soft tissue and fixed in polymethylmethacrylate. Both bone segments were then placed in aluminum holders, allowing their fixation in a linear material testing machine (MTS Corporation). One end of the tendon or LAD was fixed to a bone segment by the method to be studied. The graft was fixed parallel to the long axis of the bone. The other end of the specimen was sutured with a half Kessler technique leaving two free suture ends [3]. The suture ends were tied to a stiff wire loop that had previously been

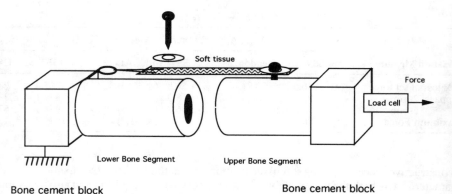

FIG. 1—*Experimental setup, SSW fixation method.*

rigidly fixed into the methylmethacrylate cylinder of the other bone segment. The bone segments were distracted by the hydraulic arm of the material testing machine along the long axis of the bones. The bone segments were distracted until the force carried by the ligament/LAD was 44.5 ($\pm$ 2) N.

After the initial force was set at 44.5 ($\pm$ 2) N the bone blocks were held in a fixed position for one minute. If the force crept below 44.5 ($\pm$ 2) N the bone blocks were further distracted to again produce a force of 44.5 ($\pm$ 2) N in the specimen. This adjustment was repeated until the force in the specimen stabilized. Stability was defined as a force reading from the load cell constant within 2 N of 44.5 N over a one-minute period. Once the force in the graft was stable, the bone segments were held in fixed positions while the second end of the graft was fixed to the second bone segment. The positions of the bone segments at this time were defined as their original positions.

Screw and Spiked Washer

To perform fixation with a screw and spiked washer, a 3.2-mm drill bit and 4.5-mm tap (4.5-mm screw system, Synthes) were used to form drill holes in both bone segments. One end of the tendon or LAD was fixed first using a 4.5-mm cortical bone screw with a spiked washer. When fixing a tendon, the tendon was doubled by looping it around the first screw. Fixation of an LAD required first threading the screw through the LAD. The screw was driven through the tendon/LAD, the immediate cortex of bone, and into the opposite cortex. The torque on the screw was not quantified but was qualitatively controlled by having the same surgeon apply the torque for each case. After the first end was fixed, sutures were placed in the other end of the tendon/LAD. The specimen was then tensioned to a stable 44.5 ($\pm$ 2) N as previously described.

Additional steps were required when fixing the second end of an LAD. During preliminary testing it was determined that threading a screw through the LAD while it was under tension caused damage to the LAD. To avoid damage, the LAD was pretensioned to a stable 44.5 ($\pm$ 2) N and the portion of the LAD that was directly over the tapped hole in the second bone segment was marked with a suture. The LAD was allowed to slacken, and the screw with spiked washer was threaded just through the LAD at the point marked by the suture. When the LAD was again pretensioned to a stable 44.5 ($\pm$ 2) N, in every case the tip of the screw aligned with the tapped hole.

For both tendons and LADs, fixation to the second bone segment was completed while holding both bone segments fixed in their original positions, the second screw being driven through the graft and fixed to bone bicortically. The distance between points of fixation was approximately 40 mm when fixing LADs and 50 mm when fixing tendons. The force in the specimen, measured by a load cell within the MTS machine, was recorded continuously during the fixation to the second bone segment. Once the force in the tendon/LAD stabilized, defined as less than a 1.5-N drop in 1 min, the sutures used to pretension the specimen were cut.

Ligament Implant Fixation Washer

A diagram of the ligament implant fixation tab (LIFT), with the ligament implant sewn in place, is shown in Fig. 2. The LIFT has a slot for the ligament implant, a hole machined to fit precisely with a cortical bone screw, and a small hole to hold the sutures with which the ligament implant is to be tensioned. Fixation using the custom designed LIFT involves first sewing the ligament implant back on to itself after it has passed through its slot in the LIFT. This was done using 7.0 braided polyester suture (Ethicon, Somerville, NJ) in a running fashion, suturing together a 16-mm length of overlapping LAD. Both ends of the LAD were fixed to LIFTs. The length of LAD between the two areas sutured together was 40 mm. Once the LAD was fixed to LIFTs on both ends, the LIFTs were grasped and the LAD was cyclically loaded from 30 N to 300 N forty times. The LAD with LIFTs attached was then ready for fixation.

One end of the LAD with LIFT was fixed to bone bicortically with a 4.5-mm cortical screw. Sutures were tied to the second LIFT and a stable force of 44.5 ($\pm$ 2) N was placed on the LAD as previously described. The second LIFT was flush against the second bone segment. A 4.5-mm drill bit was used to create a cone-shaped pit in the underlying bone using the screw hole in the second LIFT as a drill guide. The pit served to guide the 3.2-mm drill bit used to create the screw hole in the second bone segment (Fig. 3). After tapping the screw hole, a 4.5-mm cortical bone screw fixed the second LIFT to the lower bone segment. Once both ends were fixed and the force in the material was stable (defined as less than a 1.5 N drop in 1 min), the sutures used for pretensioning were cut.

Cyclic Unloading and Reloading of Fixed Tissue (or Ligament Implant)

Once fixation was complete and the pretensioning sutures had been cut, the force in the fixed material was again allowed to stabilize before cyclic unloading and reloading was begun, sta-

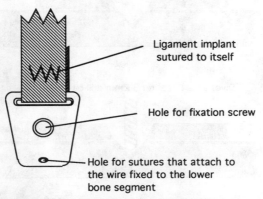

Ligament implant
sutured to itself

Hole for fixation screw

Hole for sutures that attach to
the wire fixed to the lower
bone segment

FIG. 2—*Ligament implant fixation tab (LIFT), with ligament sewn in place.*

bility being defined as less than a 1.5-N drop in 1 min. One bone segment was cyclically moved 5 mm towards the other, producing slack in the graft. The bone segment was then returned to its original position. The force in the material was continuously recorded. This movement was repeated ten times over a 10-min time period after which the force in the material was allowed to stabilize with the bone segments in their original positions. This motion was then repeated 50 times over a 5-min period, and again the force was allowed to equilibrate.

Analysis of Force Setting Accuracy

Figure 4 shows a typical continuous force recording and demonstrates the measurements extracted. The first measurement made was the initial force, the stabilized force at which fixation was begun. This was controlled during the experiment as 44.5 ($\pm$ 2) N. With fixation the force in the graft was disturbed after which some relaxation in graft force occurred. Once the force stabilized, the force after fixation was measured. The sutures used to pretension the graft were cut, and the drop in force which occurred within 1 min was measured and attributed to the loss of the sutures. After the force again stabilized, the set force was measured. After each set of cyclic unloading and reloading, the stabilized force was measured.

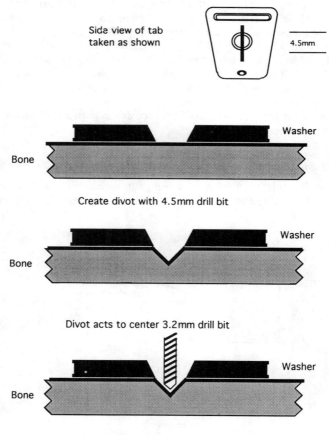

FIG. 3—*Method for centering screw for fixation.*

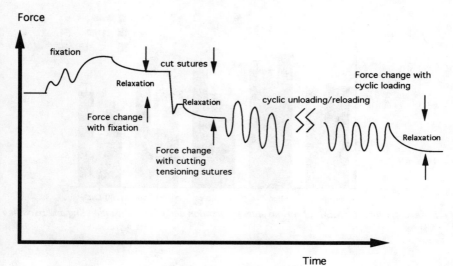

FIG. 4—*Typical continuous force recording.*

Slippage and Failure with Increasing Applied Loads

To apply increasing loads to the specimen, one bone block was cyclically moved from its original position (at a rate of 0.2 mm/s), first increasing the distance between the bone blocks, returning to its original position, and then decreasing the distance between the bone blocks, and returning to its original position. The distance moved in either direction was steadily increased, beginnng at 0.1 mm and increasing by 0.1 mm with each cycle. One measure of slippage was the change in the force remaining in the graft when the bone blocks were in their original positions. This force was measured during the portion of the cycle in which the specimen was being elongated. For the purposes of comparing applied load to resulting slippage, the applied load was defined as the peak load generated during the previous elongation of the specimen.

The second measure of slippage was the amount of specimen elongation needed to return the force in the specimen to its set level. This distance was defined as the slippage distance. This measurement was made during the elongation portion of the above cycle. Preliminary studies demonstrated that while changes in force after slippage were observed with the application of relatively small forces, large slippage distances were not observed until considerably higher loads were applied to the specimen. To apply large loads and demonstrate large slippage distances, one bone block was moved above and then below its original position (at a rate of 0.2 mm/s) by steadily increasing amounts, beginning at 1 mm and increasing by 1 mm with each cycle. This method of cyclic elongation was continued until the specimen failed, the maximum force observed being the failure load.

Results

Force Setting Accuracy

The average force ($\pm$ SEM) in the tendon/LAD for each of the three groups tested is shown at the various stages of fixation, and after cyclic unloading and reloading, in Fig. 5. The initial force was the force at which the specimen stabilized prior to fixation. This force was not exactly 44.5 N since an error of $\pm$ 2 N was allowed. The force in the specimen after it was fixed and

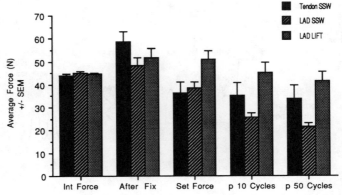

FIG. 5—*Average force (± SEM) at various stages of fixation and after cyclic unloading and reloading.*

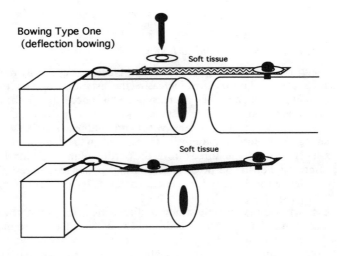

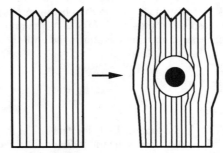

FIG. 6—*Types of bowing that occur when specimen is fixed.*

allowed time to stabilize was higher than the initial force in all cases. Based on experimental observation this increase in force is contributed to by two types of bowing which occur when the specimen is fixed. The two types of bowing are demonstrated in Fig. 6. The first type of bowing, deflection bowing, was minimized by having the tendon/LAD as flush as possible against the bone block as the second end of the tendon/LAD was fixed. The second type of bowing, compression bowing, while observed with both tendon and LAD, appeared to be more pronounced when fixing tendons.

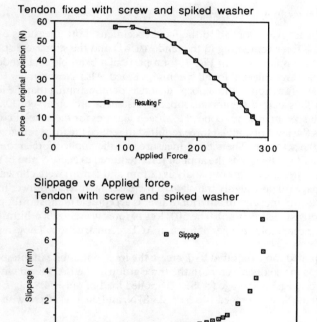

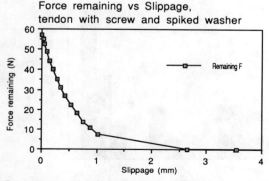

FIG. 7—*Measures of slippage for one specimen, screw, and spiked washer.*

The force was decreased in all three groups by cutting the pretensioning sutures. The greatest loss was observed in the tendon fixed with SSW, an average ($\pm$ SEM) of 16.2 ($\pm$ 0.91) N, and the least force was lost in the LAD fixed with LIFT, an average ($\pm$ SEM) of 2.0 ($\pm$ 0.32) N. With cyclic unloading and reloading the trend was for tension to be lost, but the magnitude of loss varied considerably between the groups. The average ($\pm$ SEM) force in the tendon fixed with SSW only dropped from 36.2 ($\pm$ 2.0) N to 33.6 ($\pm$ 5.9) N. The most extreme loss was observed with the LAD fixed with a screw and spiked washer where the force dropped from an average ($\pm$ SEM) of 38.3 ($\pm$ 2.6) N to 21.6 ($\pm$ 1.6) N.

Slippage with Increasing Applied Loads

As increasing loads were applied to the fixed specimens, both measures of slippage were obtained. Both the force remaining in the tendon/LAD and the slippage distance are shown as a function of the applied load in Fig. 7, for a particular example of a tendon fixed with a SSW. Similar data were collected for all specimens tested. Also shown in Fig. 7 is a plot of the force remaining as a function of the slippage distance, demonstrating that the force remaining in the specimen falls before significant slippage distances are observed. Data of this type obtained for each specimen were reduced to three measures for the sake of comparison. The first measure was the level of applied force required to reduce the force remaining in the spec-imen to 50% of the set force. The second measure was the applied force required to cause 2 mm of slippage, and the third was the applied force required to cause 5 mm of slippage. These slippage distance criteria used for our analysis (2 mm and 5 mm) were chosen assuming that distances of slippage might roughly translate to increases in anterior drawer in a ACL recon-structed knee. A 2-mm increase in anterior drawer is acceptable to most orthopaedic surgeons while a 5-mm increase clearly is not. The 50% loss of force was chosen arbitrarily since little is known regarding acceptable changes of force in ACL reconstruction. These results are shown in Fig. 8.

The average applied force required to decrease the force remaining in the specimen to 50% of the set force was markedly different in the three groups. The LAD fixed with the SSW lost 50% of its set force with an average ($\pm$ SEM) applied load of only 54.8 ($\pm$ 7.1) N, while the tendon fixed with the SSW averaged 146.5 ($\pm$ 23.8) N, and the LAD fixed with the LIFT aver-

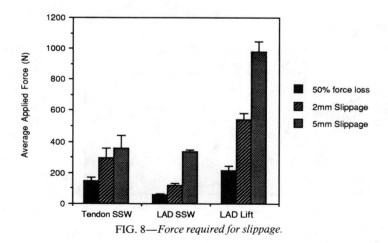

FIG. 8—*Force required for slippage.*

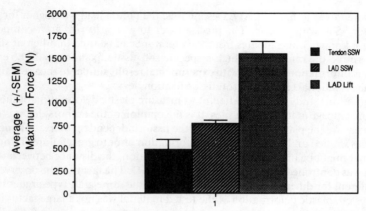

FIG. 9—*Maximum load (± SEM) for tendon SSW, LAD SSW, and LAD lift.*

aged 217.4 (± 28.5) N. Slippage of 2 mm was seen with an average of 118.3 (± 9.7) N, 293.8 (± 62.4) N, and 539.1 (± 38.8) N for the LAD fixed with SSW, tendon fixed with SSW, and LAD fixed with LIFT, respectively. At 5-mm of slippage the LAD fixed with LIFT again obtained the highest average applied loads, 978.5 (± 67.4) N, while there was little difference between the LAD fixed with SSW and the tendon fixed with SSW, with applied loads of 336.2 (± 10.8) N and 356.3 (± 82.8) N, respectively.

Failure with Increasing Applied Loads

The average maximum load (± SEM) for each of the three groups is shown in Fig. 9. The failure mode for both the LADs and tendons fixed with the SSW was to pull out from under the spiked washer. The LADs fixed with the LIFT failed within the substance of the LAD in all cases. It should be noted that the average maximum load applied to produce failure, 486.9 (± 108.4) N for the tendon fixed with SSW, 776.4 (± 31.6) N for the LAD fixed with SSW, and 1540.7 (± 139.5) N for the LAD fixed with the LIFT, was considerably higher than the applied load producing 5 mm of slippage. This is evidence that gross slippage which could render a fixed tendon/LAD biomechanically useless may occur at forces below those producing complete failure.

Discussion

The results of this study indicate that soft tissue fixation devices should be characterized by more than the load required to cause complete failure of fixation. Slippage may be critical in many surgical settings, including that of ACL reconstruction, when by setting a given length to a soft tissue graft or ligament implant the surgeon is determining the biomechanical role the graft component will play in the immediate post-operative period. Increases in the effective length of a graft component between the fixation points may decrease the force in the graft when the femur and tibia are in functional anatomical positions. Conversely, the tibia may experience more anterior displacement relative to the femur when the knee is in use due to loss of the restraining function of the graft. Clinically, slippage may result in a "properly tight" reconstruction becoming "too loose."

Several important points were demonstrated in the results of the fixation methods tested. The SSW when used to fix the tendon maintained force and slipped 2 mm at higher applied loads than when used to fix the LAD. Despite this, the failure load was higher for SSW with LAD than for SSW with tendon. The precise loads to which *in vivo* graft components are exposed is not known, but estimates from the literature can be used in different surgical settings to determine the range over which a specific soft tissue fixation would be expected to function. This information, coupled with experimental results similar to those obtained in this study, will allow rational choice of a soft tissue fixation device.

The design of this study does not attempt to measure plastic deformation of the specimen separate from slippage at the fixation sites. It is the opinion of the authors that it is difficult to accurately measure the plastic deformation of the tissue independent of fixation methods and that the tissues studied undergo little plastic deformation prior to gross failure. To decrease the variability that might be introduced by plastic deformation, the distance between the two fixation points was controlled for both the tendon and LAD. The fact that the observed slippage was very different for different fixation methods fixing the same graft type argues that for the specimens tested, plastic deformation of the tested material was not a large factor in our slippage measurement.

This study demonstrates that a great deal of variability exists between different fixation methods, and between tendon and ligament implant for the same fixation method. The results demonstrate that characterizing a fixation method by the force to complete failure is inadequate and may be misleading. Consideration of slippage and subsequent loss of tension is required in both designing and choosing a soft tissue or ligament implant fixation device.

References

[1] Hurson, B. J. and Sheehan, J. M., "The Use of Spiked Plastic Washers in the Repair of Avulsed Ligaments," *Acta Orthpedica Scandinavia,* Vol. 52, 1981, pp. 23–26.
[2] Robertson, D. B., Daniel, D. M., Biden, E. N., "Soft Tissue Fixation,"*American Journal of Sports Medicine,* Vol. 14, 1986, pp. 398–403.
[3] Kessler, I., "The Grasping Technique for Tendon Repair," *Hand,* Vol. 5, 1973, pp. 253–255.

Composite Materials

Robert A. Latour, Jr.[1] and Jonathan Black[1]

Fiber-Reinforced Polymer Composite Biomaterials: Characterization of Interfacial Bond Strength and Environmental Sensitivity

REFERENCE: Latour, R. A., Jr. and Black, J., **"Fiber-Reinforced Polymer Composite Biomaterials: Characterization of Interfacial Bond Strength and Environmental Sensitivity,"** *Biomaterials' Mechanical Properties, ASTM STP 1173,* H. E. Kambic and A. T. Yokobori, Jr., Eds., American Society for Testing and Materials, Philadelphia, 1994, pp. 193–211.

ABSTRACT: Fiber-reinforced polymer (FRP) composite materials are being developed for structural orthopaedic implant applications. The mechanical behavior, particularly the strength, of FRP composites is significantly influenced by fiber/matrix interfacial bond strength. Interfacial bond strength is known to be potentially susceptible to degradation in physiologic environments, and thus is an important area of research for the development of durable FRP composite biomaterials. A relatively simple interfacial bond strength technique has been developed by TRI/Princeton. We have further implemented and further developed this technique for addressing issues relevant to the development and evaluation of FRP composite biomaterials. In this paper, we present a detailed description of this test technique and outline the methods for sample fabrication, sample testing to determine ultimate and fatigue strength, and data analysis in sufficient detail for others to reproduce this interfacial bond strength and durability measurement technique. Potential test problems leading to erroneous test results and further development areas for this technique are also addressed.

KEYWORDS: test method, fiber-reinforced polymer (FRP) composite, interfacial bond, ultimate strength (UBS), fatigue strength, composite biomaterial

Nomenclature

a_c	crack length at which bond transitions from stable to unstable crack growth (critical)
c, m	fracture mechanics constants materials characterization
D	fiber diameter
da/dn	interfacial bond crack growth per applied load cycle
E_f	elastic modulus of fiber
F	force applied to fiber during fiber pull-out test
G_{II}	Mode II (shear) strain energy release rate
G_m	shear modulus of matrix
L	fiber embedment length within microdroplet
N	number of load cycles applied to sample to cause complete bond failure (fatigue life)
P	probability value from median rank table for appropriate sample population size
R	outer radius of matrix cylinder. See Fig. 7
r_i	radius at fiber/matrix interface = radius of fiber
u	displacement in x-direction

[1] Assistant professor and Hunter professor, respectively, Department of Bioengineering, Clemson University, Clemson, SC 29634.

u_i	displacement of fiber/matrix interface in x-direction
β	nondimensional interfacial shear stress distribution shape parameter
δ	Weibull distribution parameter
ϵ	sum of squared errors between pull-out force measured for i-th data point and predictive equation for i-th data point
μ	mean value for Weibull distribution
σ^2	variance for Weibull distribution
σ_x	normal stress in x-direction
τ	shear stress τ_{rx}
τ_i	shear stress τ_{rx} at interface ($r = r_i$)
τ_{max}	maximum interfacial shear stress

Introduction

Fiber-reinforced polymer (FRP) composite biomaterials are being investigated for a wide range of orthopaedic implant applications. As alternatives to metallic materials, FRP composites are being considered for use in fabrication of femoral components of total hip arthroplasty [1] and of fracture fixation devices [2]. Fiber reinforcement has also been investigated as a potential means of improving mechanical behavior of bulk polymers such as polymethylmethacrylate (PMMA) bone cement [3], and ultrahigh-molecular-weight polyethylene (UHMWPE) [4], and epoxies [5] for articulation components in joint arthroplasty.

As in any structural orthopaedic implant, the mechanical behavior of the FRP composite is a critical contributor to implant performance. As an anisotropic, inhomogeneous material, the mechanical behavior of FRP composites is very complex and is a function of the synergistic properties of the fiber, matrix, fiber/matrix interfacial bond, and of geometric properties such as fiber length, distribution, and orientation in the matrix. While all of these factors must be considered in the overall component design, perhaps the most difficult to address is the fiber/matrix interface. The fiber/matrix interface, an adhesive bond between the fiber and matrix, is the means by which the fiber is able to reinforce the matrix and the matrix is able to support the fibers and transfer load between them so the fibers can support compressive and shear stresses as well as tensile stresses in three dimensions. Thus, the fiber/matrix interface plays a major role in the mechanical behavior (especially fracture behavior) of a FRP composite material under all loading conditions [6]. The fact that polymer matrices are not impervious to moisture penetration is a further complication for the development and use of FRP composite materials in orthopaedic implant applications. As an adhesive bond, the fiber/matrix interface is potentially sensitive to moisture degradation, thereby making FRP composite implants potentially susceptible to environmental degradation *in vivo*. Obviously, control of interfacial bond behavior is extremely important for the development of FRP composite structural biomaterials.

While interfacial bond properties are widely acknowledged to be of critical importance for FRP composite performance, they have proven to be difficult to measure directly because they entail measurement on a micromechanics scale. Several test methods have been developed to investigate interfacial bond strength. These methods range from indirect tests that measure macroscopic composite properties which are then used to infer interfacial bond behavior [7,8], to semi-direct tests such as single fiber indentation [9], and direct tests such as pull-out tests [10] in which bond strength between single fibers and the matrix are directly measured. While single fiber indentaion and pull-out tests do provide the most direct methods of investigating interfacial bond mechanical behavior, they are typically very technically demanding tests to conduct successfully.

In 1987, a relatively simple and straightforward interfacial bond strength test method, termed the "microbond method," was first introduced by Dr. Bernard Miller of the Textile Research Institute, Princeton, NJ (TRI/Princeton) [11] for measuring the ultimate strength between single fibers and thermoset polymer matrices. Since 1985, we have worked in collaboration with Dr. Miller and TRI/Princeton to further develop this test method for use with thermoplastic matrices and have successfully used this method to investigate the effect of simulated *in vivo* environments upon both the ultimate and fatigue strength of selected fiber/matrix combinations [12]. We have found this test method to be relatively simple to perform and one that provides very reproducible quantitative bond strength data compared to other interfacial bond strength test methods considered. Thus, we believe this test method is a valuable tool for conducting both basic and applied research for the development of FRP composite implant biomaterials for structural orthopaedic and other interfacial property sensitive applications.

In this paper, we describe the procedural details of the application of this interfacial bond strength test method including sample fabrication for both thermoset and thermoplastic matrices; test methods to determine interface ultimate strength, fatigue strength, and environmental durability; and applicable methods of data analysis.

Test Methods

Overview

This technique requires the fabrication of single fiber pull-out test specimens in which a single reinforcing fiber (typically in the range of 10 μm diameter) is embedded in a polymer matrix "bead" or "microdroplet" to form an interfacial bond between the fiber and matrix which ideally is representative of the interfacial bond formed in the composite. To perform the interfacial bond strength measurement, a mechanical test machine is required with capability of applying tensile force to the fiber with load sensing capability between zero and the breaking strength of the individual fibers (i.e., 0.000 to 0.160 N, typical for high-strength carbon fiber). To measure bond strength, the polymer matrix is held by a gripping device while the test machine applies a controlled tensile load to the free end of the fiber (ramping load for ultimate strength test, sinusoidal load for dynamic fatigue test). Ultimate strength, fatigue strength, and frictional stress following debonding can be determined from the test data.

The details of these test methods are described below in three sections: sample fabrication, sample testing, and data analysis.

Sample Fabrication

Samples can be fabricated using either thermoset or thermoplastic matrices. The first step in sample fabrication is to construct an aluminum fiber holding rack on which to mount single fibers (Fig. 1). A length of about 10 cm of untwisted multifilament fiber roving is cut from a spool of the desired fiber type. Using magnification if necessary, single filaments[2] are then pulled from the roving and taped to the metal fiber rack such that the middle third of the fiber is freely suspended and slightly taught. Filaments should be spaced about 5 mm apart. Once the fibers are in place, the polymer matrix can be applied.

Thermoset microdroplets are formed on the single fibers using a fine tipped applicator to dip into the prepolymerized thermoset resin and carefully "dabbed" onto the fiber under 40 to 80× stereo microscope observation. The size of the microdroplets can be controlled by the

---

[2] This technique is unsuitable for use with multifilament fiber bundles because of the inherent difficulties of obtaining an accurate measurement of actual fiber bundle/polymer matrix interfacial bond area.

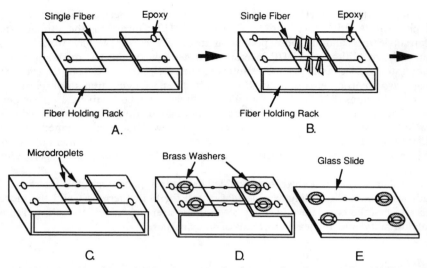

FIG. 1—*Interfacial bond sample fabrication. (a) Aluminum rack with mounted single fibers. Only two fibers illustrated for the sake of clarity. (b) For thermoplastic matrices, two "V" strips of polymer (see Fig. 2) are suspended from each fiber. If a thermoset resin is used, microdroplets are formed directly on the fiber by applying resin with fine tipped applicator. (c) Sample rack is heated to cause the thermoplastic strips to melt through the fiber leaving behind microdroplet, or if a thermoset resin is used, heat is applied for desired resin curve. (d) No. 4 brass washers bonded to each fiber end. Brass washers are used for their nonmagnetic property. (Laboratory instruments, such as tweezers, often are slightly magnetized, making them "stick" to specimens if steel washer is used). (e) Specimens are mounted on glass microscope slides for microscopic measurement of fiber diameter and embedment length.*

length of fiber wetted by the resin. The fine-tipped applicator can be made from a small diameter glass rod by heating the glass until it is red hot in a flame and then quickly drawing the ends apart to form hairlike thickness glass strands at the glass rod ends. Two droplets of resin are placed on each filament about 5 mm from the fiber midpoint. Once all microdroplets are applied, the samples are heat-treated according to the recommended curing schedule of the resin.

Thermoplastic microdroplets are formed using slightly different techniques. To form thermoplastic microdroplets on the single fibers, V-shaped pieces of polymer are cut from polymer film as shown in Fig. 2. For fibers with diameter in the range of about 10 μm, a 75-μm polymer film thickness has been found to work well. The "V" strips must be cut with the tip width within about 50 to 100 μm using a straight edge and sharp single edge razor blade under stereo microscope observation (80$\times$) using a calibrated graticule. Once cut, the V strips are hung upside-down on each single fiber about 5 mm from the fiber center. If static electricity makes the strips difficult to work with, the static charge has been found to be dissipated readily simply by pinching the "legs" of the strips in between the fingers for a few seconds. Handling of the tip of the strip must be avoided to prevent contamination of the material which will form the microdroplet. When in place, the specimens are heated in a temperature controlled oven to melt the polymer strip over the fibers, leaving behind a single microdroplet concentrically formed by surface tension about the single fiber filament.

For both thermoset and thermoplastic polymer matrices, consideration must be given to the thermal stability of the fiber as some fiber/matrix combinations may not be suitable for the application of this technique. The proper temperature program to use for specific thermoplastic polymers must be determined by trial and error; however, a peak temperature of about 175 °C above T_g has been found to work well for polysulfone, polyetheretherketone, and polycarbonate matrices. Specimens have been tested following two different heating schedules: quick quench versus slow cool. Quick quenching specimens are heated to the peak temperature, held for 5 min, and then immediately removed from the oven to cool in room temperature air. The slow-cooled specimens, on the other hand, are heated to the peak temperature, held for 5 to 20 min to form the microdroplet, and then allowed to cool down gradually from the peak temperature to the polymer T_g by simply leaving the specimens in the oven after the oven is turned off and monitoring the cool down rate. Once T_g is reached, the specimens are removed to room temperature. The quick quench specimens have typically been found to have a significantly higher bond strength than slow-cooled specimens initially, but then undergo aging with the bond strength decreasing toward the level of the slow-cooled specimens over a time frame of several months [13]. The initial high bond strength is believed to be due to differential thermal contraction induced residual interfacial stresses which relax with time tending toward the more stable (slow-cooled) bond strength levels. The slow-cooled method of sample fabrication is therefore preferred; however, it may require the use of an inert atmosphere during the heating process to prevent sample oxidation during fabrication. When severe oxidation occurs, microdroplets typically develop an amber color.

Once the microdroplets are formed, the specimens are prepared for testing. Standard #4 size brass flat washers are first placed under each fiber end and bonded to the fiber with a water-resistant epoxy such as Devcon® 2-TON epoxy. This is normally available at local hardware stores and has been found to be satisfactory for short term (1 to 3 day) immersion studies. Once the washers are bonded, the specimens are transferred to 3 in. by 2 in. (7.6 by 5.1 cm) glass microscope slides. Small strips of masking tape are used to hold the washers to the glass, such that a small amount of tension is applied to the fibers to keep the microdroplets suspended,

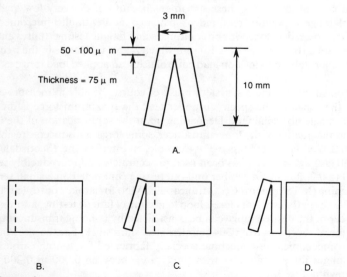

FIG. 2—*Thermoplastic V strip fabrication. (a) Dimensions of V strip cut from polymer film. Critical dimension is 50 to 100 μm tip. If too large, it will not get a single well-formed microdroplet. (b through d) Cutting sequence for V strip fabrication. (b) First cut critical dimension of tip. (c) Bend first leg to open up V. (d) Cut V from rest of film.*

thus facilitating microscopic inspection and measurement. The specimens are then numbered, the slides placed under high power magnification (500 to 1000×) and the fiber embedment length (L) and fiber diameter (D) of each specimen are measured with a calibrated graticule using both transmitted and incident light for best visualization. These measurements are used to calculate interfacial bond area ($A = \pi DL$). Ideally, measurement should be done using an image analysis system; however, measurement accuracy with a standard error of a few percent can also be obtained by eye using a suitable calibrated graticule on the microscope. Once the specimens are measured, they should be stored in a room temperature desiccator until environmental conditioning or testing, or both. If passive environmental conditioning in the form of soaking the specimens in physiologic saline is desired, a sample holding frame should be constructed which allows full immersion of the microdroplets but not the bond between the fiber and the washer at either end of the fiber, in order to ensure that the fiber does not become debonded from the washer before or during the pull-out test.

Sample Testing

Test Apparatus—This sample configuration can be used to determine both ultimate and fatigue strength of the interface, and interfacial friction following debonding. As in any mechanical strength test, the basic components needed to test these specimens are a stroke actuator, force transducer with appropriate range capability and sensitivity, sample gripping means, electronic controller and signal conditioning, and data recording device.

The stroke actuator must be able to apply controlled displacement with time. For the ultimate strength tests, the actuator must be able to apply a slow stroke rate in the range of about 0 to 100 μm/s under either open or closed-loop stroke control. For interfacial bond fatigue testing, an actuator is necessary which can operate under closed-loop load control in the load range specified for the specific specimen type being tested. Servohydraulic test machines are not believed to be commercially available which operate under both closed-loop static and dynamic load control for testing these specimens because of the very low load and stroke length control range capability required. A patented nonhydraulic micromechanical test machine [14] has been developed for both ultimate and fatigue testing. It uses an electromagnetic actuator with a stroke range of ± 1.0 mm which is able to operate in the frequency range of 0 to 10 Hz under stable closed-loop load control using an applied load range as low as 0.000 to 0.100 N.

The force transducer for the test system must, of course, be able to measure applied force accurately in the range of the specimen under test; the maximum force is dictated by the strength of the single fiber filament. Depending upon the sophistication of the test machine electronics and the quality of the force transducer, some force transducers are able to be used in the low 1 to 2 % of their rated range. For example, an Interface Inc. (Scottsdale, AZ) Model MB-5-132 5 lb (2.3 kg) load cell has been used to accurately and reproducibly sense loads in the range of 0 to 0.200 N in single fiber pull-out testing conducted on a small servohydraulic MTS test machine (MTS Systems Co., Minneapolis, MN) for stroke controlled single cycle to failure ultimate strength tests. For closed-loop load control fatigue testing, a strain gaged based force transducer in the desired range can be constructed by bonding transducer quality strain gages to thin metal sheets cut from 304 stainless steel shim stock. For the electromagnetically actuated micromechanical test machine specially fabricated for testing carbon fiber specimens, an ultralight force transducer with force range between 0.000 to 0.200 N was constructed as shown in Fig. 3.

For our work, we have developed a fixed gap microdroplet grip which is used to hold the microdroplets. The criteria of the sample grips are that they hold the microdroplet in position without severely torquing or pinching the fiber while the fiber is being debonded from the

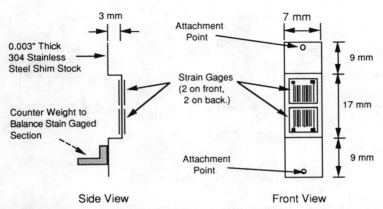

FIG. 3—*Force transducer. Schematic illustrating design of force transducer constructed for microme-chanical test machine. Load range: 0.000 to 0.200 N. Strain gages: 4500 ± 0.15% Ω, Measurements Group Inc., Model TK-060100CS-45C, full Wheatstone bridge design.*

microdroplet. After considering several designs, the design found to work best for our purposes consisted of two carefully polished square-edged stainless steel plates bonded to a substrate to form a uniform gap approximately 1.5 to 2.0 fiber diameters wide with the fiber contact surface of each grip-half being precisely even so one side will not contact the microdroplet before the other, thus avoiding microdroplet tilting upon seating (Fig. 4). Studies have shown that grip width relative to fiber diameter does influence measured mean bond strength value [15]. Therefore, to minimize experimental error, grips should be made for each fiber type of largely differing diameter to provide approximately equivalent grip gap width to fiber diameter ratio, and the same set of grips should ideally be used for testing specimens of a given fiber type. The grips can be made by constructing a polishing clamp to hold and polish one edge each of two 1.0 cm by 1.0 cm by 1.6 mm stainless steel plates. Polishing is done down to at at least a 0.3-μm size polishing abrasive following standard metallographic polishing techniques. Once polished, one plate is soldered or bonded with moisture resistant adhesive to a metal base with the polished edge toward the middle, as shown in Fig. 4. The second plate is then glued down to the base next to the first with its polished edge facing the other plate's polished edge. With the adhesive still tacky, the second plate is positioned until a uniform gap between the polished edges is formed between it and the first plate. This gap width can be controlled manually by moving the second plate while observing under about 500× microscopic magnification or by using a suitable removable precision spacer. Once both plates are secure on the base, the top surface of the grips must be finely polished to ensure that the top surfaces of the two grip halves are precisely on the same plane. If they are not, one edge will contact the microdroplet first, tilting the microdroplet, and apply a bending moment to the fiber, causing unknown changes in interfacial stress distribution and potentially breaking the fiber ahead of the microdroplet before pull-out can be achieved. Once fabricated, the grips are mounted below a grip support table with the gripping surface oriented downward.

If testing is to be conducted in a liquid environment, a fluid well is fabricated to fit over the grips such that the polished grip faces extend down below the liquid level in the fluid well to ensure full immersion of the microdroplet specimens during testing, as illustrated in Fig. 4.

The controller and signal conditioner used for the single cycle ultimate strength test must be able to control the actuator so as to apply the desired stroke rate and record the associated applied force (as a function of time) from the force transducer. For fatigue testing, the con-

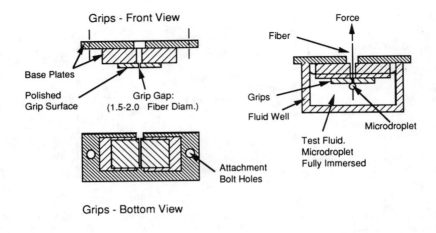

FIG. 4—*Microdroplet grip. (a) Design sketch of front and bottom view of fixed gap microdroplet grips. Critical dimension is grip gap width. (b) Illustration of grip attached to test frame with mounted specimen and fluid environment. Fluid level fully immerses microdroplet.*

troller must be designed for closed-loop control with the force transducer signal being used for feedback to be compared to a specified dynamic set point signal. The output of the controller drives the stroke actuator such that the applied load follows the desired set point. For fatigue testing, the controller must also be equipped with a cycle counter and output jacks to allow monitoring of the dynamic feedback, set-point, and actuator voltages. A schematic of the micromechanical test machine designed and constructed for this test technique is presented in Fig. 5. This apparatus is suitable for both ultimate and fatigue testing. Ultimate strength testing (but not fatigue testing) has also been conducted on servohydraulic and screw-driven mechanical testing machines equipped with a low range force transducer.

Test Procedures—The procedures for conducting an ultimate bond strength test with this sample model are relatively straightforward and simple while fatigue testing is obviously more complex. The first step for either type of test is to mount the specimen in the test machine. As

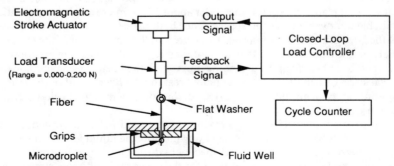

FIG. 5—*Micromechanical test machine. Schematic of basic components of micromechanical test machine for conducting either ultimate or fatigue testing of fiber/matrix interfacial bond using "microbond" sample.*

previously discussed, the specimens are fabricated with two microdroplets positioned 10 mm apart on a fiber, brass washers are bonded to each fiber end, and the washers taped to glass slides for storage. The fiber containing the interfacial bond specimen to be tested is cut halfway between the two microdroplets. A second washer is then taped to the cut end of the fiber below the microdroplet in order to act as a hang-down weight to straighten the fiber to facilitate mounting it in the test machine. The specimen is picked up with tweezers by the top washer (washer bonded to fiber) with the bottom washer hanging freely below it. The fiber is fed through the slot in the grips with the microdroplet situated below the grips and the top washer hung from the sensing element of the load transducer. A strong light is very helpful to be able to see the microdroplet on the fiber. A horizontally mounted long-range focal length microscope should be used to verify that the fiber is properly positioned and hanging freely in the grip slot.

To conduct the ultimate bond strength test, the grips are positioned about 1 mm above the microdroplet under microscopic visualization. The test machine is then set up to apply a constant stroke rate that will apply the desired interfacial bond loading rate to the specimen. When the test is started, the fiber will first be pulled freely through the slot with the force recording showing zero applied force. When the grips contact and hold the microdroplet, the force trace should then begin ramping upward, thus indicating the loading of the interfacial bond. When the ultimate strength of the fiber/matrix interface is reached, sudden and complete debonding typically occurs resulting in the applied load instantaneously dropping as strain energy is released from the specimen. The force signal should then level out to a lower near constant mean force level indicative of stick-slip interfacial friction as the fiber is pulled through the debonded microdroplet. If zero force is indicated following debonding, fiber fracture most likely has occurred rather than interfacial debonding. Observation of the microdroplet during the test using a horizontal stereo microscope is very helpful for determining if fiber pull-out actually occurs versus fiber fracture. The appearance of a good pull-out test recording is illustrated in Fig. 6. The ultimate applied force, loading rate, and frictional force following debonding can be determined from each pull-out trace. Data analysis for the calculation of ultimate bond strength (UBS) will be addressed in the next section.

Before interfacial bond fatigue strength tests can be conducted, the mean UBS value must first be determined following the ultimate strength test procedures as outlined above. While ultimate strength testing is conducted under stroke control, fatigue testing must be conducted under load control. To conduct an interfacial bond fatigue test, the specimen is loaded into the test machine as described above and, under microscopic visualization, the grips are posi-

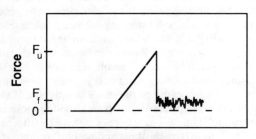

Cross-Head Displacement

FIG. 6—*Illustration of X-Y recorder plot for successful ultimate bond strength test zero applied force until microdroplet contacts grip. Force ramps upward until ultimate force reached (F_u) at which point sudden and complete debonding occurs. Force drops to low approximately constant value indicative of frictional drag force between fiber and debonded microdroplet.*

tioned such that they are just in contact with the top of the microdroplet. The load transducer signal must be monitored while positioning the grip with respect to the microdroplet to sense when contact is made and to be able to stop before excessive load is applied to the specimen. Once the microdroplet is in position, the fiber is cut between the microdroplet and the washer below the microdroplet serving as a weight to keep the fiber straight while loading the specimen into the grips. The grips are then backed away from the microdroplet until the force transducer signal stabilizes indicating a zero applied load. Both the force transducer and the fatigue cycle counter are then zeroed. The desired maximum and minimum fatigue loads to be applied to the specimen are calculated based upon the previously determined mean UBS and the desired minimum to maximum fatigue load ratio (R value). For example, if the mean UBS of the specimen type is 50 MPa and a fatigue test is to be conducted at a maximum applied average interfacial bond stress of 60% of the UBS with $R = 0.1$, the desired maximum and minimum interfacial bond stress levels to be applied during the test would be 30 MPa and 3.0 MPa, respectively. The applied force levels necessary to achieve these interfacial stress levels are calculated by multiplying the interfacial bond stress levels by the interfacial area of the specimen to be tested (assuming uniform shear stress distribution, see the subsection titled *Ultimate Bond Strength*). The applied force signal for the fatigue test can be described as the sum of static and dynamic force signals, the static level being one half the sum of the maximum and minimum applied forces, and the amplitude of the dynamic signal being one half the difference between the maximum and minimum applied forces. The first step in applying the fatigue force program is to apply the calculated static level of the force signal to the specimen while observing the force transducer signal on an oscilloscope. Once this is achieved, the desired frequency of the dynamic signal is set and its amplitude is increased from zero until the calculated maximum and minimum applied force values are achieved. Once set, the force signal program should be monitored periodically by oscilloscope to assure that it is stable. The number of fatigue cycles applied during the test are recorded by the cycle counter. Cycling is continued until either interfacial bond fatigue occurs, or a preset fatigue cycle run-out limit is reached. If bond failure occurs, sudden and complete debonding typically will occur upon the application of the last load cycle, with the force transducer subsequently sensing near zero applied load. If bond fatigue does not occur by the time the run-out limit for fatigue life is reached, the specimen can be tested to determine residual bond strength by following the methods outlined above for UBS measurement. The fatigue test data are recorded in the form of applied maximum shear stress versus the number of cycles to fiber pull-out (N). Data analysis for the calculation of fatigue strength is addressed in the next section.

If environmental sensitivity testing is to be conducted with microdroplet specimens, test methods are followed as before; however, a fluid immersion well must be attached around the sample grips to fully immerse the specimen. It has been previously observed with some fiber/matrix combinations that the loss of bond strength following saline immersion is reversible if the specimens are allowed to dry out. Therefore, if specimens are tested dry following immersion in a test liquid, it is possible that any decrease in bond strength caused by the liquid may not be detected and erroneous conclusions will result. If environmental effects are being investigated, the specimens must thus be fully saturated in the desired environment during the actual pull-out test. Fortunately, because of the small sample size of the microdroplet, diffusion times to research diffusional equilibrium with small solute molecules, such as water, are extremely rapid. For example, if an 80-μm sphere of polymer with a moisture diffusion coefficient at 37 °C of 5.0×10^{-9} cm^2/s (typical of many high-performance thermoplastic polymers such as polyetheretherketone (PEEK) [16]) is immersed in 37 °C saline, 95% diffusional equilibrium can be calculated to occur in less than 15 min. If the specimen is then removed from the liquid and exposed to laboratory air, moisture loss will occur just as rapidly. This drying effect was responsible for erroneous conclusions initially being reported concerning the effect of saline immersion upon the interfacial bond of carbon fiber/polysulfone (CF/PSF) and carbon fiber/polycarbonate samples (CF/PC) [17]. It was first reported that the interface between these materials did not undergo significant degradation following saline immersion. In the study, however, specimens were removed from saline immersion about 15 min prior to testing and tested dry. Further research subsequently then revealed that CF/PSF and CF/PC bonding does undergo significant ultimate strength degradation in saline [18,19], but the degradation is reversible upon the drying of the specimens. Since this discovery, reversible bond strength behavior has been observed by other researchers with other fiber/matrix combinations as well [20].

Data Analysis

Ultimate Bond Strength—It is well known that the interfacial stress distribution for a fiber or rod pull-out test from a matrix is nonuniform with the interfacial shear stress being concentrated toward the fiber end closest to the applied load. The geometry and gripping of the microdroplet specimens make exact theoretical modeling of the interfacial stress distribution very difficult; a full three-dimensional nonlinear finite element analysis would be necessary to properly address this problem. This type of detailed analysis is not necessary, however, as an empirical method can be implemented based upon shear-lag theory [21] to approximate the stress distribution along the interface of a given sample system.

Shear-lag theory is based upon a mechanics of materials force equilibrium approach to the fiber pull-out problem. Based upon shear-lag analysis and referring to Fig. 7, shear stress can be calculated along the interface as a function of interfacial position as described by Eq 1 (derivation presented in Appendix 1)

$$\tau_i = \frac{\beta F}{\pi D^2} \frac{\cosh[\beta(x/D)]}{\sinh[\beta(L/D)]} \; ; \text{ and } \tau_{max} = \frac{\beta F}{\pi D^2} \frac{1}{\tanh[\beta(L/D)]} \tag{1}$$

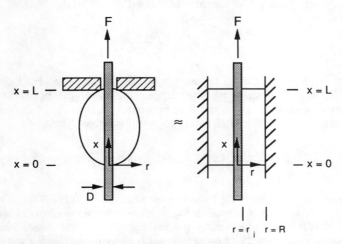

FIG. 7—*Approximation of fiber/microdroplet sample as a rod in cylinder pull-out model for application of shear-lag theory to estimate interfacial bond shear stress distribution. Boundary conditions between actual fiber/microdroplet sample and rod in cylinder are different. Thus β cannot be calculated theoretically by Eq 15 in Appendix 1, but must be empirically solved for best fit to experimental data.*

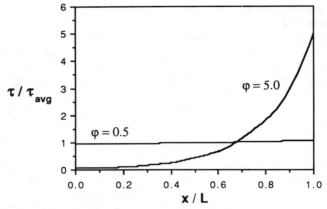

FIG. 8—*Interfacial bond shear stress distribution. Shear stress normalized by average interfacial shear stress where* $\tau_{avg} = F/(\pi DL)$ *and* $\varphi = (\beta L/D)$. *Plot is derived from Eq 1 with L = 100 μm and D = 10 μm. For low values of* φ, *shear-lag theory predicts uniform interfacial shear stress distribution equal to* τ_{avg} (= $F/\pi DL$).

where x and L are described in Fig. 7, and β is a constant for a given fiber/matrix combination which theoretically represents a nondimensional grouping of mechanical and geometric parameters (Appendix 1, Eq 5). Equation 1 is plotted in Fig. 8 as a function of fiber position to fiber embedment length ratio (x/L) for two values of the nondimensional parameter φ = $[\beta(L/D)]$. As evident from Fig. 8 and Eq 1, if φ is large, a nonuniform interfacial shear stress distribution occurs along the interface with the maximum shear stress (τ_{max}) occurring at x = L. On the other hand, if φ is small, an approximately uniform shear stress distribution is predicted over the interface. This situation can be illustrated mathematically by noting that, for small values of φ (≤ 0.50), tanh$\varphi \approx \varphi$ and τ_{max} from Eq 1 can then be expressed simply as the applied force divided by the area of the interfacial bond

$$\tau_{max} = \tau_{avg} = \frac{F}{\pi DL} \qquad (2)$$

For this condition, τ_{max} is the same as the average interfacial shear stress (τ_{avg}), thus indicating a uniformly distributed shear stress over the interface. Equation 1 can be rewritten to express the relationship between shear stress and fiber pull-out force in terms of the experimentally measurable independent variable (L/D) and dependent variable (F) as

$$F = \tau_{max}\pi D^2 \frac{\tanh[\beta(L/D)]}{\beta} \text{ ; and for small } L: F = \tau_{max}(\pi DL) \qquad (3)$$

For given values of τ_{max}, D, and β, Eq 3 can be plotted as shown in Fig. 9 (τ_{max}, = 50 MPa, D = 7 μm, and β = 0.001). As indicated in Fig. 9, a linear relationship exists between F and L/D for values of L/D between zero and some limiting value; for the values used in Fig. 9, F versus L/D is linear for $L/D \leq 25$. In order to simplify experimental testing and data analysis, it is desirable to determine what this upper limit of L/D is for a given fiber/matrix combination and ensure that specimens tested have fiber embedment lengths below the nonlinear range. This range can be fairly simply determined by fabricating specimens that span as large a L/D

ratio as the strength of a single fiber will allow (if L/D is too large, fiber fracture will occur prior to debonding). These specimens are then tested to determine the fiber pull-out force, and the F versus L/D data points plotted. From this plot, the range of L/D which will provide a linear F versus L/D relationship (and therefore approximately uniform shear stress distribution) can be determined by inspection; or, if a value of β is desired, the nonlinear form of Eq 3 can be best fitted to the experimental data points using numerical analysis and the method of least squares for multivariable, nonlinear equations [22]. For this, the square of the errors between the actually measured pull-out forces (F_k) and the theoretical pull-out forces (as predicted by Eq 3) for each data point are summed as indicated in Eq 4

$$\epsilon = \sum_{k=1}^{n} \left\{ F_k - \left[\tau_{max} \pi D_k^2 \frac{\tanh[\beta(L_k/D_k)]}{\beta} \right] \right\}^2 \qquad (4)$$

The sum of the squared errors (ϵ) is then minimized by differentiating it by τ_{max} and β, equating the differentials to zero and simultaneously solving the two resulting equations

$$\frac{d\epsilon}{d\tau_{max}} = 0 \text{ and } \frac{d\epsilon}{d\beta} = 0 \qquad (5)$$

The values of τ_{max} and β, of course, must be checked to ensure that they do represent the minimization of Eq 4 (versus a maximum or inflection point).

Once the range of the L/D ratio is determined which provides an approximately uniform shear stress distribution along the fiber/matrix interface, specimens can then all be fabricated to lie in this L/D range. Interfacial bond strength can then be determined from pull-out test data simply by dividing the measure pull-out force by the measured interfacial bond area. The mean and standard deviation of interfacial bond strength can then be simply determined for each fiber/matrix type and environmental condition investigated, and comparisons between different test groups can be statistically determined.

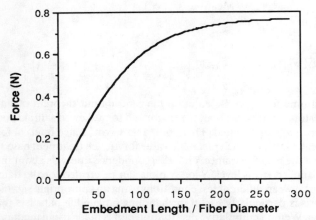

FIG. 9—*Theoretical plot of fiber pull-out force as a function of fiber embedment length (L) to fiber diameter (D). Plot derived from Eq 3 for hypothetical values of* τ_{max}, *= 50 MPa, D = 7 μm, and β = 0.001. Linear relationship exhibited for* $0 \leq L/D \leq 25$ *which is equivalent to a fiber embedment length of L = 175 μm for these conditions.*

Fatigue Strength—Fatigue data are obtained in the form of fatigue life (number of load cycles (N) applied to cause complete debonding) under a given controlled maximum peak applied load. The maximum applied interfacial shear stress is calculated from the peak applied load following methods as outlined in the preceding subsection. The fatigue data can then be presented in a standard applied stress versus the logarithm of fatigue life (log N) applied to cause fatigue failure (*S-N* fatigue plot) following ASTM Practice for Statistical Analysis of Linear or Linearized Stress-Life (*S-N*) and Strain Life (*E-N*) Fatigue (E 739) Data. This method of analysis, however, can only be properly applied for normally distributed fatigue life data with constant variance and with no run-outs. Fatigue life distribution data, however, are often skewed and contain run-outs. In such situations, a two-parameter Weibull distribution [23–25] can be used to analyze fatigue life data in which Weibull distribution parameters are calculated for each sample treatment group (treatment group is defined as the set of a given sample type tested under a given fatigue load level and given test environment). The Weibull distribution parameters for a given set of data are calculated from the Weibull cumulative distribution function equation [26]

$$P(x < a) = 1 - \exp\{-\alpha a^\delta\} \tag{6}$$

This equation can be linearized to the form

$$\log \ln \left[\frac{1}{1 - P} \right] = \log \alpha + \delta \log (a) \tag{7}$$

The Weibull distribution parameters, α and δ, are determined by plotting the log N fatigue life ($a = \log N$) versus the appropriate tabled median rank cumulative probability value (P) for the sample size of the treatment group [27]. A best fit line is fitted to this data by linear least squares regression, and from this plot, log α = y-axis intercept, and δ = slope of the plot. Once these parameters are determined, the mean and variance for the sample group can be calculated from the following equations [26]

$$\text{Mean:} \ \mu = \alpha^{-1/\delta} \Gamma \left[1 + \frac{1}{\delta} \right] \tag{8}$$

$$\text{Variance:} \ \sigma^2 = \alpha^{-2/\delta} \left\{ \Gamma \left[1 + \frac{2}{\delta} \right] - \left(\Gamma \left[1 + \frac{1}{\delta} \right] \right)^2 \right\} \tag{9}$$

where Γ is the gamma function. Based upon the central limit theorem of statistical analysis [28], a series of estimated means about the true mean for a skewed sample population will be approximately normally distributed. Therefore, a 95% confidence interval for a normal distribution can be calculated for each mean life value for a given treatment based upon a normal distribution. Once the mean, variance, and 95% confidence intervals about the mean are calculated for each applied stress level, *S*-log *N* plots can be created for the data. Comparisons can then be made between different test conditions using an appropriate significance test. This method of analysis is particularly useful for handling fatigue life data sets that contain run-outs. In this case, a Weibull cumulative distribution plot is made using median rank values for the total sample size tested (fatigued plus run-out specimens). Fatigue life values, however, are plotted only for the specimens that have successfully fatigued (fully debonded). A line is then least squares fitted to the distribution plot and, as before, the y-axis intercept and slope of the

TABLE 1—*Example of ordered fatigue life data for a Weibull cumulative distribution plot.*

N^a	$\log(N) = a$	$\log a$	P^b	$\log \ln (1/(1-P))$
16	1.21	0.082	0.109	−0.937
156	2.19	0.340	0.265	−0.511
210	2.32	0.365	0.421	−0.261
5731	3.76	0.575	0.578	−0.064
9119	3.96	0.597	0.734	+0.123
13 246	4.12	0.614	0.890	+0.345

$^a N$ = Ordered fatigue life values for set of specimens testing under given treatment.
$^b P$ = median rank values from Johnson [27].

best fit line used to determine the Weibull distribution parameters, α and δ, and the mean, variance, and 95% confidence interval for the data set are then calculated from Eqs 8 and 9.

This method is illustrated in the following example set of fatigue data which was obtained by Latour and Black [15] from an interfacial bond fatigue study for CF/PSF specimens tested in physiologic saline at an interfacial shear stress level set at 27% of its dry bond strength level. The fatigue life data for the set of six specimens tested are presented in Table 1 along with the analytical manipulations to put the data in the form necessary to plot the Weibull cumulative distribution shown in Fig. 10. The Weibull distribution parameters, α and δ, are calculated from a linear regression least squares fit line to the data plot. These parameters are then used in Eqs 8 and 9 to calculate that the mean and variance of the logarithm of fatigue life are 3.01 and 2.19, respectively. If the cut-off limit for this fatigue study had been set at 10 000 cycles ($\log N = 4$), following which the fatigue test would be suspended, then the last data point in Table 1 would have been a run-out. In this situation, the data would be exactly as given in Table 1 with the median rank value based upon all six specimens but with the exception that only the first five median rank values (P) would be plotted in the cumulative distribution plot

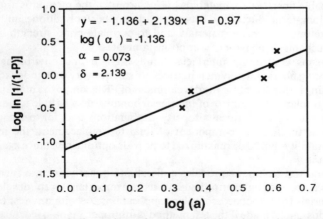

FIG. 10—*Hypothetical Weibull cumulative distribution plot based upon data from Table 1 and Eq 7. The Weibull distribution parameters (α and δ) are determined from the slope (slope = δ) and y-axis intercept (y-intercept = log [α]) of a linear regression line fitted to the plotted data points and then used to estimate the mean and variance of the fatigue life by Eqs 8 and 9.*

with estimated values of α and δ determined from the linear regression line fitted to the available data and used to estimate the mean and variance.

The interfacial bond fatigue behavior can also be characterized by a fracture mechanics based analysis. A fracture mechanics model of interfacial bond fatigue has been developed for this purpose [29] which relates interfacial bond crack propagation to the strain energy release rate similar to models previously developed and applied to characterize adhesive bond fatigue between two flat substrate materials [30]. This analysis is based upon the relationships

$$\frac{da}{dn} = c(G_{\mathrm{II}})^m; \frac{1}{c}\int_0^{a_c}(G_{\mathrm{II}})^{-m}da = N \tag{10}$$

where G_{II} is a function of the change in sample compliance per change in crack length. Latour et al. [29] reported on the development of an approximate expression for G_{II} for the fiber/microdroplet sample model. Using the strain energy release rate expression, Eq 10 can be integrated and the constants c and m derived from the fatigue test data for a given fiber/matrix combination and test environment.

Discussion and Concluding Remarks

The single fiber/microdroplet sample model has gained increased popularity since it was first reported in the literature in 1987. Since this time, over 45 publications have appeared in the composite science and engineering literature concerning the development and use of this test technique [20].

We believe that this test technique provides a very valuable tool for the development of fiber-reinforced polymer implant materials for orthopaedic applications. This method can be applied as a useful screening test to evaluate candidate FRP composite fiber/matrix combinations, and as a basic science tool to directly evaluate the effectiveness of fiber surface treatments or processing time-temperature profiles, or both, to optimize interfacial bonding and durability in the *in vivo* environment.

This method has most recently been applied to investigate the interfacial bond behavior between absorbable fiber/matrix materials [31]. Currently, the method is also being applied to investigate long-term durability between carbon fiber/polysulfone and carbon fiber/polyetheretherketone composite materials, and to correlate bond strength behavior to the macroscopic mechanical behavior of composite laminates.

The mechanisms controlling interfacial bond strength and environmental resistance between reinforcing fibers and polymer matrices are still not very well understood. We believe this understanding is important for the development of FRP composite materials: For absorbable composite implants, the control of interfacial bonding may be able to be applied toward controlling the rate of mechanical property degradation; and for permanent structural implants, such as the femoral component of total hip replacement, the interfacial bond strength and durability should be maximized to provide optimal resistance against fatigue failure of the implant.

The microbond test technique provides a direct and quantitative test method to address these material science and engineering issues which are important for the development of FRP composite materials for orthopaedic implant applications. As with any test technique, erroneous conclusions can be made if the test method is improperly employed. Over the past eight years, we have been working with and developing this technology with associated analytical methods for characterization of interfacial bond strength between fiber/matrix combinations of interest for the development of FRP composite materials for orthopaedic applications. The details of the sample fabrication, testing, and data analysis for the technique presented in this paper have been found to provide reproducible results that we believe accurately reflect actual interfacial bond strength conditions in composite materials.

Acknowledgments

The authors gratefully acknowledge Dr. Bernard Miller and the rest of the staff of TRI/Princeton for their valuable assistance in helping us to apply the microbond test method to address problems pertinent to the development of FRP composite materials for orthopaedic implant applications. The authors would also like to thank the National Science Foundation (NSF Grant ECE-86119897) and Osteonics Corp., Allendale, NJ, for providing the funding to conduct the research and development work.

APPENDIX 1

Shear-Lag Theory Derivation

A. Force equilibrium for element representing cross-section of fiber surrounded by matrix

$$\sum F_x = 0 = \left(\left[\sigma_x + \frac{d\sigma_x}{dx} \, dx \right] - \sigma_x \right) \pi r_i^2 + \tau_i(2\pi r_i) \, dx \tag{11}$$

B. Rearranging force equilibrium equation and differentiating with respect to x

$$\frac{d^2\sigma_x}{dx^2} + \frac{2}{r_i} \frac{d\tau_i}{dx} = 0 \tag{12}$$

C. Applying boundary conditions as shown in rod in cylinder model for Fig. 7

$$\text{At } r = r_i, u = u_i$$

$$\text{At } r = R, u = 0$$

$$\tau = G_m \frac{du}{dr}; \int_{u_i}^{0} du = \frac{1}{G_m} \int_{r_i}^{R} \tau \, dr; \text{ with } \tau = \frac{r_i}{r} \tau_i; u_i = \frac{-r_i\tau_i}{G_m} \ln \left[\frac{R}{r_i} \right] \tag{13}$$

D. Plug Eq 13 into stress-strain relation

$$\sigma_x = E_f \frac{du_i}{dx} = \frac{-r_i E_f}{G_m} \ln \left[\frac{R}{r_i} \right] \frac{d\tau_i}{dx}; \frac{d\tau_i}{dx} = \frac{-G_m}{r_i E_f \ln \left[\frac{R}{r_i} \right]} \sigma_x \tag{14}$$

E. Plug Eq 14 into Eq 13

$$\frac{d^2\sigma_x}{dx^2} - \frac{2G_m}{r_i^2 E_f \ln\left[\dfrac{R}{r_i}\right]} \sigma_x = 0; \text{ or } \frac{d^2\sigma_x}{dx^2} - \left[\frac{\beta}{D}\right]^2 \sigma_x = 0; \text{ with } \beta^2 = \frac{8G_m}{E_f \ln\left[\dfrac{R}{r_i}\right]} \quad (15)$$

F. Solving differential Eq 13

$$\sigma_x = A \cosh(\beta x) + B \sinh(\beta x) \quad (16)$$

G. Apply boundary conditions and referring to Fig. 7

At $x = 0$, $\sigma_x = 0$

At $x = L$, $\sigma_x = F/(\pi r^2)$

Solution:

$$\sigma_x = \frac{4F}{\pi D^2} \frac{\sinh(\beta x/D)}{\sinh(\beta L/D)} \quad (17)$$

$$\tau_i = \frac{-\beta F}{\pi D^2} \frac{\cosh(\beta x/D)}{\sinh(\beta L/D)} \quad (18)$$

(NOTE: If positive force applied (tensile force), shear stress acts on the positive r-surface on fiber in the negative x-direction, and vice versa. For the sake of simplicity, Eq 1 presents absolute magnitude of τ_i and thus the negative sign is dropped from the equation.)

References

[1] Skinner, H. B., "Composite Technology for Total Hip Arthroplasty,"*Clinical Orthopaedics and Related Research,* Vol. 235, 1988, pp. 224–236.
[2] Ali, M. S., French, T. A., Hastings, G. W., et al., "Carbon Fiber Composite Bone Plates. Development, Evaluation, and Early Clinical Experience," *Journal of Bone and Joint Surgery* (British), Vol. 72-B, 1990, pp. 586–591.
[3] Vainionpaa, S., Kilpikari, J., Laiho, J., et al., "Strength and Strength Retention *In Vitro* of Absorbable, Self-reinforced Polyglycolide (PGA) Rods for Fracture Fixation," *Biomaterials,* Vol. 8, 1987, pp. 46–48.
[4] Wright, T. M., Fukubayashi, T., and Burstein, A. H., "The Effect of Carbon Fiber Reinforcement on Contact Area, Constant Pressure, and Time-Dependent Deformation in Polyethylene Tibial Components," *Journal of Biomedical Materials Research,* Vol. 15, 1981, pp. 719–730.
[5] Plitz, W. and Walter, A., "Tribology of Carbon Fiber Reinforced Epoxy Resin Acetabular Cups," *Abstracts of the First World Congress of Biomechanics,* 30 August 1990–4 September 1990, La Jolla, CA, Vol. II, p. 345.
[6] Drzal, L. T., "Fiber-Matrix Interphase Structure and Its Effect on Adhesion and Composite Mechanical Properties," in *Controlled Interphases in Composite Materials,* H. Ishida, Ed., Elsevier Science Publishing Company Inc., NY, 1990, pp. 309–320.
[7] Hull, D., "Measurement of Bond Strength," in *An Introduction to Composite Materials,* Cambridge University Press, NY, pp. 48–57.
[8] DiBenedetto, A. T., Nicolais, L., Ambrosio, L., and Groeger, J., "Stress Transfer and Fracture in Single Fiber/Epoxy Composites," in *Composite Interfaces,* H. Ishida and J. L. Koenig, Eds., Elsevier Science Publishing Company Inc., NY, 1986, pp. 47–54.
[9] Mandell, J. F., Grande, D. H., Tsiang, T.-H., and McGarry, F. J., "Modified Microdebonding Test for Direct *In Situ* Fiber/Matrix Bond Strength Determination in Fiber Composites," *Composite Materials: Testing and Design (Seventh Conference), ASTM STP 893,* J. M. Whitney, Ed., American Society for Testing and Materials, Philadelphia, 1986, pp. 87–108.

[10] Broutman, L. J., "Measurement of the Fiber-Polymer Matrix Interfacial Strength," in *Interfaces in Composites, ASTM STP 452,* American Society for Testing and Materials, Philadelphia, 1969.

[11] Miller, B., Muri, P., and Rebenfeld, L., "A Microbond Method for Determination of the Shear Strength of a Fiber/Resin Interface,"*Composites Science and Technology,* Vol. 28, 1987, pp. 17–32.

[12] Latour, R. A. Jr., Black, J., and Miller, B., "Fracture Mechanisms of the Fiber/Matrix Interfacial Bond in Fiber Reinforced Polymer Composites," *Surface and Interface Analysis,* Vol. 17, 1991, pp. 477–484.

[13] Black, J., Latour, R. A. Jr., and Miller, B., "Failure of Desiccator Storage to Maintain Interfacial Bond Strength in Some Thermoplastic/Fiber Systems," *Journal of Adhesion Science Technology,* Vol. 3, 1989, pp. 65–67.

[14] Latour, R. A. Jr. and Black, J., *Miniature Closed-Loop Dynamic Universal Mechanical Testing Machine,* U.S. Patent 4,858,473, 22 August 1989, licensed to Dynatek Laboratories, Galena, MO.

[15] Latour, R. A. Jr., "In Vitro Simulation of In Vivo Dynamic Micromechanical Failure of Structural Composite Biomaterials," Doctoral dissertation, University of Pennsylvania, Philadelphia, December 1989 (University Microfilms International DA9015125, Ann Arbor, MI).

[16] Grayson, M. A. and Wolf, C. J., "The Solubility and Diffusion of Water in Poly(Aryl-Ether-Ether-Ketone) (PEEK)," *Journal of Polymer Science: Part B: Polymer Physics,* Vol. 25, 1987, pp. 31–41.

[17] Latour, R. A. Jr., Black, J., and Miller, B., "Durability of Fiber/Thermoplastic Composite Biomaterials: Passive Exposure to Physiologic Saline," *Transactions of the Society for Biomaterials,* Vol. 11, p. 470, 1988.

[18] Latour, R. A. Jr., Black, J., and Miller, B., "Interfacial Bond Degradation of Carbon Fiber-Polysulfone Thermoplastic Composite in Simulated *In Vivo* Environments," *Transactions of the Society for Biomaterials,* Vol. 13, 1990, p. 69.

[19] Latour, R. A., and Black, J., "Development of FRP Composite Structural Biomaterial: Ultimate Strength of the Fiber/Matrix Interfacial Bond in *In Vivo* Simulated Environments, *Journal of Biomedical Materials Research,* Vol. 26, 1992, pp. 593–606.

[20] TRI/Princeton, "Adhesion and Fiber Composites," *Progress Report No. 18, 7/1/91–12/31/91,* Princeton, NJ, March 92.

[21] Piggott, M. R., "Debonding and Friction at Fiber-Polymer Interfaces. I: Criteria for Failure and Sliding," *Composites Science and Technology,* Vol. 30, 1987, pp. 295–306.

[22] Hoffman, J. D., "Least Squares Approximation," Numerical Methods for Engineering and Scientists, McGraw-Hill, Inc., NY, 1992, pp. 144–155.

[23] Weibull, W., "A Statistical Distribution Function of Wide Applicability, *Journal of Applied Mechanics,* September 1951, pp. 293–297.

[24] Weibull, W., "Statistical Design of Fatigue Experiments," *Journal of Applied Mechanics,* March 1952, pp. 109–113.

[25] Little, R. E. and Jebe, E. H., "Fitting the P-N Curve to Ordered Life Data," in *Statistical Design of Fatigue Experiments,* ch. 12, John Wiley & Sons, NY, 1975, pp. 221–234.

[26] Miller, I. and Freund, J. E., "The Weibull Distribution," Section 4.9, in *Probability and Statistics for Engineers,* Prentice-Hall, Inc., Englewood Cliffs, NJ, 1984, pp. 121–123.

[27] Johnson, L. G., *The Statistical Treatment of Fatigue Experiments,* Elsevier Science Publishing Co., NY, 1964, pp. 3–48.

[28] Snedecor, G. W. and Cochran, W. G., "Frequency Distribution of Sample Means," *Statistical Methods,* 8th ed., ch. 4, Iowa State University Press, Ames, IA, 1989, pp. 44–48.

[29] Latour, R. A. Jr., Black, J., and Miller, B., "Fatigue Behavior Characterization of the Fiber-Matrix Interface," *Journal of Material Science,* Vol. 24, 1989, pp. 3616–3620.

[30] Mall, S. and Johnson, W. S., "Characterization of Mode I and Mixed-Mode Failure of Adhesive Bonds Between Composite Adherends," *Composite Materials: Testing and Design (Seventh Conference), ASTM STP 893,* J. M. Whitney, ed., American Society for Testing and Materials, Philadelphia, 1986, pp. 322–334.

[31] Leadbetter, K. J., Latour, R. A. Jr., Johnson, R. A., and Shalaby, S. W., "Micromechanical Testing of Interfacial Bonding in Absorbable Composites," *Biomaterials' Mechanical Properties, ASTM STP 1173,* H. E. Kambic and A. T. Yokobori, Jr., Eds., American Society for Testing and Materials, Philadelphia 1994, pp. 256–264 (this publication).

K. A. Jockisch,[1] S. A. Brown,[1]* and A. Moet[2]

The Use of Small-Scale Flexure Test Specimens to Evaluate the Mechanical Properties of Polymer Composites for Biomaterials Applications

REFERENCE: Jockisch, K. A., Brown, S. A., and Moet, A., "**The Use of Small-Scale Flexure Test Specimens to Evaluate the Mechanical Properties of Polymer Composites for Biomaterials Applications,**" *Biomaterials' Mechanical Properties, ASTM STP 1173*, H. E. Kambic and A. T. Yokobori, Jr., Eds., American Society for Testing and Materials, Philadelphia, 1994, pp. 212–224.

ABSTRACT: Miniflexbars (MFBs), 1 by 5 by 30 mm, which are tested in three-point bending, have been used to study the mechanical properties of polymer composites. Chopped carbon fiber reinforced polyetheretherketone (PEEK) injection-molded bendbars, 6 by 12 by 120 mm, were chosen for analysis. MFBs were cut parallel and perpendicular to the mold fill direction from four sections of the standard size bendbar. Results of the flexure testing indicated that the strength of the MFBs was significantly decreased from the strength of the standard size bendbar. Strength also varied with position of the MFB in the standard size bendbar. To better understand these results, several factors were evaluated. Upon cutting the MFBs from the injection-molded bar, residual stresses were relieved. The decrease in strength, however, could not be associated entirely with the release of residual stresses. Local fiber orientation was examined with light microscopy. Results from this analysis indicated that flexure testing of MFBs is sensitive to local variation in microstructure. Evaluation of an injection-molded chopped fiber composite bendbar using MFBs has indicated that these small-scale specimens can provide valuable information about the mechanical properties of polymer composites. With this understanding, MFBs can be used, with caution, in the development of *in vitro* and *in vivo* accelerated degradation test methods as well as other biomaterials applications.

KEYWORDS: composite, small-scale, polyetheretherketone (PEEK), flexure testing, orthopaedic materials

The potential benefits that may be derived from the incorporation of polymer composites in a variety of orthopaedic applications are beginning to be exploited. This is primarily due to the inherent nature of composites which enables the designer or manufacturer to compose a material that meets mechanical requirements. High-strength composites with stiffnesses near that of bone have been the impetus for the use of composites in fracture fixation plates [1,2] and total joint replacement [3,4]. Emphasis has been placed on carbon fiber reinforced thermoplastic composites primarily because of the good biological response to carbon and the resistance of thermoplastic polymers to degradation in an aqueous environment. Other advantages of thermoplastic matrix composites include the ability of thermoplastic materials to be

[1] Departments of Biomedical Engineering and [2]Macromolecular Science, Case Western Reserve University, Cleveland, OH 44106.
* To whom all correspondence should be addressed.

contoured [5] and the ease of processing that can be attained, especially with chopped fiber composites that are injection molded.

The use of composite materials in orthopaedic applications requires in-depth characterization of the mechanical properties of the material. Composite evaluation is not a straightforward task since mechanical and material properties of composites are critically dependent on processing conditions. As a consequence of processing, most composites exhibit local variation in microstructure. The ensuing anisotropy or heterogeneity, or both, results in a distribution of mechanical properties within the composite. Therefore, choosing specimens for testing can be quite difficult. One option is to have test specimens be individually molded. These specimens, however, run the risk of being quite different from the material that is used in a device. Another option is to cut specimens from a mother piece or from the device itself. If specimens are cut from representative sections, and the microstructure of these specimens is known, much information can be gained as to how a device may behave mechanically.

The objective of this study was to evaluate the use of small-scale flexure test specimens cut from a composite part as a method for characterizing the mechanical properties of polymer composites. Within this objective are four pertinent considerations. The first is the specification for small-scale specimens. A small specimen size is necessary so that local variations in mechanical properties can be detected. Keeping specimens small is also advantageous for statistical analysis, since many specimens can be tested. Also, for orthopaedic applications, small specimens can be readily used in aging experiments both *in vitro* and *in vivo,* even possibly accelerating these tests [6]. The potential benefit of the use of small-sized fracture toughness specimens has already been shown in the evaluation of bone cement and dental restorative materials [7].

A second consideration of the above objective is the condition for flexure test specimens. Flexure testing was chosen for two reasons: (1) the specimen shape is very simple, and (2) flexure tests are easy tests to execute. In addition, the use of small-scale flexure test specimens has been validated for testing bone cement and acrylic [8].

The third consideration in the objective is the need to cut the specimens from a composite part. A consequence of many composite processing methods is the introduction of residual stresses in the composite parts. In injection-molded materials, residual stresses are usually compressive near specimen surfaces and of a greater magnitude than the tensile stresses in the interior of the specimen [9]. By cutting specimens from molded parts, residual stresses may be relieved, and consequently effect flexure test values. Therefore, in order to evaluate the use of cut specimens for mechanical characterization of composites, residual stress analysis is required.

Finally, in order to implement our objective it was necessary to determine what polymer composite system to use for evaluation of the method. Injection-molded 30% chopped carbon fiber reinforced polyetheretherketone (CFRPEEK) was chosen. Although local variation in mechanical properties is observed with some continuous fiber composites as a consequence of generated internal stresses and morphological changes [10], heterogeneity is more readily apparent with chopped fiber composites, particularly those that are injection molded. Anisotropy in material properties of injection-molded short-fiber-reinforced thermoplastics is primarily related to flow-induced fiber orientation. The pre-eminence of fiber orientation in determining mechanical properties has been upheld by recent studies that have predicted properties with computer modeling based solely on fiber orientation [11,12]. Since fiber orientation plays such a key role in the ultimate mechanical properties of an injection-molded composite, and is easy to evaluate with microscopy, this investigation concentrated on evaluating an injection-molded composite.

The selection of CFRPEEK was based on its potential for a variety of medical applications. PEEK is one of the few matrix materials being considered for orthopaedic applications. A good short-term biological response to CFRPEEK has been demonstrated both *in vitro* [13] and *in vivo* [14]. Results from short-term environmental testing of continuous CFRPEEK in saline solution at elevated temperatures are also promising [15]. Additionally, the influence of microstructure on various properties of injection-molded CFRPEEK has been shown. Specifically, differences in thermoelastic properties were found in injection-molded dogbone tension specimens containing three distinct layers of fiber orientation [16]. This layering was also observed in injection-molded pin edge gated discs, with resulting anisotropic fracture properties [17].

Materials

Poly(etheretherketone) reinforced with 30% chopped carbon fiber (IM CFRPEEK) (450CA30, ICI) was injection molded (Dexter Composites, Cleveland, OH) into a mold with a side gate. High modulus 7-μm-diameter fibers (Hercules AS4) were used to reinforce the PEEK matrix.

Methods

Microstructure

Local microstructure of the IM CFRPEEK bars was evaluated using reflected light microscopy. Two bars were sectioned with a band saw into four equal sections (A,B,C,D). Each of these sections was cut in half either through the thickness or through the width, with a slow-speed saw and diamond wafering blade (Buehler-Isomet). The sections were then sanded and polished using metallographic technique, and viewed with a dissecting scope (Bausch and Lomb Stereozoom VB-73) and with a reflected light microscope (Ziess-Photo One) for global fiber orientation and distribution.

Density

The density of selected specimens (Z MFBs, see below) was determined using Archimedes principle in accordance with ASTM D 792, Test Methods for Specific Gravity (Relative Density) and Density of Plastics by Displacement. A density determination kit (Mettler) was used in conjunction with an analytical balance (Mettler AE163). The specimens were conditioned (as suggested by ASTM D 792) by being immersed in boiling distilled water and then being placed under vacuum to avoid the entrapment of air bubbles by surface irregularities.

Flexure Testing

The injection-molded bendbar was cut into miniflexbars (MFBs) as illustrated in Fig. 1. One bendbar was cut into sections A, B, C, and D using a bandsaw. Each section was then cut through the width (in the X-Z plane, perpendicular to the Y axis) using a diamond blade on a low-speed saw (Buehler). As-cut Y-MFBs were approximately 1 by 6 by 30 mm. The edges of each MFB were lightly sanded with 240 grit carborundum paper. The surface MFBs, which were the first or the last cut (and therefore may have been cut irregularly), were sanded to uniform dimensions only on the cut (not the surface) side. Another bendbar was also cut into sections A, B, C, and D. Each section was then cut through the thickness into Z-MFBs. Z-MFBs were cut in the X-Y plane perpendicular to the Z-axis. As-cut z-MFBs were approximately 1 by 5 by 30 mm. Once again the surface sections were sanded to uniformity on the cut side if necessary.

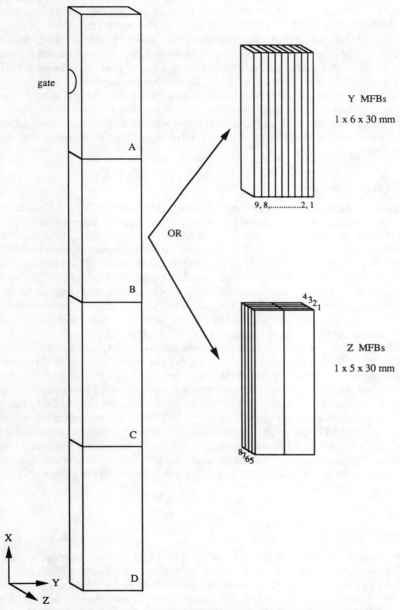

FIG. 1—*Sectioning of 30% CFRPEEK injection-molded bendbar into MFBs.*

MFBs were tested in three-point bending. Other than the choice of specimen size (1 by 5 by 30 mm), ASTM D 790, Test Methods for Flexural Properties of Unreinforced and Reinforced Plastics, was followed using a testing jig with a constant support span of 16.07 mm. Radius of curvature of the loading nose and supports was 1.2 mm. The MFBs were tested with a screw-driven mechanical test machine (SCOTT-CRE/1000) at a strain rate of 0.01 mm/mm-min (0.5 mm/min cross-head rate). An extensometer (MTS model 632-118-20) was used to measure deflection. The extensometer was attached to the moving loading nose and the stationary supports. Y and Z MFBs were tested to failure using a 245-N load cell. The edge MFBs were tested with the surface side down (in tension). X-Y plots were recorded.

Maximum flexural stress, axial strain at maximum stress, and flexural modulus were calculated from the curves. Strain was analyzed at maximum stress for consistency, since the load deflection traces after the point of maximum stress was reached varied between specimens. Results of flexure testing were statistically analyzed using the BMDP Statistical Software package (1988 release).

Residual Stress Measurements

To determine if residual stresses are relieved upon cutting the MFBs, and to determine an approximate magnitude of these stresses, a technique was employed using strain gages. Strain gages have been previously used for directly determining the residual stress distribution in molded plastic pipes [18]. A single 120-Ω gage (Micro Measurements Compression/Tension EA-13-125-BB-120) was bonded with extra solder tabs (M-bond 200) to the surface of an injection-molded CFRPEEK bendbar. This bar served as a control. Another CFRPEEK bendbar was gaged similarly. The gage on the control bendbar was hooked into a quarter bridge circuit using a strain gage conditioner (2120A, Measurements Group). The bridge was balanced and the gage calibrated. The gage on the other bendbar replaced the control gage in the circuit. Any difference (usually slight) between the output for the two gages was noted.

The ends of the test bendbar were cut on a bandsaw so that the gaged section would be able to be cut on the diamond saw. Once the ends were cut, the output of the gage was tested against the control gage. Any change in microstrain was noted. The lead wires were removed from the solder tabs of the test bendbar. On the diamond saw, approximately 1 mm (similar to the depth of a MFB) was cut from the bendbar. The resulting slice, with the gage still attached, was air dried, and the lead wires reattached to the solder tabs of the gage. Once again the output of this gage was compared with that of the control gage. Any change in microstrain was noted. The block that remained after slicing was then gaged and the entire process repeated. Microstrain measurements were obtained for three sequential slices through the thickness of the bendbar. To consider possible viscoelastic effects, each slice was remeasured after two weeks.

Results

Microstructure

The general pattern of fiber distribution in the 6 by 12 by 120 mm bendbar is indicated in Fig. 2. This distribution pattern was found to be repeated in different CFRPEEK bendbars from the same processing lot. Arrows indicate locations where the reflected light micrographs (Fig. 3.) were taken. For ease in terminology, those fibers aligned parallel with the X axis are denoted as X fibers, parallel with the Y axis as Y fibers, and parallel with the Z axis as Z fibers. The following observations pertain to the fiber orientation observed in the X-Y plane, although similar observations are also evident in the X-Z plane. Note that in Section A, where the gate is located, the fibers are not aligned at the surface. Reflected light micrographs of the corners

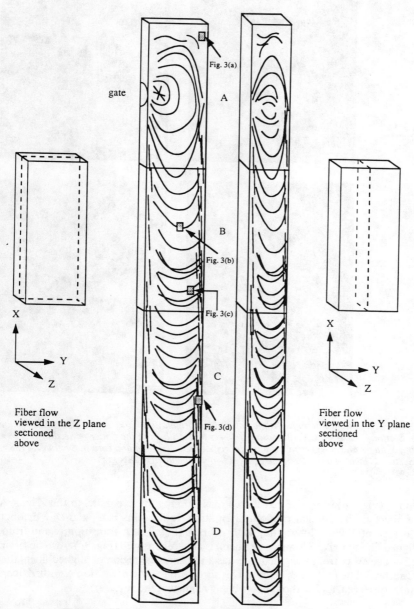

FIG. 2—*Fiber flow in 30% CFRPEEK injection-molded bendbar.*

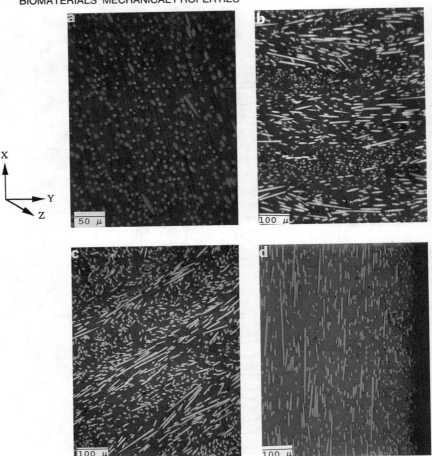

X
Y
Z

FIG. 3—*Reflected light micrographs indicating fiber orientation in the 30% CFRPEEK bendbar. (a) Corner of Section A (256×). (b) Alternating Y fibers and Z fibers in the center of Section B (128×). (c) Alternating Y fibers and Z fibers in a transition region between edge and core in Section B (128×). (d) Edge of Section C located away from the gated side of the bendbar (128×).*

of Section A (Fig. 3a) illustrate that there are also many fibers parallel to the Z axis. At the gate, the fibers are in a planar random orientation. In Sections B, C, and D, a distinct flow pattern is seen of Y fibers alternating with Z fibers (Fig. 3b). A transition region from edge (fully aligned fibers) to core (transverse fibers) is apparent as well (Fig. 3c). Also observed was that the surface away from the gated side has a thicker edge region of aligned fibers than the opposite surface. The bottom of Section D is similar to the top of Section A with Z fibers predominantly observed, and without fibers being aligned at the surface.

Density

The results of the density experiments are shown in Table 1. The average density of the composite was 1.4140 g/cm³. A significant difference was found for density between Sections A&D and Sections B&C, with sections A&D having the lower density.

Flexure Testing

Trends in ultimate flexural stress with position of the MFB in the bendbar are indicated in Fig. 4. The lines in each graph connect individual data points. Three features can be observed in these graphs. First, the strengths in Sections B, C, and D are greater for MFBs located at the edge of the intact bendbar than those in the core of the bendbar. This is most readily seen for the Z MFBs, although it is apparent for the Y MFBs as well. Second, the strengths of the MFBs are greater for those MFBs located away from the gate. For the Z MFBs, "away" is considered to be MFBs 1,2,3, and 4 and "near" is considered to be MFBs 5,6,7, and 8. For the Y MFBs, away MFBs are 1,2,3, and 4 and near MFBS are 6,7,8, and 9. The graphs of the Y MFBs show an increasing trend as the distance from the gated side of the intact bendbar is increased. Finally, the strengths of the MFBs tend to be greater for those MFBs located in Sections B and C compared to those in Sections A and D.

Means and standard deviations are listed in Table 2. (For all statistical analysis MFBs, AZ3, BZ6, and CZ8 were deleted from analysis because they were cut less than 0.8 mm thick.) Sample groups are defined as the following: All MFBs includes both the Y MFBs and Z MFBs; A&D includes all MFBs in Sections A and D from both the Y MFBs and Z MFBs (the Y and Z MFBs were combined since a significant difference was not found between these two groups for stress, strain, or modulus, Table 3.); B&C includes those MFBs in Sections B and C. The MFBs in Sections A and D were grouped together, and the MFBs in Sections B and C were grouped together due to the similar microstructure between these groups as previously discussed. This grouping also increased the sample size which facilitated statistical analysis.

In Table 2, the average flexural stress for all MFBs (both Y and Z) is 280.0 ± 37.9 MPa. This is significantly less than 314.0 ± 3.8, the average strength of intact injection-molded bendbars tested in three-point bend [5]. This strength is indicated in Fig. 4 by the dotted line at 314 MPa.

Statistical differences between group means were determined at $p \leq 0.05$ using Student's t-test for the groups listed in Table 2. The pooled test was used if Levene's test for equality of variances was not significant, otherwise the t-test using separate variances was used. Ten comparisons between group means were made within the data set; therefore, the Bonferroni correction for multiple comparions was applied. Using this conservative correction, a p-value $\leq$ 0.005 is required for significance at the 0.05 level.

TABLE 1—*Density of Z MFBs.*

	N	Density, g/cm^3 Avg.	Std.
Z MFBs	32	1.4140	0.0014
AZ	8	1.4141	0.0019
BZ	8	1.4145	0.0009
CZ	8	1.4146	0.0011
DZ	8	1.4129	0.0009
BZ,CZ[a]	16	1.4146	0.0010
edge	8	1.4146	0.0011
core	8	1.4146	0.0009
AZ,DZ[a]	16	1.4135	0.0016
edge	8	1.4135	0.0021
core	8	1.4136	0.0009

[a] $P = 0.0451$ (separate variances).

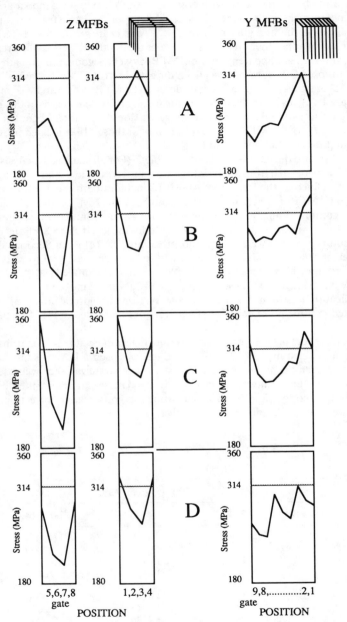

FIG. 4—*Trends in ultimate flexural stress with position of the MFB bendbar.*

TABLE 2—*Means and standard deviations for sample groups.*

	N	Stress (MPa)	Strain (%)	Modulus (GPa)
All MFBs	65	280.02 (37.93)	3.21 (0.54)	13.50 (3.05)
Y MFBs	33	281.78 (29.80)	3.27 (0.56)	13.66 (2.90)
Z MFBs	32	278.20 (45.24)	3.14 (0.52)	13.34 (3.24)
AD	33	266.93 (35.25)	3.58 (0.48)	11.82 (2.51)
away	15	291.84 (23.10)	3.33 (0.36)	13.50 (0.33)
near	16	244.47 (30.86)	3.78 (0.47)	10.31 (2.03)
edge	12	272.64 (38.72)	3.39 (0.35)	12.20 (2.68)
core	21	263.67 (33.65)	3.69 (0.51)	11.60 (0.51)
BC	32	293.52 (36.30)	2.82 (0.26)	15.24 (2.56)
away	16	305.87 (28.09)	2.74 (2.13)	16.18 (2.11)
near	14	280.38 (42.94)	2.88 (0.31)	14.25 (2.88)
edge	12	324.46 (20.62)	2.65 (0.16)	17.19 (1.44)
core	20	274.95 (30.59)	2.92 (0.26)	14.08 (2.39)

The results of statistical analysis are indicated in Table 3. Significant differences were found between Sections A&D and B&C for stress, strain, and modulus. Significant differences were also found between Sections A&D and B&C for the groups that are more descriptively defined. For instance, stress, strain, and modulus differ significantly for the A&D MFBs located near the gated side versus the B&C MFBs located in similar positions. This is also true for the A&D edge MFBs versus the B&C edge MFBs. Strain and modulus are significant between the A&D and B&C sections for those MFBs located away from the gated side, as well as for those MFBs located in the core. Within Section B&C a significant difference was found between edge MFBs and core MFBs for stress strain and modulus. A significant difference was not found between the MFBs located away from the gated side and those MFBs located near the gated side,

TABLE 3—*P-values for differences in group means using Student's t-test with separate variances.*

Group	Stress	Strain	Modulus
Y vs Z	0.7073	0.3314	0.6740
AD vs BC	0.0039[a]	0.0000[a]	0.0000[a]
BC			
Away vs near	0.0615	0.1723	0.0503
Edge vs core	0.0001[a]	0.0029[a]	0.0019[a]
AD			
Away vs near	0.0000[a]	0.0058	0.0001[a]
Edge vs core	0.7183	0.0595	0.8671
AD vs BC			
Away	0.2245	0.0000[a]	0.0017[a]
Near	0.0031[a]	0.0000[a]	0.0003[a]
Edge	0.0005[a]	0.0000[a]	0.0000[a]
Core	0.1618	0.0000[a]	0.0005[a]

[a] Significant at 0.05 level using Bonferroni's correction for multiple comparisons.

TABLE 4—*Residual strain/stress measurements in the CFRPEEK bendbar. Results are given as microstrain/stress. Microstrain was determined from the strain gage recordings. Stress was calculated using the microstrain measurements and Hooke's law. Percent error was determined as (residual stress/average stress) × 100. For Slice #1 avg. modulus and avg. stress recorded for the BC edge MFBs were used in the calculations. For Slices #2 and #3 avg. modulus and avg. stress recorded for BC core MFBs were used in the calculations.*

| | | Strain (μ strain)/Stress MPa | | |
Slice	Thickness, mm	Reading 1	Reading 2	% Error[a]
#1	1.2	+730/+12.56	+750/+12.90	3.9
#2	1.2	+1650/+23.23	+1640/+23.09	8.4
#3	0.9	−250/−3.52	−420/−5.91	2.1

[a] Residual stress/avg. stress × 100.

although the *p*-values are quite low. Within Sections A&D a significant difference was found between the away MFBs and the near MFBs for stress and modulus; however, a significant difference was not found between edge and core MFBs.

Residual Stresses

The results of residual stress measurements are given in Table 4. Slices #1 and #2 experienced positive strain when cut, and Slice #3 experienced negative strain. The average flexural modulus of the BC edge MFBs for Slice #1 and the average flexural modulus of the BC core MFBs for Slices #2 and #3 were used in Hooke's law ($\sigma = E\epsilon$) to determine approximate axial stress relieved. As seen in Table 4, the outer 2.4 mm of the bendbar is in residual compression, and the core is in residual tension.

Discussion

By looking back at the fiber orientation in Figs. 2 and 3, and considering statistical differences found in the flexure testing data, a correlation between microstructure and mechanical properties can be observed. First and most obviously, the aligned surface fibers in Sections B and C provide extra strength, since the fibers are aligned perpendicular to the fracture plane, whereas in the core region the fibers are either at an angle, or parallel to the fracture plane. In Section A, where there is little alignment of surface fibers, the edge/core strength trend is not observed. This also gives evidence that the surface finish, which is present on the edge MFBs in Section A, is not important for increasing the strength of the composite.

The differences, especially in Sections A and D, between those MFBs located near the gate and those located away from the gate, can also be related to differences in fiber orientation and distribution. In Section A, it is apparent that the fibers are more heavily distributed away from the gate as compared to near the gate. This asymmetry is most likely due to the location of the gate on the side of the bar.

The overall differences between Sections A&D and Sections B&C, although predominantly orientation effects, may also be fiber volume fraction effects as indicated by the decrease in density for the fibers in Sections A and D. Density in a composite is a function of the volume fraction of matrix material and the volume fraction of reinforcing material, carbon fibers. The density of the carbon fibers is approximately 1.77 g/cm³. However, since PEEK is a semicrystalline thermoplastic, matrix density depends on the volume fraction of crystalline material which has a density of 1.4006 g/cm³ and the volume fraction of amorphous material which has a density of 1.2626 g/cm^3 [*19*]. Therefore, the differences in density observed in Table 1 could be a consequence of a change in matrix crystallinity or in a change in the fiber volume fraction, either of which are microstructural changes.

The impact of released residual stresses on the values of MFB flexural strength seems to be minor. Although values have been recorded in Table 4, the absolute magnitudes can only be used as guides due to the assumptions involved in calculating the stress. These assumptions include: (1) stress is only relieved in the axial direction, (2) the gates are aligned perfectly with the axis (this is difficult since there is a slight bend in the bar) and (3) the stress can be calculated using Hooke's law. Also, the viscoelastic nature of the material is unknown. Despite these assumptions it can be concluded that there are residual stresses that may cause an error of between 2.1% and 8.4%. These stresses are small, however, and cannot account for the differences observed between MFBs or between the overall average strength of the MFBs and the intact bendbar.

Although the release of residual stresses cannot explain why the average strength of all the MFBs is less than that of the intact bendbar, fiber orientation effects can. An examination of Fig. 4 indicates that the strength of the edge MFBs in Sections B and C are similar to the ultimate flexural strength of the intact bar [*5*]. This is not surprising since in three-point bending the properties of the surface of the bendbar at the middle of the bar are critical for ultimate flexural strength. The surfaces of the edge MFBs in Sections B and C are similar to the surface of the central section of the intact bendbar (where it was tested). Therefore, one hypothesis for the decrease in strength is that in effect, three-point bend testing of the intact bendbar is almost the same as three-point bend testing the edge MFBs of Sections B and C. Because of the differences found between the MFBs and standard size specimens, data obtained using the MFBs should not be substituted (or used with great caution) for standard specimen size data for other engineering applications.

These results indicate that the MFBs are sensitive to local microstructural differences described globally as edge or core, Sections A&D or Sections B&C, and away from the gated side or near the gated side. In many of the same sample groups both stress and modulus were significantly different. This implies that both elastic behavior (as described by modulus) and plastic behavior (as described by ultimate stress) of the composite are effected by local microstructure and can be detected by the MFBs.

Conclusions

Flexural properties of injection-molded 30% chopped carbon fiber reinforced PEEK have been characterized using small-scale flexure test specimens. These specimens were used to better understand the relationship between local microstructure and mechanical properties. As a consequence of this characterization, these small-scale specimens may be used in subsequent degradation studies or other applications.

References

[*1*] McKenna, G. B., Bradley, G. W., Dunn, H. K., and Statton, W. O., "Mechanical Properties of Some Fiber Reinforced Polymer Composites After Implantation as Fracture Fixation Plates," *Biomaterials,* Vol. 1, 1980.

[*2*] Gillette, N., Brown, S. A., Dumbleton, J. H., and Pool, R. P., "The Use of Short Carbon Fiber Reinforced Thermoplastic Plates for Fracture Fixation," *Biomaterials,* Vol. 6, 1985, pp. 113–121.

[*3*] Skinner, H. B., "Composite Technology for Total Hip Arthroplasty,"*Clinical Orthopaedics and Related Research,* Vol. 235, 1988, pp. 224–236.

[*4*] Maggee, F. B., Weinstein, A. M., Longo, J. A., et al., "A Canine Composite Femoral Stem: An *In Vivo* Study," *Clinical Orthopaedics and Related Research,* Vol. 235, 1988, pp. 237–252.

[5] Mason, J. J., Brown, S. A., and Moet, A., "An Evaluation of the Use of Infrared Heating for Contouring 30% Short-Fiber-Reinforced PEEK," *Journal of Materials Science: Materials in Medicine,* Vol. 3, 1992, pp. 88–94.

[6] Wagner, H. D., "Statistical Concepts in the Study of Fracture Properties of Fibers and Composites," in *Application of Fracture Mechanics to Composite Materials,* K. Friedrich, Ed., Elsevier, 1989, pp. 39–77.

[7] Pilliar, R. M., Vowles, R., and Williams, D. F., "Note: Fracture Toughness Testing of Biomaterials Using Mini-Short Rod Specimen Design," *Journal of Biomedical Materials Research,* Vol. 21, 1987, pp. 145–154.

[8] Brown, S. A. and Bargar, W. L., "The Influence of Temperature and Specimen Size on the Flexural Properties of PMMA Bone Cement," *Journal of Biomedical Materials Research,* Vol. 18, 1984, pp. 523–536.

[9] Nimmer, R. P. and Tantina, G. G., "Design for Ultimate Strength with a Chopped Glass-Filled Phenolic Composite: Critical Flaw Sensitivity, Residual Stress, Fiber Orientation," *Recent Advances in Composites in the United States and Japan, ASTM STP 864,* J. R. Vinson and M. Taya, Eds., American Society for Testing and Materials, Philadelphia, 1985, pp. 556–582.

[10] Lawrence, W. E., Manson, J.-A. E., and Seferis, J. C., "Thermal and Morphological Skin-Core Effects in Processing of Thermoplastic Composites," *Composites,* Vol. 21, 1990, pp. 475–480.

[11] Ranganathan, S. and Advani, S. G., "Characterization of Orientation Clustering in Short-Fiber Composites," *Journal of Polymer Science, Part B: Polymer Physics,* Vol. 28, 1990, pp. 2651–2672.

[12] Matsuoka, T., Takabatake, J.-I., Inoue, Y., and Takahashi, H., "Prediction of Fiber Orientation in Injection Molded Parts of Short-Fiber-Reinforced Thermoplastics," *Polymer Eng. Sci.,* Vol. 30, No. 16, 1990, pp. 957–966.

[13] Wenz, L. M., Merritt, K., Brown, S. A., and Moet, A., "*In Vitro* Biocompatibility of Polyetheretherketone and Polysulfone Composites," *Journal of Biomedical Materials Research,* Vol. 24, 1990, pp. 207–215.

[14] Jockisch, K. A., Brown, S. A., Bauer, T. W., and Merritt, K., "Biological Response to Chopped-Carbon-Fiber-Reinforced PEEK," *Journal of Biomedical Materials Research,* Vol. 26, No. 2, 1992, pp. 133–146.

[15] Maharaj, G. R., Strait, L. H., Gavens, A. J., and Jamison, R. D., "Characterization of Creep and Environmental Effects on Composite Materials for Human Hip Prostheses," *Proceedings of the 8th International Conference on Composite Materials,* Honolulu, HI, 15–19 July 1991.

[16] Bozarth, M. J., Gillespie, J. W., and McCullough, R. L., "Fiber Orientation and Its Effects Upon Thermoelastic Properties of Short Carbon Fiber Reinforced Poly(etheretherketone) (PEEK), *Polymer Composites,* Vol. 8, No. 2, 1987, pp. 74–81.

[17] Friedrich, K., Walter, R., Voss, H., and Karger-Kocsis, J., "Effect of Short Fibre Reinforcement on the Fatigue Crack Propagation and Fracture of PEEK-Matrix Composites," *Composites,* Vol. 17, 1986, pp. 205–216.

[18] Chaoui, K., Moet, A., and Chudnovsky, A., "Strain Gage Analysis of Residual Stress in Plastic Pipes," *Journal of Testing and Evaluation,* Vol. 16, No. 3, 1988, pp. 286–290.

[19] Blundell, D. J. and Osborne, B. N., "The Morphology of Poly(aryl-ether-ether-ketone)," *Polymer,* Vol. 24, 1983, pp. 953–958.

Jeremy L. Gilbert[1] and De Rei Dong[1]

A Numerical Time-Frequency Transform Technique for the Determination of the Complex Modulus of Composite and Polymeric Biomaterials from Transient Time-Based Experiments

REFERENCE: Gilbert, J. L. and Dong, D. R., **"A Numerical Time-Frequency Transform Technique for the Determination of the Complex Modulus of Composite and Polymeric Biomaterials from Transient Time-Based Experiments,"***Biomaterials' Mechanical Properties, ASTM STP 1173*, H. E. Kambic and A. T. Yokobori, Jr., Eds., American Society for Testing and Materials, Philadelphia, 1994, pp. 225–244.

ABSTRACT: A numerical time-frequency transform technique is described that can be used to determine the complex modulus of a material as a function of frequency from stress relaxation experiments. This technique uses analog-to-digital data acquisition techniques to obtain the time domain response over several decades of time. Numerical filtering techniques are then applied to reduce spurious noise. An exponential interpolating function is fit to the relaxation data and this function is then transformed into the frequency domain with the use of piece-wise integration of the Laplace transform. The error associated with the numerical transform technique is found to be very small (on the order of 10^{-4}%) when analyzing ideal behavior.

An experimental apparatus is developed and used in conjunction with this technique and initial tests of poly(methyl methacrylate) (PMMA) and polyethylene (PE), and PMMA/GF composites reveal that relaxation peaks (maximums in the loss modulus) associated with molecular transitions in the polymers can be detected with this method. Modulus-temperature-frequency plots indicate that the methodology is able to detect changes in peaks with increasing or decreasing temperature and that some of these peaks appear to correlate with known molecular transitions.

KEYWORDS: complex modulus, Laplace transform, stress relaxation, viscoelasticity, numerical methods, dynamic mechanical properties, poly(methyl methacrylate) (PMMA), composites

The dynamic mechanical properties of viscoelastic materials are of great concern in biomaterials applications. Diverse phenomena such as orthodontic band relaxation, cold flow of ultrahigh molecular weight polyethylene (PE), and creep and fatigue fracture of acrylic bone cement are just a few examples where the viscoelastic behavior of a biomaterial impacts on its performance. The viscoelastic response of a tissue, polymer, or composite material to an applied stress depends on the long-range and short-range molecular motions of the polymeric chains in the material in question. These motions result in time (or frequency) dependent primary transitions (glass transition or melting point) or secondary transitions (short chain segment motions or side group rotations) which can impact on the performance of the biomaterial over time. For instance, it has been shown [1] that the fatigue behavior of polymers and

---

[1] Associate professor and graduate student, respectively, Division of Biological Materials, Northwestern University, Chicago, IL 60611.

composites can be affected by the presence and frequency of secondary relaxation processes in the polymer. Thus, it is essential to understand the effect of primary and secondary transitions of viscoelastic materials on their durability, subjected to the variable loading associated with long-term implantation in specific medical applications.

Tests to assess the viscoelastic behavior of materials have centered on the use of dynamic mechanical analysis techniques (DMA) which determine the complex modulus of composite and polymeric biomaterials [2,3]. These techniques typically apply a small amplitude, sinusoidally varying forcing function (cyclic strain), and measure the response function (cyclic stress) and phase lag (or loss tangent, tan δ). In turn, these data yield critical information about the elastic storage and viscous dissipation of energy in the material and the molecular processes that result in the relaxation processes observed. These tests are usually performed over a range of temperatures at a set frequency and are used to determine the primary (glass transition) and secondary relaxation processes (also known as β, γ . . . relaxations).

There are several limitations with these techniques relating to the geometry of the specimen, loading configurations, range of moduli measurable, and the limited range of frequencies that can be analyzed. Also, temperature increases during testing can result in modification of the polymer or composite by continued curing, volatilization of diluent or residual monomer, stress relief, and modification of structure via heat treatment. While DMA is still the technique of choice in characterization of polymer dynamic behavior, the advent of analog-to-digital computer data acquisition techniques and post-collection numerical analysis has provided a new means of assessing dynamic mechanical behavior.

This paper describes a novel method that can be used in place of these frequency based tests that uses the properties of time-frequency transforms (i.e., Laplace transforms) to take transient-time (i.e., stress relaxation or creep) data and transform them into the frequency domain. The strength of this technique is that a frequency range from 0.0001 Hz to 100 Hz can be analyzed from a single transient time test in the course of 15 min. Another strength of this transform technique is that a relatively simple stress relaxation or creep test methodology can be used. Therefore, a wide range of geometries, loading patterns, and moduli can be assessed. The errors associated with the data collection and analysis techniques will be discussed.

This technique can provide valuable information about primary and secondary relaxation processes in polymers and composites, both of which may play significant roles in their fatigue and degradation behavior [1]. Examples of the viscoelastic behavior of Poly(methyl methacrylate) (PMMA), PE, and some PMMA-based experimental composites will be presented.

The nondestructive nature of this test provides a means of assessing the change in complex stiffness of a material or structure due to fatigue damage, fluid absorption, or other material degradation mechanisms. Thus, a single specimen can be monitored throughout its test lifetime.

Mathematical Development

The mechanical analog will be discussed in this paper; however, it must be kept in mind that this method can be applied to any relaxation experiment irrespective of what is to be measured (e.g., dielectric relaxation, electrochemical impedance, etc.).

The technique to be used to convert the data from a time domain to a frequency domain is a numerical Laplace transform method. The Laplace transform is of the form

$$F(s) = \mathcal{L}[f(t)] = \int_0^\infty f(t)e^{-st}dt \qquad (1)$$

where $s = a + i\omega$ in the limit as $a \to 0$, and $i = \sqrt{-1}$. In the limit as $a \to 0$, $s = i\omega$ and Eq 1 becomes

$$F(\omega) = \int_0^\infty f(t)e^{-i\omega t}dt \tag{2}$$

Thus, it can be seen that the Laplace transform expression is derived from a "unilateral Fourier transform," multiplied by a convergence factor. An advantage of the Laplace transform is that it is particularly well suited for situations where step-type forcing functions are found (as in our situation). The specifics of the Laplace transform and its applications will not be presented at this point. However, a development of the expressions for use in our measurements will be given.

Generalized Laplace Transform of Stress-Strain Data

In linear systems terminology, where one is considering a system's response, the ratio of the Laplace transform of the output to the Laplace transform of the input is known as the transfer function for the system [4]. In the case of time dependent mechanical testing, the transfer function is the complex modulus ($E^*(\omega)$).

$$E^*\omega = \frac{\mathcal{L}[\sigma(t)]}{\mathcal{L}[\varepsilon(t)]} = E' + iE'' \tag{3}$$

where $\mathcal{L}$ denotes the Laplace transform of the functions. It should be noted that the creep compliance and the complex modulus can be related to one another in the frequency domain as follows

$$E^*(\omega) = \frac{1}{J^*(\omega)}, \qquad J' + iJ'' = \frac{E' - iE''}{E'^2 + E''^2} \tag{4}$$

This relationship demonstrates that there is a direct mathematical link between creep and stress relaxation experiments.

If Eq 2 is substituted into Eq 3 for both stress and strain and the real and imaginary parts are separated, then the following generalized equations for the storage and loss moduli result

$$E'(\omega) = \frac{\int_0^\infty \sigma(t) \cos \omega t \, dt \int_0^\infty \varepsilon(t) \cos \omega t \, dt + \int_0^\infty \sigma(t) \sin \omega t \, dt \int_0^\infty \varepsilon(t) \sin \omega t \, dt}{\left(\int_0^\infty \varepsilon(t) \cos \omega t \, dt\right)^2 + \left(\int_0^\infty \varepsilon(t) \sin \omega t \, dt\right)^2} \tag{5}$$

$$E''(\omega) = \frac{\int_0^\infty \sigma(t) \cos \omega t \, dt \int_0^\infty \varepsilon(t) \sin \omega t \, dt - \int_0^\infty \sigma(t) \sin \omega t \, dt \int_0^\infty \varepsilon(t) \cos \omega t \, dt}{\left(\int_0^\infty \varepsilon(t) \cos \omega t \, dt\right)^2 + \left(\int_0^\infty \varepsilon(t) \sin \omega t \, dt\right)^2} \tag{6}$$

These equations can be used when an arbitrary strain path is chosen and the stress response is measured. The only limitation on this equation is that the time frame for the collection must be long enough to include all of the relaxation frequencies. Equations 5 and 6 have been presented elsewhere in the development of electrochemical impedance techniques [5].

Laplace Transform of Stress Relaxation Experiments

Stress relaxation experiments represent a special case of the generalized Laplace transform previously described. From Fig. 1 we see that in a stress relaxation experiment, a step-in-strain input is applied and the output, or response function, is how the stress decays over time. The time dependent (or relaxation) modulus is thus just

$$E(t) = \frac{\sigma(t)}{\varepsilon_0 u[t]}, \qquad u[t] = \begin{matrix} 0 \text{ if } t < 0 \\ 1 \text{ if } t > 0 \end{matrix} \qquad (7)$$

where ε_0 is the magnitude of the applied strain, $u[t]$ is known as the unit step function, and σ is the stress response. To get the complex modulus as a function of frequency we need to expand upon Eq 3.

To find the Laplace transform of the forcing function we need to know the Laplace transform of a step function

$$\mathcal{L}[\varepsilon_0 u[t]] = \frac{\varepsilon_0}{s} \qquad (8)$$

Now, the transfer function $E^*(s)$ is of the form

$$E^*(s) = \frac{1}{\varepsilon_0} s\mathcal{L}[\sigma[t]] \qquad (9)$$

but

$$s\mathcal{L}[\sigma(t)] = \mathcal{L}[\sigma'(t)] + \sigma_0 \qquad (10)$$

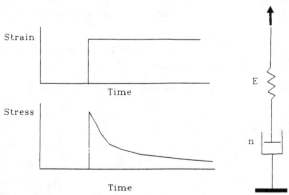

FIG. 1—*Schematic of a stress relaxation experiment where an instantaneous step in strain is applied to a Maxwell element model and the stress response is monitored.*

where $\sigma'(t)$ is the time derivative of the stress function and σ_0 is the stress at $t = 0$. The complex modulus (or transfer function) is then

$$E^*(\omega) = \frac{1}{\varepsilon_0} \int_0^\infty \sigma'(t) e^{-i\omega t} dt + \frac{\sigma_0}{\varepsilon_0} \qquad (11)$$

Therefore, we have an expression that will determine $E^*(\omega)$ as a function of frequency based on measurements of a time-based experiment where the forcing function is a step function in strain. Breaking the complex modulus up into its real and imaginary components yields

$$E'(\omega) = \frac{1}{\varepsilon_0} \int_0^\infty \sigma'(t) \cos \omega t \, dt + \frac{\sigma_0}{\varepsilon_0} \qquad (12)$$

and

$$E''(\omega) = -\frac{1}{\varepsilon_0} \int_0^\infty \sigma'(t) \sin \omega t \, dt \qquad (13)$$

Equations 12 and 13 are the foundation upon which the present analysis is based.

To demonstrate that one does, in fact, obtain the frequency spectrum of the complex modulus from a Laplace transform of a stress relaxation experiment, we employ a Maxwell element model subjected to a step in strain (as shown in Fig. 1). The solution to the differential equation describing Maxwell behavior of the stress during stress relaxation is

$$\sigma = \sigma_0 e^{-bt}, \qquad b = \frac{1}{\tau} = \frac{E}{\eta} \qquad (14)$$

where E is the modulus, η is the viscosity, and b is the characteristic relaxation frequency (i.e., the inverse of the time constant) for the model. Substituting Eq 14 into Eq 11, integrating and separating real and imaginary components yields

$$E'(\omega) = \frac{\sigma_0}{\varepsilon^0}\left(1 - \frac{b^2}{\omega^2 + b^2}\right), \qquad E''(\omega) = \frac{\sigma_0}{\varepsilon_0}\frac{\omega b}{\omega^2 + b^2} \qquad (15)$$

If these equations are plotted over ω, then the expected curves for storage and loss modulus are obtained (Fig. 2). Furthermore, it should be noted that a single discrete characteristics relaxation frequency (or time constant) results in what appears to be a distributed frequency spectrum in the loss modulus curve (Fig. 2).

Next, we must determine how one can acquire the data and apply this integral numerically to arrive at a full description of the frequency response. To do this, we will acquire data at a rate that depends on when we are sampling. For the very early part of the experiment we will sample at the highest rates possible and as time progresses, we will slow the acquisition. This will be done by increasing the sampling interval by one order of magnitude as the decade of time increases. This process minimizes the number of data points collected yet still provides all of the data necessary for the transform. We will show that this uneven sampling technique is valid and does yield accurate results for the discrete Laplace transform. If the sampling rate is kept constant during data collection at twice the maximum frequency to be analyzed, as is required for fast Fourier transforms [6], then up to 10^8 data samples will be collected for seven

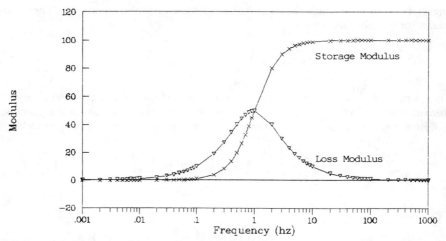

FIG. 2—*Analytic solution of the complex modulus of the Maxwell model using a Laplace transform of the exponential decay solution to stress relaxation. Note the peak in E" is distributed several decades about b and that its height is 0.5 a. (E = ae^{-bt}, where b=1 and a = 100).*

decades of time, making the numerical integration of the transform untenable with present desk-top computational capabilities.

Piece-Wise Integration Technique

Since it is the derivative of the response function that is needed in the Laplace integral (see Eqs 12 and 13), noise in the signal will be amplified in the derivative. To minimize this effect, software filtering, using a novel exponential running average method, is applied to the data. Once the data have been smoothed, piece-wise polynomials are fit to adjacent data points. These piece-wise functions could be cubic (i.e., cubic splines) or exponential or any other function that yields a continuous second derivative. Several functions were investigated; however, it appears that piece-wise exponentials yielded the most stable results upon integration. Therefore, this paper will describe the technique based on piece-wise exponential fitting of the data.

The post-filtered data from the stress relaxation experiment can be fitted with a series of piece-wise exponential functions fit between adjacent data points. This choice of function is suitable, since the nature of the process is one of exponential decay where the characteristic relaxation frequencies (or time constants) are changing over the course of data collection, as different molecular relaxation processes are taking place at different times. If one assumes a fitting function between adjacent data points of the form

$$\sigma = a_j e^{-b_j t} \tag{16}$$

for the *j*th interval of the stress data set, then the coefficients a_j and b_j can be found by inserting the *t*'s and σ's at the end points of the interval and solving for *a* and *b*.

$$b_i = \frac{\ln(\sigma_{i+1}) - \ln(\sigma_i)}{t_i - t_{i+1}}, \qquad a_i = \sigma_i e^{b_i t_i} \tag{17}$$

Once these coefficients have been found, the Laplace transform can be piece-wise integrated over each interval and the sum of the resultant terms will be the total Laplace transform; that is, the Laplace transform can be broken up as follows

$$\mathcal{L}[f(t)] = \int_0^\infty f(t)e^{-i\omega t}dt = \sum_{j=1}^{N\to\infty} \int_{t_j}^{t_{j+1}} f_j(t) \, e^{-i\omega t}dt + \text{trunc.error} \qquad (18)$$

where the truncation error results from relaxation processes occurring outside of the data collection window.

Taking the derivative of the stress and substituting into the expression for the Laplace transform one gets

$$E^*(\omega) = \frac{1}{\varepsilon_0} \sum_{j=1}^{N\to\infty} \int_{t_j}^{t_{j+1}} - b_j a_j e^{-(b_j+i\omega)t} \, dt + \frac{\sigma_0}{\varepsilon_0} \qquad (19)$$

If one integrates this equation across the jth interval and sums up each interval, the following equations for storage and loss modulus result

$$E'(\omega) = \frac{\sigma_0}{\varepsilon_0} + \frac{1}{\varepsilon_0} \sum_j \frac{a_j b_j}{b_j^2 + \omega^2} (b_j(\cos \omega t_{j+1}e^{-b_j t_{j+1}} - \cos \omega t_j e^{-b_j t_j})$$
$$- \omega(\sin \omega t_{j+1}e^{-b_j t_{j+1}} - \sin \omega t_j e^{-b_j t_j})) \qquad (20)$$

and

$$E''(\omega) = -\frac{1}{\varepsilon_0} \sum_{j=1}^{N\to\infty} \frac{a_j b_j}{b_j^2 + \omega^2} (\omega(\cos \omega t_{j+1}e^{-b_j t_{j+1}} - \cos \omega t_j e^{-b_j t_j})$$
$$+ b_j(\sin \omega t_{j+1}e^{-b_j t_{j+1}} - \sin \omega t_j e^{-b_j t_j})) \qquad (21)$$

These expressions are the central ones used in the numerical calculation of the Laplace transform and yield the loss and storage moduli of the material obtained from a stress relaxation experiment. It should be noted that it is not necessary that the sampling interval be uniform to use these expressions since the data are fit with interpolating functions.

Experimental Methods

Computer Experiments

To assess the performance of the numerical transformation technique, several computer generated stress relaxation data were analyzed. First, a comparison of the analytic results and the numerically derived results was made for the Maxwell model. Then, a second term was added to the relaxation expression that approximated a sinusoidal noise of 10% of the maximum signal to determine the effects of such noise on the response spectra.

Mechanical Tests

The stress relaxation experiments were performed on two different instruments. The first was a custom built three-point bend apparatus and the second was an electrohydraulic mechanical test system (Instron model 1350, Canton, OH). The three-point bend device used a solenoid as the displacement actuator for the center loading point. When the circuit was energized the solenoid thrust the actuator at a high rate of speed to the desired adjustable displacement which was measured with a linear variable differential transformer (LVDT). A calibrated load cell consisting of a LVDT and a metal plate measured the resultant load versus time response. Both the displacement and load were measured with analog-to-digital computer acquisition techniques (Kiethley model 570, and SOFT500 Programming installed in an IBM XT compatible). All acquisition and analysis software were written by the authors. The highest rate of acquisition used was 0.01 s/sample (i.e., 100 Hz). This maximum frequency was determined by the solenoid rate (about 0.01 s/full scale displacement). A triggering technique was used to initiate data collection at the onset of loading so that an accurate accounting of the time could be effected.

The electrohydraulic test machine was also used for testing of specimens in tension. In this case the gain of the machine was placed as high as possible to obtain a high rate of motion of the actuator without overshoot. The rate of displacement achieved by the actuator was approximately 0.01 s/full scale (i.e., full scale displacement was reached in about .01 s). Total collection time for both experimental apparati was 25 min (1500 s). Therefore, the smallest valid frequency is 6.7×10^{-4} Hz and the maximum frequency 50 Hz. It should be noted, however, that extrapolation of the exponentials at either end allows one to extrapolate beyond these limits with the understanding that relaxation processes outside of the data window would still not be observed.

Test materials investigated include an experimental uniaxial graphite fiber reinforced poly(methyl methacrylate) (GF/PMMA) composite, neat PMMA, and a medium density polyethylene (PE, Subortholen™). The experimental CF/PMMA composites were made in the laboratory using high-strength graphite fiber (Hercules, Inc., Wilmington, DE). The composite was fabricated using a solutionized thermoforming technique currently under development. This technique results in composites with a fiber volume fraction of about 35% and ultimate strengths of about 1400 MPa [8].

The neat PMMA and PE were tested using three-point bending over a temperature range of 25 to 85 °C (six temperatures). Five specimens per temperature were tested for the polymers. The PMMA/CF composites were tested in tension at room temperature and the effects of applied strain range were investigated. Strains from 0.1 to 0.4% were investigated for three composite specimens, while a constant maximum strain of about 1% were applied to the three-point bend specimens.

Results

Computer Experiments

The numerical integration technique yields virtually identical results as the exact solution. Figure 3 shows the difference between the analytic and numerical results for the Maxwell model. It is evident that the difference between the two is extremely small with a maximum error of about 8×10^{-5}%. Also, the single valued time constant yields a loss peak that is distributed over about four orders of magnitude of frequency with a peak height of 0.5, the maximum storage modulus (as the analytic expression predicts, see Fig. 2).

When a sinusoidal noise component is added, the time dependent modulus and its transform show evidence of its presence. Figure 4 shows the time transient response again in uneven sampling intervals with a characteristic peak at 0.0015 Hz and 10% noise at 60 Hz. Figure 5 shows the corresponding transformed data. Two observations can be made. First, at the frequency of the noise (60 Hz), there is a spike in both the loss and storage modulus values. Second, the storage modulus is raised by the magnitude of the noise signal across the entire frequency range.

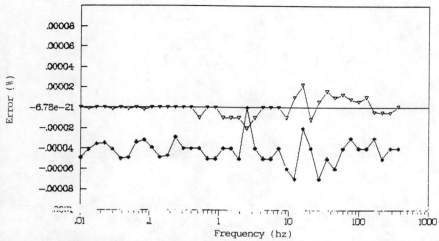

FIG. 3—*The difference between the numerical and analytic solutions to the Maxwell model. Note that the error is very small (on the order of 10^{-4}). Thus, little error is introduced as a result of the piece-wise integration techniques.* ▼—*loss modulus,* #—*storage modulus.*

Mechanical Tests

Poly(methyl methacrylate)—A typical plot of the time dependent moduli for PMMA is shown in Fig. 6. Transformation of these curves yields the storage modulus, loss modulus, and loss tangent for the average of the five specimens per temperature. The corresponding transformed storage and loss moduli for PMMA at 46 °C are shown in Fig. 7 which plots the mean and standard deviation of the five tests as a function of frequency. It should be noted that the standard deviations for these tests are small compared to the signal. It is evident from Fig. 6 that complete relaxation has not yet occurred by the end of the test, thus the low frequency peak may not actually reflect all of the low frequency behavior.

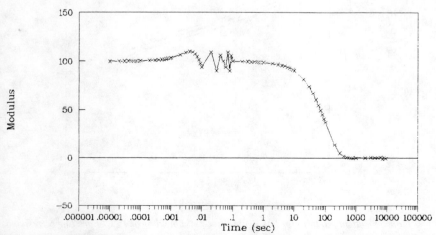

FIG. 4—*Computer generated relaxaton curve for a Maxwell model with a characteristic frequency of 0.0015 Hz and a 10% noise component at 60 Hz.*

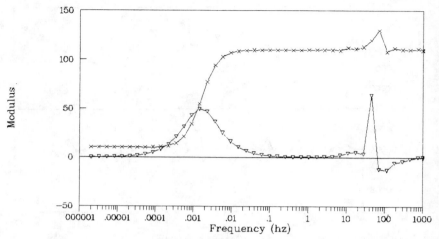

FIG. 5—*Storage and loss moduli for the stress relaxation curve in Fig. 4. Note that the storage modulus is raised by 10% and both peaks show the presence of the 60 Hz noise in their spectra. ▽—loss modulus, ✕—storage modulus.*

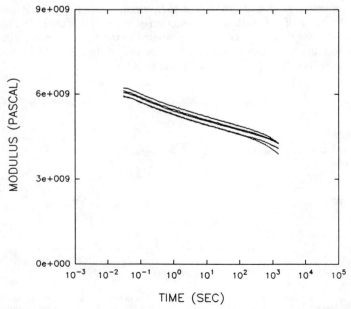

FIG. 6—*Time dependent modulus for PMMA in three-point bending at 46°C. Each line corresponds to one test.*

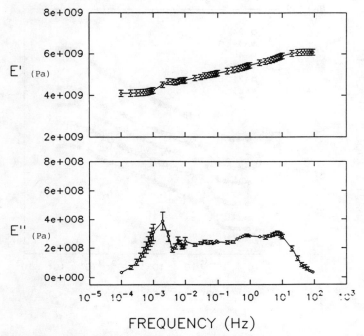

FIG. 7—*The mean and standard deviation of the storage and loss modulus for PMMA at 46 °C. Note that the variance is small compared to the mean.*

The means of the complex modulus of all tests for PMMA at all temperatures investigated are plotted in Fig. 8. The storage modulus varies from 7 GPa to 5 GPa at 24 °C down to about 4 GPa to 2.5 GPa at 83 °C (Fig. 8a). The loss modulus (in Fig. 8b) has several features of interest. First, there are at least three characteristic frequencies present in this figure (manifested as peaks in the curves) which vary when the temperature changes. The low frequency peak (at about 2×10^{-3} Hz) increases with increasing temperature while the two higher frequency peaks (one at about 0.7 Hz and the other at about 8 Hz) appear to decrease with increasing temperature. There may also be a small peak in the 10^{-2} to 10^{-1} frequency range which appears little changed with temperature. Also, all loss tangent curves appear to intersect at about 0.04 Hz.

The loss tangent is shown in Fig. 8c. This plot clearly shows the low-frequency peak increasing with temperature while the other peaks remain approximately constant. The three-dimensional relationship between frequency, temperature, and loss tangent is shown in Fig. 9. From this figure it is clear that the loss tangent monotonically increases with temperature for the low frequency component and is relatively constant for the higher frequency peaks with a slight increase at the higher temperatures. A constant frequency section through this plot shows the loss tangent to be increasing smoothly with temperature, as would be expected in this temperature range from dynamic mechanical analysis techniques.

Polyethylene—The results of time-frequency transform of the PE data for all six temperatures investigated are shown in Fig. 10. From the plot of loss tangent versus frequency (Fig. 10c) it can be seen that several peaks are present. The three-dimensional relationship between loss modulus, temperature, and frequency can be seen in Fig. 11. Three features are worthy of

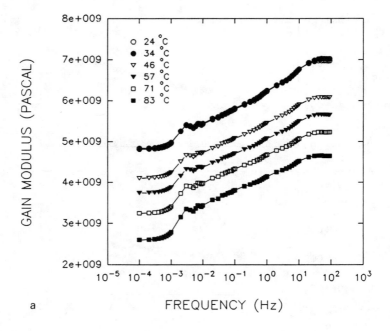

a

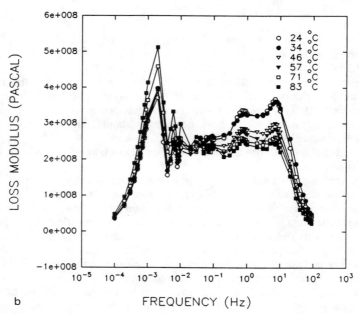

b

FIG. 8—*The mean storage, loss moduli, and loss tangent for PMMA at 24, 35, 46, 57, 71, and 83 °C.* (a) *Storage modulus.* (b) *loss modulus,* (c) *tan* δ. *Note the peaks evident in the loss modulus and tan* δ *curves and their variation with temperature.*

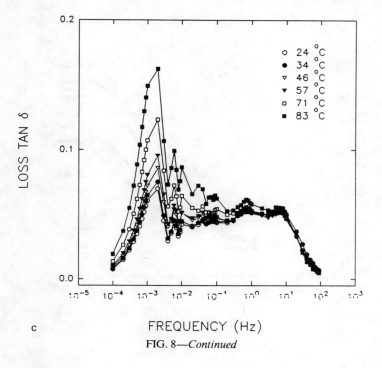

c

FIG. 8—*Continued*

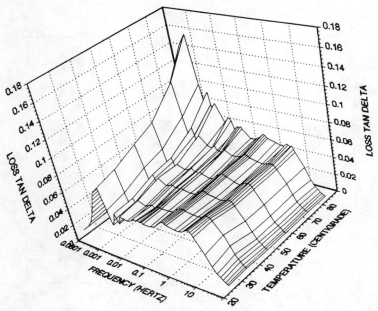

FIG. 9—*Plot of the loss tangent as a function of temperature and frequency for PMMA. Note the upward trend with temperature at any constant frequency.*

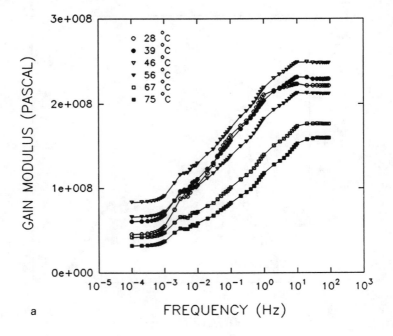

a

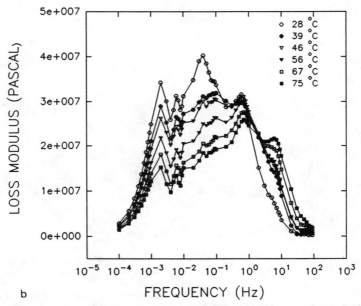

b

FIG. 10—*Storage and loss moduli, and loss tangent for PE specimens tested at 28, 39, 46, 56, 67, and 75 °C. (a) Storage modulus, (b) loss modulus,(c) loss tangent.*

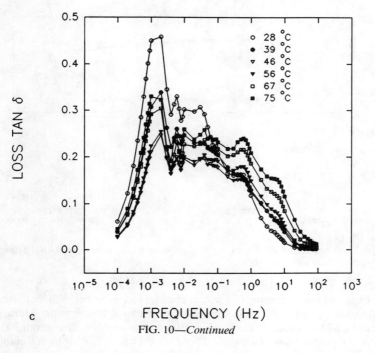

c

FREQUENCY (Hz)

FIG. 10—*Continued*

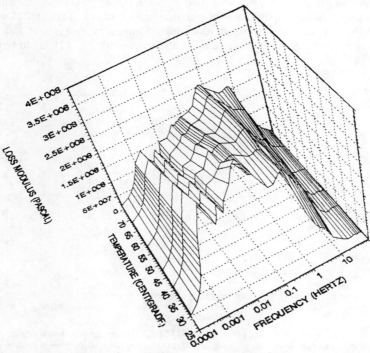

FIG. 11—*Loss modulus as a function of frequency and temperature for PE. Note the decrease of the 0.04 Hz peak and an increase in the 6 Hz peak with increasing temperature.*

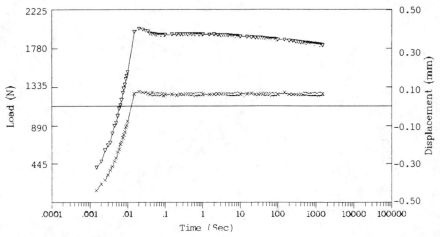

FIG. 12—*Stress relaxation data from a PMMA/CF composite (strain = 0.4%). Triangles are load response and the x's are the stroke input.*

mention. First, the higher frequency peak, at about 6 Hz, increases with increasing temperature. Second, the peak at 0.03 Hz decreases with increasing temperature. Third, as with the PMMA curves, all loss modulus curves (Fig. 10*b*) appear to intersect at about 2 Hz.

PMMA/CF Composites—The transient time response for the PMMA/CF composite specimens is shown in Fig. 12 (strain = 0.4%). Also shown in this figure is the displacement of the actuator which reaches its maximum level with minimal overshoot at about .015 s.

The PMMA/CF composites exhibited much higher storage moduli (about 45 to 60 MPa) and much lower loss tangents than the neat PMMA specimens (Fig. 13). It can be seen from

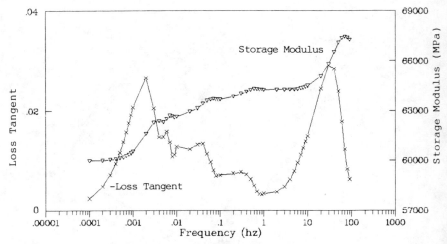

FIG. 13—*Storage modulus and loss tangent for PMMA/CF composite test shown in Fig. 15. Note the decrease in magnitude in the low-frequency peaks and a shifting of the high-frequency peak to 30 Hz compared to the neat resin.*

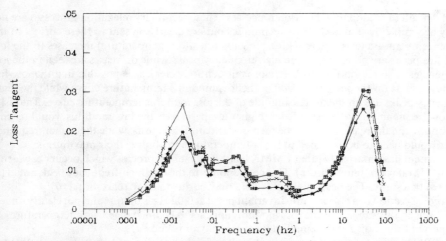

FIG. 14—*Plot of loss tangent versus frequency for PMMA/CF composites tested at different strain ranges. Note the similarity in appearance with little change in magnitude.*

Fig. 13 that the magnitude of the low-frequency peaks are reduced compared to the neat resin while the peak at 8 Hz has not dropped significantly and has shifted to a higher frequency (see Fig. 8c for comparison).

Comparison of the results of the different strain magnitudes indicates that there is little effect of strain magnitude on the complex moduli for the strain range from .1 to .4% (Fig. 14).

Discussion

Computer Results

It is clear from the computer experiments that this numerical Laplace technique is valid for transforming time-domain data into the frequency domain. The use of exponential fitting of the response and piece-wise integration of the Laplace transform allows for uneven sampling intervals to be used with little loss of information. When the data are compared to the analytic results for a Maxwell model, there is very good agreement.

Sinusoidal noise has a definite effect on the resultant frequency spectra for the complex modulus. This includes raising the storage modulus by an equal amount at all frequencies (vertical offset). Also, if the frequency is outside the transition region (i.e., away from a characteristic relaxation frequency) then a spike in both the storage and loss curves will be evident. If the frequency of the noise coincides with the signal, then the ability to distinguish between actual signal and artifact becomes more difficult. However, if the noise is made small either by increasing the signal or post-collection numerical filtering, then these effects can be minimized. Clearly, further quantification of the noise effects and their minimization is required to refine this technique.

Mechanical Results

PMMA—The results for the PMMA specimens appear to correspond to what is to be expected in an amorphous polymer. The low-frequency peak (10^{-3} Hz) most likely corresponds to the primary (or glass) transition in the polymer, while the higher frequency peaks are the result of secondary relaxation processes. These secondary relaxation processes are not easily accessible by standard DMA techniques but are clearly present in these curves. In the higher temperature tests (approaching the glass transition temperature) increases in the loss modulus peaks are observed for the high-frequency peaks while decreases are seen in the low frequencies. The reason for this behavior is not entirely clear. It is possible that the low-frequency peak is on the increasing side of the loss modulus-temperature curve while the high-frequency peaks are on the decreasing side of the loss modulus-temperature curve. That is, if the low-frequency curve is extended to higher temperatures, the loss modulus would reach a maximum and decrease, as would be seen in standard DMA tests, while the higher frequency peaks would need to be extended to lower temperatures to observe their maximums.

Sternstein has reported [7] that PMMA has a β relaxation process which occurs between 1 and 10 Hz (at room temperature). This corresponds to the one high-frequency peak noted (at 8 Hz) in this study. The peak at about 0.7 Hz may be due to an α' relaxation [10].

The observation of a temperature invariant point at 0.02 Hz is unique and not clearly understood. It is in this range that the loss modulus appears to be unchanged with temperature. At the present time, no clear explanation for this behavior is known.

The PMMA/CF composite specimens had peaks that corresponded to the neat PMMA; however, the low-frequency peaks (indicative of the main chain molecular motions) were reduced in the composite while the high-frequency peak (8 Hz) was relatively unchanged but shifted to higher frequencies (about 30 Hz). This indicates that this peak is most likely associated with side group motion which appears to be unchanged in magnitude but increased in frequency in the presence of the carbon fibers. The primary relaxation processes, however, do appear to be reduced by the carbon fibers.

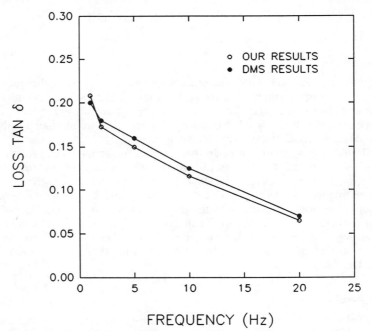

FIG. 15—*Plot of the loss tangent obtained from the Laplace transform and a standard DMA versus frequency for the PE at T = 75 °C. Note that there is very good agreement between techniques.*

Polyethylene—The PE data also present some interesting results. It appears that a high-frequency peak (at about 5 to 7 Hz) is developing as the temperature increases from 28 °C to 75 °C for these specimens as well as the decrease of a lower frequency peak (at .04 Hz) with increasing temperature. These transitions are most likely the result of changes in crystallinity of the polymer with temperature [*3*].

The results from this analysis were checked by dynamic mechanical analysis performed in another study in our laboratory [*9*]. A dynamic mechanical analyzer was used to test the material at four frequencies through a range of temperatures. Comparison of the loss tangent obtained from the Laplace transform technique and the DMA show very good agreement as can be seen in Fig. 15.

One observation from these results that is unexpected is that there is very little shift in peak frequencies with temperature. If one assumes that each peak in the loss tangent curve (of which there are at least three in PMMA) is the result of characteristic chain motion events (i.e., main chain sliding, side chain rotation, etc.) then it is expected that these peaks would shift with temperature as the time-temperature superposition principal requires. However, this does not appear to be the case for PMMA or PE in this temperature range. This may be due to the limited temperature range investigated for each polymer. Clearly, more work is needed to clarify this behavior. However, the methodology is supported by the fact that the curves presented are shown to be repeatable, and consistent for each temperature.

Summary and Conclusion

This paper has presented a numerically based technique to obtain the frequency-based complex modulus of a viscoelastic material from a stress relaxation experiment. A computer-based data acquisition system and a numerical Laplace transform methodology have been shown to result in frequency-based information. An assessment of the associated sources of error was presented as were some preliminary results on PMMA, PE, and PMMA/CF composite specimens. This technique has several advantages in that it can be applied to a range of sample geometries and loading conditions as well as it having the ability to assess very low frequencies which are not easily accessible with current DMA techniques. The initial results for PMMA and PE present mechanical spectra that are related to the characteristic relaxation processes in the materials as a function of frequency, and reveal several features that deserve further study. However, initial results indicate that this technique can resolve not only primary transitions but secondary transitions in viscoelastic materials and may serve as a sensitive means of evaluating dynamic mechanical properties at specific temperatures.

Acknowledgments

Support for this work was provided in part by Grant NIDRR H133E 80013, and the Republic of Taiwan student traineeship grant.

References

[*1*] Hertzberg, R. W. and Manson, J. A., *Fatigue of Engineering Plastics,* Academic Press, New York, 1980, p. 90.
[*2*] Ward, I. M., *Mechanical Properties of Solid Polymers,* J. Wiley and Sons, Chichester, 1979.
[*3*] Rodriguez, F., *Principles of Polymer Systems,* Hemisphere Publishing Co., New York, 1982.
[*4*] Wylie, C. R., *Advanced Engineering Mathematics,* McGraw-Hill, New York, 1975.
[*5*] Macdonald, D. D. and McKubre, M. C. H., "Electrochemical Impedance Techniques in Corrosion Science," *Electrochemical Corrosion Testing, ASTM STP 727,* F. Mansfeld and U. Bertocci, Eds., American Society for Testing and Materials, Philadelphia, 1981, pp. 110–149.

[6] Press, W. H., Flannery, B. P., Teukolsky, S. A., and Vetterling, W. T., *Numerical Recipes,* Cambridge University Press, 1989.

[7] Sternstein, S. S., "Transient and Dynamic Characterization of Viscoelastic Solids," Ch. 7, *Polymer Characterization,* American Chemical Society, 1983, pp. 136.

[8] Wills, R. D., Gilbert, J. L., and Lautenschlager, E. P., "Novel Processing Technique for PMMA/CF and PC/CF Composites for Orthotic Applications," presented at the 7th World Congress of International Society for Prosthetics and Orthotics, Chicago, June 1992.

[9] Chiu, C. H. and Healy, K. E., Division of Biological Materials, Northwestern University, unpublished data.

[10] Roberts, G. E. and White, E. F. T., *The Physics of Glassy Polymers,* Ch. 3, R. N. Haward, Ed., Halsted Press, New York, 1973, pp. 183–185.

Russell P. Wong[1,2] *and Roberto S. Benson*[1]

Fracture Behavior of Polyurethane-Calcium Chloride Blends

REFERENCE: Wong, R. P. and Benson, R. S., **"Fracture Behavior of Polyurethane-Calcium Chloride Blends,"** *Biomaterials' Mechanical Properties, ASTM STP 1173,* H. E. Kambic and A. T. Yokobori, Jr., Eds., American Society for Testing and Materials, Philadelphia, 1994, pp. 245–255.

ABSTRACT: Two polyurethanes and their respective 1, 5, and 10 wt.% $CaCl_2$ blends were studied. The normalized strain energy ($\mathcal{F}$) was used to characterize the fracture susceptibility of films made from the polyurethane-calcium blends. The low normalized strain energy is correlated with ease of fracture. The normalized strain energy to failure for all the Biomer®-calcium chloride blends throughout the entire range of crack lengths was less than observed for the pure Biomer. The normalized strain energy values obtained for the Biomer-1 wt.% $CaCl_2$ were comparatively lower than all other Biomer blends. At concentrations of 5 and 10 wt.%, there was some evidence that increase in the normalized strain energy to failure could be attributed to plasticization and crack arresting behavior of the calcium chloride dissolved in the matrix. The normalized strain energy values for calcium chloride blended with Pellethane® were different above and below the critical crack length. For initial crack lengths less than the critical length, the normalized strain energy for the Pellethane-calcium chloride blends were less than for pure Pellethane. At cracks larger than the critical length, the Pellethane-calcium blends displayed greater normalized strain energy to failure. The addition of a small amount of calcium chloride to Biomer and Pellethane leads to a reduction in the normalized strain energy which can be associated with lower fracture toughness. Pellethane appeared to be more susceptible than Biomer to the deterioration of its fracture properties.

KEYWORDS: polyurethane, calcium chloride, internal elastic energy, fracture toughness, normalized strain energy

Historically, catastrophic failures of engineered structures have motivated research into understanding materials defect propagation. Defects propagate with the conversion of elastic energy to crack surface energy. Above a critical stress value the energy of the system cannot be dissipated quickly enough by a reduction in the system entropy and the creation of a crack surface (propagation of defects) becomes more energetically efficient for storage of the excess strain energy. As a result of fundamental studies, engineers have developed fracture mechanics testing methods. Their belief is that knowledge of the tendency of a material to propagate a crack can be used during the materials selection process of design.

Because failure occurs at the point where the failure stress is reached first, stress risers, i.e., holes, sharp angles, notches, grooves, and inclusions, greatly weaken the strength of a structure by causing stress to reach critical values at lower loads. Clinical studies as well as *in-vivo* studies have demostrated that calcium salts can be incorporated into polyurethane implants [1]. The

[1] Research engineer and associate professor, respectively, Materials Science and Engineering, University of Tennessee, Knoxville, TN 37996-2200.
[2] Present affiliation: Senior research engineer, Monsanto Chemical Co., Plastic Division, Springfield, MA 01151.

incorporation of calcium salts has been associated with failure of implants, especially when cracks were observed on the surface [2]. The simultaneous presence of cracks and calcium deposits on the surface of an implant suggest a possible interdependence between calcification and changes in fracture behavior of the materials. The present work examines the effect of the interaction of calcium salt on the fracture behavior of biomedical polyurethanes. A series of blends consisting of polyurethane with known concentrations of calcium chloride was used to simulate a degree of calcium incorporation into the implants.

Theory of Fracture

The fracture behavior of a material can be characterized through its fracture toughness, J, a measure of the strength of the crack tip singularity in nonlinear fracture mechanics. The application of the J-integral to materials testing was first recognized by Rice [3], proposed by Paris [4], and demonstrated by Landes and Begley [5]. Hashemi and Williams [6,7] have used the J method to characterize the fracture toughness of several polymers with rubbery phases. Huang and Williams [8] also applied the same method to study toughened nylons.

The fracture toughness of a material is determined from the change in internal elastic energy with crack growth.

$$J = -[dU/da] = (\partial U/\partial a)_l$$

In practice the fracture toughness for a given material can be determined from the total change in internal energy for specimens with various initial crack lengths. All specimens must be elongated to a predetermined displacement, l. Under these conditions, the fracture toughness can be expressed as

$$J = (\partial U/\partial a)_l$$

where U is the total change in internal elastic energy and is measured from the total area under the stress versus strain curves up to the predetermined strain using the expression given below

$$U = \int_0^{\epsilon_b} \sigma d\epsilon$$

U can be calculated using a direct numerical integration.

Because of the large strain energy absorbed by polyurethanes for short cracks, the strain energy for crack propagation alone could not be determined directly. As a result, in the present study it was not possible to directly determine true fracture toughness J, but rather a pseudo-fracture toughness $\mathcal{F}$. This pseudo-fracture toughness is really a normalized strain energy that was calculated from the following expression

$$\mathcal{F} = (U)(W)(l_0)/(W - a)$$

where a is the initial crack length of the specimen, and W and l_0 are the width and the initial length of the specimen, respectively. The units of $\mathcal{F}$ are the same as J. The pseudo-fracture toughness or normalized strain energy, $\mathcal{F}$, is analogous to the Rivlin-Thomas [9] tearing energy. As in the case of Rivlin-Thomas tearing energy, the lower normalized strain energy is correlated with ease of fracture of the material.

Experimental

Samples

In this study, samples of medical grade polyurethanes Biomer® (Ethicon, Inc.) and Pelle-thane® 2363-80A (Dow Chemical Co.)-calcium chloride (1, 5, and 10 wt.%) blends were examined. Pellethane is a poly(ether)urethane and Biomer is a poly(ether)urethane-urea. Biomer was received in a solution of dimethyl acetamide; Pellethane 2363 was in pellet form.

Thin films of Biomer and Pellethane-calcium chloride blends were cast from 20 wt.% solutions of dimethyl acetamide (DMAC). All films were cast on clean glass plates using a casting knife. The solvents were driven off in a forced air oven at 80°C. A multiple specimen J-integral method was used in the fracture characterization. In the multiple specimen J-integral method one specimen is completely fractured to determine the ultimate displacement and the remaining test specimens are given different initial crack length prior to fracturing under tensile mode. J is calculated from the area under each tensile curve. Crack growth is measured from the surface for each J-specimen. A plot of J as a function of crack extension can be constructed. The test specimens had dimensions of 3.8 cm by 3.8 cm by t cm, the thickness (t) was within 2.54×10^{-3} to 5.08×10^{-3} cm and measured using a micrometer. Initial crack lengths ranging from 0.25 to 1.0 cm were carefully introduced into the films. For each crack length eight specimens of each material were tested. The films were drawn at a strain rate of 20% per second on a microcomputer-based tensile tester. The change in internal elastic energy upon fracture was measured as the total area under the stress versus strain to failure curve using a direct numerical integration of the data by trapezoidal approximation [10]. Normalized strain energy plots were used to estimate the instability or critical crack length. The instability or critical crack length is considered the limit for constant crack propagation rate. Beyond the instability length the crack propagation rate increases.

Tensile Mechanical Testing Instrument

A microcomputer-based tensile tester consisting of two JASTA Pulse Power step motor driven linear actuators (drawing in opposite directions) were used to draw the films. The actuators were mounted on columns which move the motor vertically. The flat film clamps were designed to allow measurements on film specimens having a maximum width of 8 cm. The front edges of the clamps were machine-rounded to avoid formation of pressure-cut on the specimens and the subsequent failure. None of the specimens tested in this work using the rounded front edge grips failed near the clamps. The actuators were capable of applying a maximum of 89 N of thrust while achieving stroke speeds of 12.7 cm/s. At slower speeds, each actuator can apply up to 800 N of thrust. Each actuator was precisely positioned by steps of 6.35×10^{-6} meters; with two actuators acting in concert, the positioning precision was 12.7×10^{-6}. The actuators were controlled by a Step Pak motor controller Model MCU-2 and power supply PSU-2. The power supply was used to control the maximum work that could be done by each actuator.

Results and Discussion

The Mode I (tensile) mechanical fracture tests were performed on the polyurethane films blended with different amounts of calcium chloride. A second order polynomial (parabolic) curve fit was calculated with the stress versus strain data and plotted in the form of a solid line. A representative plot (Fig. 1) shows the stress as a function of strain for Biomer with varying crack lengths. The area under these curves representing the strain energy to failure, U, were plotted as a function of the initial crack length, a. Composite plots of strain energy versus ini-

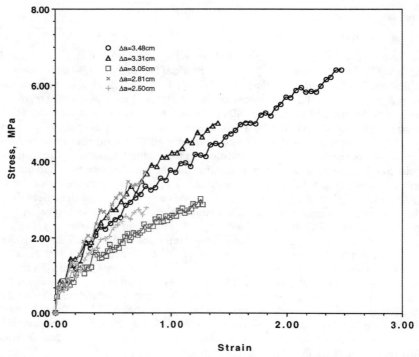

FIG. 1—*Stress versus strain data for pure Biomer films with varying crack growth to failure.*

tial crack length for the Biomer-calcium chloride blends a is given in Fig. 2. The strain energy curves were recalculated to account for the length of the uncracked ligament in an attempt to formulate J-integral curves that could be used to assign critical conditions to the fracture behavior. The strain energy to failure had significant contributions from two material properties. The first was tensile drawing in which the material absorbed strain energy in the form of molecular orientation or deformation. The increase in molecular orientation was determined using FTIR dichroism [11]. The second material contribution was strain energy absorbed through the propagation of a crack. The energy absorbed during crack growth was the desired quantity, J. The separation of the overall strain energy into two contribution permits corrections for the fact that deformation (non-crack propagating) energy was more dominant at shorter crack lengths than at longer crack lengths. The strain energy for crack propagation in the polyurethane-calcium chloride blends was determined using the normalized strain energy, $\bar{J}$.

The pure specimens of Biomer displayed rubber elastic type behavior during tensile testing to fracture. This was true even at longer initial crack lengths where one might not expect an unstable crack growth dominated tensile behavior to continue to display rubber elastic properties. This behavior can be observed in Fig. 1. The variation of the normalized strain energy with crack length for pure Biomer given in Fig. 3 indicates a steady decrease in $\bar{J}$ with increasing initial crack length. The lengths at which the crack becomes unstable were estimated from the intersect of two tangents drawn on the plot of $\bar{J}$ versus initial crack length and are summarized for all blends in Table 1. The pure Biomer critical crack length was estimated to occur for values exceeding 5 mm.

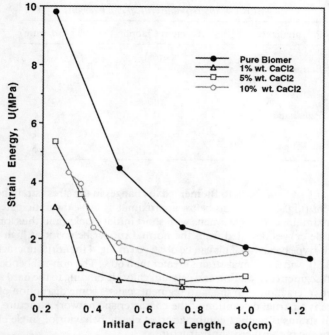

FIG. 2—*Strain energy versus initial crack length of pure and CaCl₂ blended Biomers.*

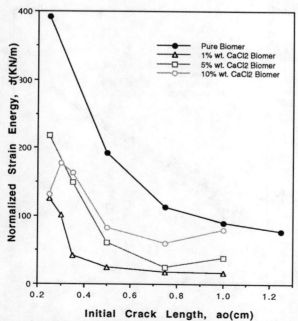

FIG. 3—*Comparison plots of normalized strain energy to failure versus initial crack length for Biomer blended with various calcium chloride concentrations.*

TABLE 1—*Approximate critical crack lengths.*

Polyurethane	Calcium Chloride	a_c (mm)
	(wt.%)	
Biomer®	0	5
	1	3.5
	5	5
	10	4
Pellethane®	0	5.5
	1	4
	5	4.5
	10	6.5

The addition of 1 wt.% of $CaCl_2$ to Biomer led to changes in the stress-strain behavior of the cracked specimens (Fig. 4). At strains below approximately 60%, the anticipated rubber type curvature was maintained. For specimens with short initial cracks (and thus longer strains to failure), the tensile curves deviated from the normal rubber behavior at high strains into a more linear elastic type behavior. This can be observed in Fig. 4 for initial uncracked ligaments values of 3.55, 3.50, and 3.45 cm at strains greater than 60%. The non-rubber behavior can be attributed to soft segment orientation and calcium chloride binding to the hard segments. The calcium chloride interaction with the hard segments causes some disruption of the domains [11]. Since there is a partial disruption of the characteristic network structure, the observed response to high strains is really a combination of elastic behavior of single chains and the rubbery behavior the physical crosslink structure.

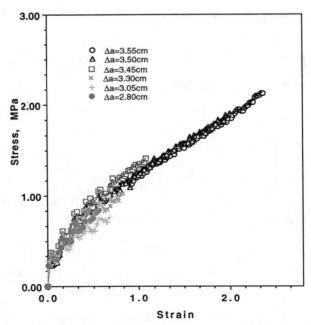

FIG. 4—*Stress versus strain data for Biomer blended with 1 wt.% calcium chloride with varying crack growth to failure.*

The Biomer-1 wt.% calcium chloride blend exhibits the lowest normalized strain energy within its group (Fig. 4). The strain energy to failure fell sharply between 3 and 3.5 mm, leading to a considerably lower critical crack length than observed for pure Biomer (Table 1). The rapid decrease in the strain energy indicates that blending low concentrations of calcium chloride into Biomer weakens the interaction which stabilizes the domain-matrix morphology of the polymer. The domain-matrix morphology of polyurethanes is predicated on the presence of hydrogen bonding within the hard segments domains and any disruption of the hydrogen bonding, e.g., the presence of calcium chloride which can interact with the carbonyl oxygen partial negative charge, leads to partial or total destruction of the overall morphology. The studies on the disruption of hard segment hydrogen bonding caused by blending calcium chloride were performed by Wong [11] using Fourier Transform Infrared (FTIR) spectroscopy. The study noted that the addition of calcium chloride led to the appearance of the infrared absorption band for free N-H stretching vibration at 3450 cm^{-1} and the shifting of the infrared absorption band associated with the stretching of the hydrogen bonded carbonyl in the urea group at 1640 cm^{-1}. The new absorption band at 3450 cm^{-1} indicates that previously hydrogen bonded N-H functional groups are no longer interacting with the carbonyl groups. The shift of the urea carbonyl band to lower wavenumber was interpreted as resulting from increased hindrance to stretching motion due to interaction with calcium chloride.

The stress-strain curve for the Biomer-5 wt.% calcium chloride blend indicates a certain degree of plasticization (Fig. 5). The fracture process involved more steady tearing to failure along these curves rather than the stretching followed by immediate failure observed for pure Biomer and Biomer-1 wt.% calcium blend. The upswing in the stress-strain curves observed above 150% strain is indicative of reduction in free volume which normally accompanies strain orientation. An increase in the molecular orientation of Biomer-5 wt.% calcium chloride

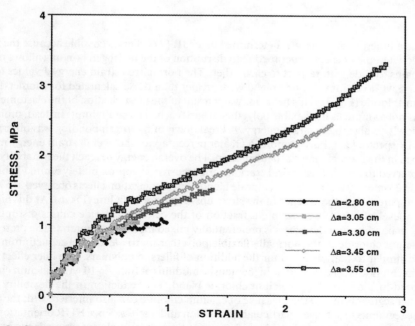

FIG. 5—*Stress versus strain data for Biomer blended with 5 wt.% calcium chloride with varying crack growth to failure.*

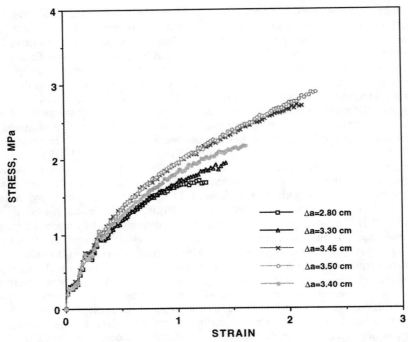

FIG. 6—*Stress versus strain data for Biomer blended with 10 wt.% calcium chloride with varying crack growth to failure.*

blend as a function of strain was determined by FTIR [*11*]. This is possible because the initial breakdown in the domain structure due to disruption of the hydrogen bonding allows molecular chains to slide with respect to each other. The normalized strain energy J values for the Biomer-5 wt.% calcium chloride blend were greater than those calculated for Biomer-1 wt.% calcium chloride (Fig. 3). This behavior was a result of the plasticization of the elastomer; failure was not as rapid as the flexible polyether group reached its strain limit. Instead, molecules slide slowly to absorb the strain energy. A breakdown of hydrogen bonding was observed in the FTIR spectra [*11*]. Furthermore, a greater percentage of the overall strain energy may be absorbed in the form of material deformation. The overall energy to reach the instability point was observed to increase as critical crack length occurred at approximately 5 mm (Table 1).

In the Biomer-10 wt.% calcium chloride blend, the plasticization effects observed at 5% were not as apparent with the absence of the stress upswing prior to failure (Fig. 6). At this high (10 wt.%) a level of salt concentration, a fraction of the calcium chloride causes disruption of hydrogen bonding and the excess is preferentially mixed into the soft matrix. The presence of the calcium chloride in the normally flexible polyether matrix leads to a reduction in chain motion similar to that observed for the addition of fillers to polymers. The filler effect of the calcium chloride is reflected in the higher tensile modulus of Biomer-10 wt.% calcium chloride compared to Biomer-5 wt.% calcium chloride blend. The reduction in the flexibility of the polyether segments due to the presence of calcium chloride can also interfere with the ability of these segments to achieve a particular orientation under stress. Since FTIR orientation studies of polymers have shown that a high chain orientation region always preceeds the crack tip during propagation, the inability of chains to assume a favorable orientation is associated with crack arresting. In the case of Biomer-10 wt.% calcium chloride blend, the salt hindered the polyether segment orientation causing failure to be more abrupt. The normalized strain energy associated with fracture of Biomer-10 wt.% calcium chloride blend is given in Fig. 3. There also appeared to be a broad distribution of stress levels, depending on the initial crack length. This may be due to the variations in the stress fields surrounding the crack tip which varied with local salt concentration. The strain energy values obtained for crack lengths below the critical value of the Biomer-10 wt.% calcium chloride blend were comparable to those observed for the Biomer-5 wt.% calcium chloride blend. When the initial crack lengths were greater than the critical value, the strain energy values of the Biomer-10 wt.% calcium chloride blend exceeded those for Biomer-5 wt.% calcium chloride blend. For the Biomer-10 wt.% calcium chloride blend, the large salt aggregates probably aided in arresting crack propagation. The critical crack length was estimated to be approximately 4 mm (Table 1).

Fracture experiments were also conducted on pure Pellethane 2363 and Pellethane-calcium chloride blends. Pure Pellethane had a rubbery behavior with no observable non-rubber elastic effects prior to failure. The stress levels to achieve similar elongation were much lower than those measured for Biomer and the films failed much more rapidly than pure Biomer. Plots of the strain energy to failure U, as a function of initial crack length for pure Pellethane 2363 and Pellethane-calcium chloride blends are given Fig. 6. The comparison of the normalized strain energy for Biomer and Pellethane is given in Fig. 7. Inspection of Fig. 7 clearly shows that for a given crack length, a lower energy is required to cause failure in Pellethane as compared to Biomer. This observed difference in the fracture behavior between Biomer and Pellethane can be attributed to differences in the chemical nature and size of the hard domains of

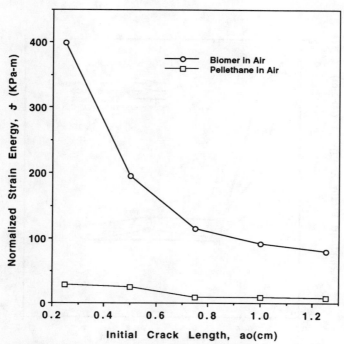

FIG. 7—*Normalized strain energy, 𝔍 versus initial crack, a_o for Biomer and Pellethane.*

polyetherurethanes and polyetherurethane-ureas. The larger domains present in the polyetherurethane-urea have better reinforcing properties and thus may hinder chain motion during uncoiling leading to requirement of higher energy for Biomer than Pellethane to produce similar deformation. In addition, the presence of urea groups along the polyetherurethane-urea means an increase in the relative number of hydrogen bonding in stabilizing the domains. Since the hydrogen bonds serve as the crosslinks between the chains and higher crosslink density leads higher tensile strength in elastomers, then higher stress levels for the same amount of deformation should be expected for polyetherurethane-urea (Biomer) as compared to polyetherurethane (Pellethane). For pure Pellethane, the transition between stable and unstable conditions is very broad and the critical crack length was estimated at 4.5 mm (Fig. 7).

The fracture behavior of the Pellethane-calcium chloride blends is best understood when the regions above and below the critical crack length on the normalized strain energy curve (Fig. 8) are considered separately. Below the critical length the normalized strain energies for the Pellethane-calcium chloride blends are lower than for pure Pellethane. The lowest normalized strain energy is obtained for the Pellethane-5 wt.% calcium chloride blend. The value of the normalized strain energy for the Pellethane-10 wt.% calcium chloride blend is highest for the blends. The general behavior of reduction in normalized strain energy with addition of calcium chloride is also observed in this region but with minimum value achieved at a concentration of 5 wt.% instead of 1 wt.% calcium chloride. This behavior seems to be very consistent with the filler effect and disruption of hydrogen bonding used to explain the behavior of the Biomer-calcium chloride blends. The fact that the minimum normalized strain energy in Pellethane-calcium chloride blends is obtained at higher concentration of calcium chloride (5 wt.%) may be due to higher molecular weight combined with a higher degree of hydrogen bonding. Above the critical length, there is very little difference between the values of the nor-

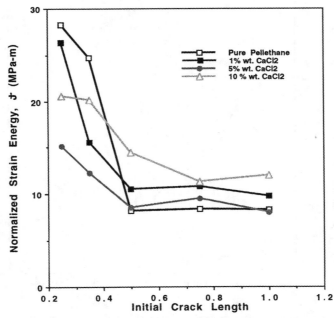

FIG. 8—*Comparison plot of normalized strain energy to failure versus initial crack length for Pellethane blended with various calcium chloride concentrations.*

malized strain energy of the Pellethane-calcium chloride blends. The exact reason for this behavior remains unclear. The Pellethane-10 wt.% calcium chloride shows a slightly higher value of normalized strain energy which may be due to the strong filler effect of the calcium chloride. The transition between stable and unstable crack propagation was estimated for the Pellethane-calcium chloride blends with 1, 5, and 10 wt.% at 4.0, 4.5, and 6.5, respectively (Table 1).

The fracture results indicate that calcium chloride has two roles in effecting changes in mechanical properties. At the lower concentration (1 wt.%), there is a significant reduction in the strain energy to failure. The reduction in the strain energy to failure is due primarily to the addition of calcium chloride which disrupts the hard domain. At higher concentrations (5 and 10 wt.%), a portion of the calcium chloride disrupts the hydrogen bonding between hard segments and the excess is dispersed in the matrix assuming a role similar to a filler. In general, the domains disruption leads to increased viscous flow of the polyurethane chains which is reflected in the overall lowering of the modulus and strength.

Conclusions

The addition of small quantities of calcium salts (1 wt.%) will reduce the fracture toughness of polyurethanes due to disruption of hydrogen bonding. At high concentrations (10 wt.%), the presence of the calcium chloride tends to make the precracked polyurethanes less susceptible to fracture. Pellethane appeared to be more susceptible than Biomer to the deterioration in fracture toughness due to the addition of calcium chloride.

Acknowledgments

The authors gratefully acknowledge the support of the Whitaker Foundation and the Center for Materials Processing at the University of Tennessee, Knoxville.

References

[1] Lo, H. B., Herold, M., Reul, H., et al., " A Tricuspid Polyurethane Heart Valve as an Alternative to Mechanical Prostheses or Bioprostheses,"*Transactions of the American Society of Artificial Internal Organs,* Vol. 35, 1988, p. 839.
[2] Stokes, K. B., Berthelson, W. A., and Davis, M. W., "Metal Catalyzed Oxidative Degradation of Implanted Polyurethane Devices," *Polymeric Materials Science and Engineering,* Vol. 53, 1985, p. 6.
[3] Rice, J. R., "A Path Independent Integral and the Approximate Analysis of Strain Concentrations by Notches and Cracks," *Journal of Applied Mechanics,* Vol. 35, 1968, p. 379.
[4] Paris, P. C., "Fracture Mechanics in the Elastic-Plastic Regime," *Flaw Growth and Fracture, ASTM STP 631,* American Society for Testing and Materials, Philadelphia, 1977.
[5] Begley, J. A. and Landes, J. D., " The J-Integral as a Fracture Criterion," *Fracture Toughness (Proceedings of the 1971 National Symposium on Fracture Mechanics), Part II, ASTM STP 514,* American Society for Testing and Materials, Philadelphia, 1972.
[6] Hashemi, S. and Williams, J. G., "A Fracture Toughness Study on Low Density and Linear Low Density Polyethylenes," *Polymer,* Vol. 27, No. 3, 1986, p. 384.
[7] Hashemi, S. and Williams, J. G., "Fracture Characterization of Tough Polymers Using the J-Method," *Polymer Science and Engineering,* Vol. 26, 1986, p. 760.
[8] Huang, D. D. and Williams, J. G., "J-Testing of Toughened Nylons,"*Journal of Materials Science,* Vol. 22, No. 7, 1987, p. 250.
[9] Rivlin, R. S. and Thomas. A. G., "Rupture of Rubber. I. Characteristic Energy for Tearing," *Journal of Polymer Science,* Vol. 10, 1953, p. 291.
[10] *Engineering Mathematics Handbook,* 2nd ed., J. J. Tuma, Ed., McGraw-Hill, New York, 1979.
[11] Wong, R. P., "The Effects of Calcification on the Structure and Properties of Biomedical Polyurethanes," Ph.D. dissertation, The University of Tennessee, 1991.

Karen J. Leadbetter,[1] *Robert A. Latour, Jr.,*[1] *Russell A. Johnson,*[1] *and Shalaby W. Shalaby*[1]

Micromechanical Testing of Interfacial Bonding in Absorbable Composites

REFERENCE: Leadbetter, K. J., Latour, R. A. Jr., Johnson, R. A., and Shalaby, S. W., "**Micromechanical Testing of Interfacial Bonding in Absorbable Composites,**" *Biomaterials' Mechanical Properties, ASTM STP 1173,* H. E. Kambic and A. T. Yokobori, Jr., Eds., American Society for Testing and Materials, Philadelphia, 1994, pp. 256–264.

ABSTRACT: A new approach is described, involving microdroplet fiber composites, to study absorbable fiber-reinforced composites with physicochemically hybridized interfaces. Both an Instron Dynamic Test Machine and a micromechanical testing machine are successfully used to monitor variation in interfacial bond strength resulting from changes in certain key processing variables, and a comparison is made between the two test methods. It is concluded that these procedures are able to discern small interfacial adhesion strength differences and can contribute effectively to the establishment of an optimal filler-matrix interface.

KEYWORDS: absorbable, composite, fracture fixation, polymer, interface

Many cases of fracture fixation, particularly load-bearing, demand a high-strength, sufficiently stiff material in order to avoid further damage by a material failure and subsequent bone refracture. Not only the obvious immediate detrimental effects of implant failure are of concern, but also the further unnecessary strain placed on the patient by a follow-up surgery. The first available option was a durable metallic or ceramic implant which afforded the necessary strength to avoid such problems. Indeed, so stiff are many such implants that they actually may undermine bone formation and even weaken it as a result of the large bone/implant modulus mismatch and subsequent bone resorption. For these reasons, polymeric implants with much lower moduli come under great scrutiny. Unreinforced polymeric orthopedic devices are relatively low modulus options and are viewed as unsatisfactory in load bearing applications. Mixed with an appropriate reinforcement phase, however, the resulting composite may be quite effective.

The mechanical strength of a composite is governed by, among other factors, the interface or the area between the matrix and reinforcement. Many attempts have been made to optimize the mechanical properties of polymeric composites through enhanced interfacial bonding. This is undertaken by controlling filler orientation, filler shape and size, surface treatments of fillers, and the addition of "binding" or coupling agents. Only a few attempts, primarily those involving the "self-reinforced" composites, have been made to characterize composites comprised of physically and chemically similar components [1]. The absorbable polymers are chosen to be studied because they demonstrate high chemical reactivity and will clearly show any bonding dependencies upon processing variables.

---

[1] Graduate student, assistant professor, graduate student, and professor, respectively, Bioengineering Department, Clemson University, Clemson, SC 29634-0905.

The research idea is to choose a few of the key processing variables governing interfacial interactions in a physicochemically hybridized absorbable composite system and to see if their effect on interfacial bond strength is measurable and predictable. The primary focus of this study is to ascertain that changes in interfacial bond strength due to varying processing time, processing temperature, and simulated *in vivo* aqueous conditions are indeed measurable quantities. The two composite systems under scrutiny are a polydioxanone (PDS) matrix reinforced with poly(glycolic acid) (PGA) fibers and a partially aromatic oxalate copolymer reinforced also with PGA fibers. These components are chosen for their physicochemical compatibility; a composite with effective wetting and interfacial bond formation may be readily formed via ester-ester interchange [2].

Materials and Equipment

The PDS matrix material was obtained in pellet form from Ethicon, Inc. and the PGA was obtained as suture grade from Davis and Geck. The second matrix was a partially aromatic oxalate copolymer made in the laboratory; its composition and key properties are noted in the next section. The major equipment included a Carver heat press, Napco (E series) vacuum oven, Instron Dynamic Test Machine (1320), and a miniature mechanical test machine [3]. For aging studies, a phosphate buffer with a pH of 7.28 was used [4].

Procedures

PGA/PDS Microdroplet System

The initial microdroplet fiber composites were processed with three variables in mind: processing time, processing temperature, and post-processing soak in phosphate buffer.

First, PDS films were compression-molded by sandwiching about 0.05 g of PDS between aluminum foil and metal plates, for one minute at 121°C and 7000 kg pressure. The film, approximately 130 μm in thickness, was then cut into V-shaped specimens (Fig. 1) with an approximately 500-μm tip dimension.

The PGA sutures were scoured in acetone and dried under vacuum. Single filaments retrieved from the suture core were then taped onto tabs on a metal frame, where the tabs served to protect the filaments from heat damage. The polymeric V's were suspended (Fig. 2), two per filament, in the mid-section of the fiber, each frame holding approximately 20 filaments. The frame was placed in an oven (preheated to the appropriate temperature) for the appropriate processing time period, followed by a quick air quench to room temperature. The legs of the polymeric V's melted in the oven and detached, embedding the remaining polymer as a droplet on the fiber.

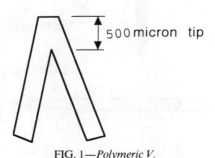

500 micron tip

FIG. 1—*Polymeric V.*

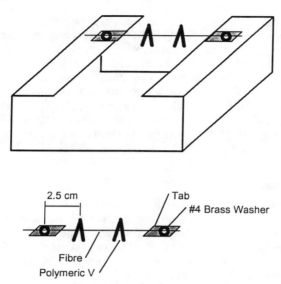

FIG. 2—*Microdroplet processing.*

After processing and cooling, a #4 brass washer was glued under each fiber end with epoxy, 2.5 cm from the closest droplet. The samples were then stored in an Argon environment for a 15-h time period to allow curing of the glue. Following this, the samples were removed from the frame and taped on glass slides. The embedment length of the dry samples and the fiber diameter were measured immediately under the microscope, and the remainder of samples placed in buffer solution for later measurement and testing. The processing times were five

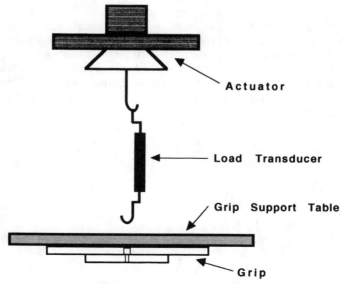

FIG. 3—*Miniature mechanical tester.*

and ten minutes, the processing temperatures 121°C and 131°C, and the treatment in 7.28 pH buffered environment entailed 24-h soaking at 37°C. Approximately 30 droplets were processed in this manner for each possible combination, of which there are 2^3 or eight variations.

PGA/Oxalate Microdroplet System

A PGA/oxalate study was run in the same fashion. The partially aromatic oxalate copolymer (OX-6/T-6) [90/10 poly(hexamethylene oxalate-co-hexamethylene terephthalate, T_m = 70°C, η,35°C/CHCl$_3$, = 0.31] was synthesized in our laboratory [5]. The only distinctions between the oxalate experiment and the PDS experiment were the film processing temperature of 70°C and the microdroplet processing temperatures of 70° and 90°C.

Inert Processing Environment

To determine the effects of inert processing, PGA/PDS microdroplet specimens were processed at 121°C for 5 min in a dry, argon environment, prior to their exposure to the aqueous degrading environment.

Composite Testing

The microdroplets themselves were in the embedment range of 0.075 to 0.150 mm and the fiber diameter was consistently 0.012 mm. The original microdroplet studies, those systems processed in a normal or so-called "reactive" environment, were tested on the miniature composite test machine [6] as shown in Fig. 3. The specimen was attached to a hook that was attached to the load transducer which, in turn, was connected to the actuator, an audio speaker. A function generator output a signal to the controller; the controller then output a voltage which caused the actuator to cycle up and back. Just below the specimen hook was a grip support table by which the grip was attached and held in position. The grip support table is a platform that allows grip height adjustment. The specimen was attached to the hook and positioned through the slit in the grip. The force transducer signal was zeroed, through both oscilloscope and voltmeter monitoring, and the table moved down until contact was made with the droplet. The function generator was triggered, the speaker pulled up, and the droplet was sheared from the filament. The output was recorded on an xy plotter measuring applied force versus time.

The microdroplets formed in Argon environment were tested on the Instron Dynamic Test Machine, using the same cycle frequency as that of the miniature mechanical test machine. A 50-lb (~22.7-kg) load cell was used in this case. It was necessary to construct special holders to clamp the grip in place and hold the specimen in the appropriate position. The grip itself was fabricated by gluing with epoxy two 0.8-cm by 1.0-cm by 0.1-cm stainless steel pieces to a 4.0-cm by 1.8-cm by 0.2-cm metal base with a center gap (Fig. 4). The gap between the two pieces was uniformly 25 μm.

Statistical Analysis

The results were analyzed using the SAS®^{2} statistical package (1985). The analysis was based on the assumption of a normal distribution, and treated as an unbalanced design with unequal specimen sizes.

---

^{2} SAS Institute, Cary, NC.

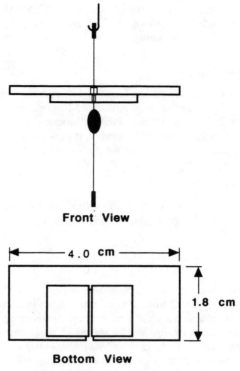

Front View

Bottom View

FIG. 4—*Microdroplet grip.*

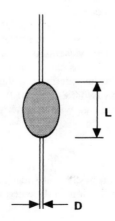

BOND STRENGTH = FORCE / (ΠDL)

FIG. 5—*Microdroplet.*

TABLE 1—*Bond strength data for PGA/PDS single fiber composites in reactive atmosphere.[a]*

Processing Time (min)	Processing Temperature (°C)	Aqueous Environment Level[b]	Bond Strength (MPa)	S[c]	N[d]
5	121	0	15.3	4.1	57
5	121	1	5.7	3.2	56
5	131	0	13.6	2.8	63
5	131	1	7.3	2.3	28
10	121	0	11.8	3.5	59
10	121	1	5.6	2.3	51
10	131	0	11.6	3.7	30
10	131	1	5.9	2.3	32

[a] Debonding forces obtained with micromechanical test machine.
[b] Aqueous environment: Level 0 = none, Level 1 = 24 h at 37°C, pH 7.28.
[c] Sample standard deviation.
[d] Number of specimens.

Results and Discussion

Comparison of Oxalate Versus PDS System

The microdroplet pull-out force is measured on the micromechanical tester by shearing the droplet from the fiber, where the bond strength is the measured force divided by the contact surface area (Fig. 5). The initial microdroplet system examined is made of a PGA fiber and PDS matrix and was processed in a reactive environment. The experimental variables in the first set of pull-out tests are processing time, processing temperature, and exposure to a buffer solution. The results are given in Table 1 and statistical data shown in Table 2. The sources of variability are processing time (T), processing temperature (TT), and aging time in phosphate buffer (PP). As can be seen, both processing time and exposure to aqueous environment are significant factors affecting bond strength. An increase in either of these two variables causes a decrease in bond strength.

As a means of system comparison, an oxalate matrix, an AA-BB type polyester, was chosen to replace the PDS. The same detailed study was run giving the results in Table 3 and statistical data in Table 4. Comparing the two systems shows the much higher strength of the PGA/PDS

TABLE 2—*Statistics for PGA/PDS single fiber composites in reactive atmosphere.[a]*

Source	DF[b]	F[c] Value	Pr[d] > F
T	1	26.16	.0001
TT	1	0.00	.9867
PP	1	426.1	.0001
T*TT	1	0.01	.9131
T*PP	1	8.61	.0036
TT*PP	1	7.78	.0056
T*TT*PP	1	4.54	.0337

[a] Null hypothesis (H_0): The source of variability is zero.
[b] Degrees of freedom.
[c] Fisher test statistic.
[d] Probability of incorrectly rejecting the null hypothesis and concluding that the source of variability in question is significant.

TABLE 3—*Bond strength data for PGA/Oxalate single fiber composites in reactive atmosphere.*[a]

Processing Time (min)	Processing Temperature (°C)	Aqueous Environment Level[b]	Bond Strength (MPa)	S[c]	N[d]
5	70	0	4.6	1.6	33
5	70	1	4.2	1.6	41
5	90	0	4.0	1.4	31
5	90	1	3.6	1.4	50
10	70	0	4.1	1.6	29
10	70	1	4.6	1.7	29
10	90	0	4.8	1.7	30
10	90	1	2.6	0.9	57

[a] Debonding force obtained with micromechanical test machine.
[b] Aqueous environment: Level 0 = none, Level 1 = 24 h at 37°C, pH 7.28.
[c] Sample standard deviation.
[d] Number of specimens.

system. The strength of the oxalate system decreased significantly with increased processing temperature. Interestingly, the aging of the oxalate-based composites was less noticeable than that of PDS composites in a buffered medium, as reflected in a 10 to 20% and 50 to 60% loss of interfacial strength, respectively.

Comparison of Inert and Reactive Processing

PGA/PDS specimens were processed at 121°C for 5 min in a dry, argon environment and subsequently exposed to the degrading aqueous medium for 24 h. Bond strengths were calculated, with the micromechanical test machine debonding force values, for 32 specimens, giving an average of 8.7 MPa and standard deviation of 2.3. Nine of these values, included directly into the average without mathematical approximation, are minimal bond strength values; that is, the stroke range on the micromechanical test machine was insufficient to shear the droplet, and the bond strength included in the calculation corresponds to the highest force value recorded on the plot.

TABLE 4—*Statistics for PGA/Oxalate single fiber composites in reactive atmosphere.*[a]

Source	DF[b]	F[c] Value	Pr[d] > F
T	1	0.14	.7079
TT	1	11.87	.0007
PP	1	12.12	.0006
T*TT	1	0.08	.7796
T*PP	1	1.77	.1846
TT*PP	1	16.17	.0001
T*TT*PP	1	14.87	.0001

[a] Null hypothesis (H_0): The source of variability is zero.
[b] DF is degrees of freedom.
[c] F is Fisher test statistic.
[d] Pr is the probability of incorrectly rejecting the null hypothesis and concluding that the source of variability in question is significant.

TABLE 5—*Statistics comparing micromechanical test machine and Instron tensiometer: 5 min processing at 121°C, 24 h aging.*[a]

Machine	Mean Bond Strength (MPa)	S[b]	N[c]
Micromechanical Tester	8.7	2.3	32
Instron Dynamic Tester	5.7	2.3	56

[a] Aqueous environment, 37°C, pH 7.28.
[b] S is the standard deviation.
[c] N is the number of specimens.

The 8.7 MPa average bond strength, Case #1, is compared to the average bond strength obtained from Case #2, specimens processed for 5 min at 121°C, in a reactive environment, and exposed to aqueous environment for 24 h. Twenty-one specimens were tested in Case #2, resulting in an average 5.7 MPa bond strength with a standard deviation of 2.2. Only one specimen was not sheared when tested. The results are analyzed using a one-tailed t-test with the null hypothesis, H_o, that the mean bond strength from Case #1 equals the mean bond strength from Case #2. The alternative hypothesis, H_a, is that the mean bond strength of Case #1 is greater than that of Case #2. The data are significant at the 0.5% level, rejecting H_o and favoring H_a.

The bond strength increase, from inert processing, results in a large number of bonds which simply cannot be broken on the micromechanical tester. Therefore, in this case the Instron tensiometer is preferred over the micromechanical tester, for it has a larger stroke capacity and, thus, avoids a censored distribution of results and subsequent error in mathematical approximations.

Comparison of Results from the Instron Tensiometer and the Micromechanical Test Machine

Results of a study, comparing bond strength data obtained on the Instron tensiometer and the micromechanical test machine, are shown in Table 5. The values are from systems processed at 121°C for 5 min in inert environment and exposed to 37°C phosphate buffer for 24 h. A statistical analysis rejects the null hypothesis, H_0, that the two means are equal. The data speak against H_o ($p < 0.005$) and favor the alternative hypothesis, indicating that the Instron, in fact, consistently records lower values than those of the micromechanical test machine. Both machines were set to a stroke cycle frequency of 0.05 Hz and, with different stroke lengths, it is possible that they are not performing with identical shearing speeds as is desired. Another possibility is that the two different load cells have different sensitivities and, therefore, contribute to the varied results between machines. That is, the Instron load cell is of approximately 223 N capacity, the micromechanical tester is of approximately 0.20 N capacity, and the debonding forces average about 0.03 N. This means that the forces measured on the Instron are in the lower 0.013% of the load cell range and, thus, may contribute to the discrepancies between the results from the two machines.

Conclusions

Although the pattern of potential bonding is effectively masked by the characteristics of the absorbable systems and the processing conditions, the test methods are effective in detecting small changes between specimen groups. Used in combination with other quantitative and qualitative analyses, the micromechanical testing provides critical information towards the establishment of an optimal interface.

Acknowledgments

The authors wish to thank Davis & Geck and Ethicon for supplying the materials for this project, Dr. Dan Edie, Dr. Dennis Powers, and Dr. Len Stefanski, for their technical assistance, and the Department of Bioengineering, Clemson University and the Shriners Hospital for Crippled Children for supporting the project.

References

[1] Vainionpaa, S., Kilpikari, J., Laiho, J., et al., "Strength and Strength Retention in Vitro, of Absorbable, Self-Reinforced Polyglycolide (PGA) Rods for Fracture Fixation," *Biomaterials*, Vol. 8, January 1987, pp. 46–48.
[2] Shalaby, S. W., Schipper, E., and Koelmel, D., "Methyl P-(- Acetoxyalkoxy) Benzoate and Method of Preparation," U.S. Patent 4,433,161 (to Ethicon Inc.), Feb. 21, 1984.
[3] Latour, R. A., Black, J., and Miller, B., "Fracture Mechanisms of the Fiber/Matrix Interfacial Bond in Fiber-Reinforced Polymer Composites," *Surface and Interface Analysis*, Vol. 17, No. 7, June 16, 1991, pp. 477–484.
[4] Shalaby, S. W. and Jamiolkowski, D., "Synthetic Absorbable Devices of Poly(alkylene oxalates)," U.S. Patent 4,205,399 (to Ethicon Inc.), 1980.
[5] Johnson, R. A., "Effect of Chemical Composition on Biologically Relevant Properties of Oxalate-Based Absorbable Polyesters," M.S. thesis, Clemson University, 1992.
[6] Latour, R. A. and Black, J., Miniature Closed-Loop Dynamic Universal Mechanical Testing Machine, U.S. Patent 4,858,473, August 22, 1989.

Urologic Materials

Mutsumi Uchida,[1] *Yoichiroh Imaide,*[1] *and Hiroki Watanabe*[1]

Chemical Components and Mechanical Properties of Urinary Calculi

REFERENCE: Uchida, M., Imaide, Y., and Watanabe, H., **"Chemical Components and Mechanical Properties of Urinary Calculi,"** *Biomaterials' Mechanical Properties, ASTM STP 1173,* H. E. Kambic and A. T. Yokobori, Jr., Eds., American Society for Testing and Materials, Philadelphia, 1994, pp. 267–274.

ABSTRACT: As part of a research project on the intracorporeal destruction of urinary calculi with a small dose of explosives, a study of the correlation between the chemical components and the mechanical properties of urinary calculi was made. Compressive strength, tensile strength, and modulus of elasticity under dry and wet conditions were measured to find the mechanical properties of urinary calculi. All urinary calculi in the dry condition could be classified into two groups with a borderline of 6.5 MPa for compressive strength, 1.5 MPa for tensile strength, and 600 MPa for modulus of elasticity, and most of the calculi fell below the borderline. The chemical composition of calculi belonging to the high-strength calculus group was mostly a mixture of calcium phosphate and calcium oxalate. The strength of calculi in the wet condition was less than that in the dry condition.

KEYWORDS: urinary calculi, chemical components, mechanical properties, high-strength calculus group, low-strength calculus group

Urolithiasis, which can be classified into renal, ureteral, and bladder calculi depending on position, is probably as old as mankind itself and has often caused colicky pain, fever, and macrohematuria. The calculi have a variety of sizes and shapes. Some 70 to 80% of small urinary calculi, those below approximately 7 mm in diameter, are spontaneously passed through the urinary tract. However, conventional open surgery has been performed on patients with big urinary calculi, those over 10 mm in diameter.

Recently, minimal invasive surgery for the treatment of urinary calculi, such as percutaneous nephroureterolithotomy (PNL), transurethral ureterolithotripsy (TUL), and extracorporeal shock wave lithotripsy (ESWL), has made rapid progress in the field of urology. We started a research project for the intracorporeal destruction of urinary calculi with a small dose of explosives in 1975 and named this technique Microexplosion Lithotripsy (MEL). As part of this project, a study of the correlation between the chemical components and the mechanical properties of urinary calculi was made.

Materials and Methods

Forty-one urinary calculi removed by open lithotomy from patients at Kyoto Prefectural University of Medicine were employed in this study. The chemical components of all the calculi were analyzed using an infrared spectrophotometer and X-ray diffraction apparatus at the National Chemical Laboratory for Industry, MITI. Urinary calculi preserved in air after sur-

---

[1] Department of Urology, Kyoto Prefectural University of Medicine, Kyoto, Japan 602.

TABLE 1—*Materials.*

41 Urinary Calculi: Chemical Components
  In wet and dry conditions, 8 calculi:
    compressive strength
    modulus of elasticity
  In dry condition only, 33 calculi:
    compressive strength
    tensile strength
    modulus of elasticity

gical removal on operation were immersed in physiologic saline for 48 h and were then left to dry for 22 days. Stones under immersion were defined as urinary calculi in the wet condition and those after the drying period in the dry condition. In all, 33 calculi were used in the dry condition and 8 in both dry and wet conditions. Compressive strength, tensile strength, and modulus of elasticity were measured. Measurements for compressive strength and modulus of elasticity were performed on 41 calculi and those for tensile strength on 33 calculi (Table 1).

To measure compressive strength, the specimen was abraded into a cube 1 cm in diameter using a sheet of sandpaper, attached to a multi-material tester (Fig. 1). The load cell was adjusted to 500 kg, the full scale 10 kg and 25 kg, at a load speed 0.5 mm/min. The compressive strength was calculated from the load weight and the measured size of the broken surface when the specimen split. To measure tensile strength, the specimen was shaped into a cube and

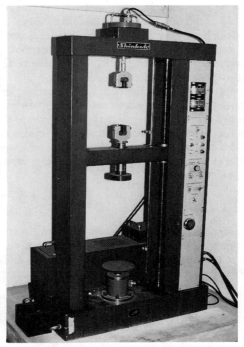

FIG. 1—*Multi-material tester.*

TABLE 2—*Results of chemical components.*

Ca phosphate, Ca oxalate	16 (39%)
Ca phosphate, Ca oxalate, Struvite	11 (27%)
Ca phosphate, Struvite	8 (20%)
Uric acid	2 (5%)
Ca phosphate	1 (2%)
Ca oxalate	1 (2%)
Unknown	2 (5%)

pieces of wire were attached to each end using a tough adhesive agent. The wire was attached to the same test system and the specimen was pulled at a load speed of 1.0 mm/min for the tensile strength study. The tensile strength was calculated from the load weight and the measured size of the broken surface when the specimen broke. The modulus of elasticity was calculated from the results of the compressive strength study.

Results

Chemical Components

The chemical components of 41 urinary calculi were studied with the following results.

Mixed components of calcium oxalate and calcium phosphate were most frequently observed, in 16 calculi (39%). Mixed components of calcium phosphate, calcium oxalate, and struvite were observed in 11 calculi (27%), mixed components of calcium phosphate and struvite in 8 calculi (20%), uric acid in 2 calculi (5%), calcium oxalate in 1 calculus (2%), and calcium phosphate in 1 calculus (2%). The chemical components of the remaining 2 calculi (5%) were undetermined (Table 2).

Compressive Strength

Forty-one calculus specimens were used to measure the compressive strength in the dry condition. In all, 14 calculi were broken during the study and the compressive strength was measured for 27 calculi. Of these 27 calculi, 8 were used for the measurement of compressive strength in both dry and wet conditions.

The compressive strength in the dry condition varied from 1.1 MPa to 17.6 MPa (mean strength 4.3 MPa) and that in the wet condition from 0.7 MPa to 3.6 MPa (mean strength 1.9 MPa) (Table 3).

TABLE 3—*Results of compressive strength.*

41 Calculi → 14 Calculi (broken during the study)	No. of Calculi	MPa	Mean ± SD
In dry condition	27	1.1–17.6	4.3 ± 3.7
In wet condition	8	0.7–3.6	1.9 ± 1.1
Ratio wet to dry condition	8		
Range 0.32–1.04			
Average 0.67			

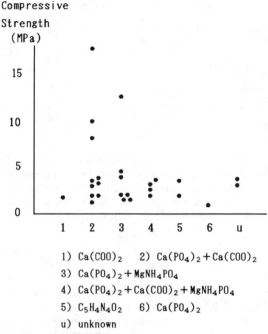

1) $Ca(COO)_2$ 2) $Ca(PO_4)_2 + Ca(COO)_2$
3) $Ca(PO_4)_2 + MgNH_4PO_4$
4) $Ca(PO_4)_2 + Ca(COO)_2 + MgNH_4PO_4$
5) $C_5H_4N_4O_2$ 6) $Ca(PO_4)_2$
u) unknown

FIG. 2—*Correlation between chemical components and compressive strength.*

The compressive strength of 23 out of the 27 calculi (85%) was less than 6.5 MPa and that of the remaining 4 calculi (15%) was above 6.5 MPa (Fig. 2). Of the 4 calculi with high compressive strength, 3 had mixed components of calcium phosphate and calcium oxalate. The compressive strength in the wet condition was lower than that in the dry condition and the ratio of wet to dry conditions was from 0.32 to 1.04 (mean ratio = 0.67).

Tensile Strength

Thirty-three calculus specimens were used to measure the tensile strength in the dry condition. Of these, 8 were broken during the study and the tensile strength was measured for 25 calculi.

The tensile strength varied from 0.1 MPa to 3.4 MPa (mean strength 0.7 MPa) (Table 4). The tensile strength of 23 out of the 25 calculi (92%) was less than 1.5 MPa and the remaining 2 calculi, which showed great compressive strength, had much greater tensile strength than the others (Fig. 3). The chemical composition of the 2 high tensile strength calculi was a mixture of calcium phosphate and calcium oxalate.

TABLE 4—*Results of tensile strength.*

33 Calculi → 8 Calculi (broken during the study)		
	No. of Calculi	MPa	Mean ± SD
In dry condition	25	0.1–3.4	0.7 ± 0.9

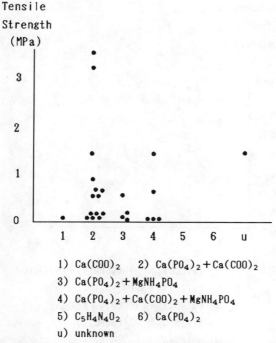

FIG. 3—*Correlation between chemical components and tensile strength.*

Modulus of Elasticity

Forty-one calculus specimen were used to measure the modulus of elasticity in the dry condition. Of these, 13 were broken during the study and the modulus of elasticity was measured for 28 calculi. Of these 28 calculi, 8 were used for the measurement of the modulus of elasticity in both dry and wet conditions.

The modulus of elasticity in the dry condition varied from 50 MPa to 880 MPa (mean modulus of elasticity 280 MPa) and that in the wet condition from 40 MPa to 240 MPa (mean modulus of elasticity 150 MPa) (Table 5). The modulus of elasticity of 26 out of the 28 calculi (93%) was less than 600 MPa and of the remaining 2 calculi was above 600 MPa. The chemical

TABLE 5—*Results of modulus of elasticity.*

41 Calculi → 13 Calculi (broken during the study)		
	No. of Calculi	MPa
In dry condition	28	50–880
In wet condition	8	40–240
Ratio wet to dry condition	8	
Range 0.26–1.10		
Average 0.66		

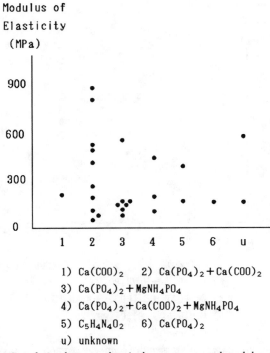

1) $Ca(COO)_2$ 2) $Ca(PO_4)_2 + Ca(COO)_2$
3) $Ca(PO_4)_2 + MgNH_4PO_4$
4) $Ca(PO_4)_2 + Ca(COO)_2 + MgNH_4PO_4$
5) $C_5H_4N_4O_2$ 6) $Ca(PO_4)_2$
u) unknown

FIG. 4—*Correlation between chemical components and modulus of elasticity.*

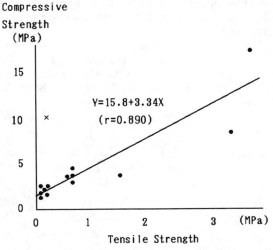

FIG. 5—*Correlation between tensile strength and compressive strength.*

composition of the calculi with a high modulus of elasticity was a mixture of calcium phosphate and calcium oxalate (Fig. 4). The modulus of elasticity in the wet condition was lower than that in the dry condition and the ratio of wet to dry was from 0.26 to 1.10 (mean ratio = 0.66).

Correlation Between Compressive Strength and Tensile Strength

The correlation between the compressive strength and the tensile strength was studied on 14 calculi in which both kinds of strength were measured in the dry condition. As shown in Fig. 5, except for one calculus (marked X in the figure), both tensile and compressive strength were proportional to each other for all calculi. A best fit approximation ($R = 0.89$) for this data yields a slope expressed as $Y = 3.34X + 15.8$.

Discussion

A research project for MEL was started in our clinic in 1975 [1]. An explosive has a powerful natural energy that is caused by two actions [2]: shock waves and gas generated by the detonation. The destruction process of urinary calculi in MEL is thought to be as follows. When a shock wave comes in contact with the surface of a urinary calculus (Fig. 6), compressive stress occurs on the surface as a result of the difference in acoustic impedance. At the point where the peak pressure of the shock wave exceeds the compressive strength of the calculus, a mechanical crack occurs in zone A. The transmitted shock wave is consecutively reflected to the opposite side and tensile stress occurs in zone B. Zone B cracks above the limit of the tensile strength of the calculus. The cracked calculus is separated into debris by the expanded gas (Fig. 6). In order to find the explosive dose suitable for the destruction of urinary calculi, the correlation between the chemical components and the mechanical properties of urinary calculi was studied in this paper.

The chemical components of urinary calculi were calcium oxalate; calcium phosphate; a mixture of calcium phosphate and calcium oxalate; a mixture of calcium phosphate and struvite; a mixture of calcium phosphate, calcium oxalate, and struvite; and uric acid. Of these components, the mixture of calcium phosphate and calcium oxalate was most frequently observed, in 16 calculi (39%).

The mechanical properties of urinary calculi including the compressive strength, the tensile strength, and the modulus of elasticity were studied along with the chemical composition.

The compressive strength in the dry condition varied from 1.1 MPa to 17.6 MPa and the average compressive strength was 4.3 MPa. The tensile strength in the dry condition varied from 0.1 MPa to 3.4 MPa and the average tensile strength was 0.7 MPa. These values were

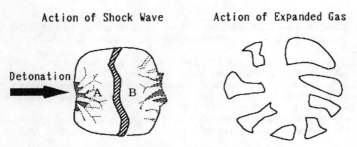

FIG. 6—*Destruction process of urinary calculi in MEL.*

almost equal to that of tuff, the weakest of the building stones. With all calculi, except for one marked X in Fig. 5, in which both kinds of strength were measured, a clear correlation was observed between the compressive strength and the tensile strength. The specimen marked X might have had an internal crack before measurement.

The modulus of elasticity of all calculi in the dry condition varied from 50 MPa to 880 MPa and the average modulus of elasticity was 280 MPa.

All calculi could be classified into two groups with a borderline of 6.5 MPa for compressive strength, 1.5 MPa for tensile strength, and 600 MPa for modulus of elasticity, and most of the calculi fell below the borderline. Therefore, it seems more reasonable to classify the calculi into two groups: a high-strength calculus group and a low-strength calculus group. The chemical composition of the calculi that belonged to the high-strength calculus group was mostly a mixture of calcium phosphate and calcium oxalate.

Since urinary calculi in the normal situation are actually suspended in urine, it is necessary to study these mechanical properties in the wet condition. The compressive strength and the modulus of elasticity were therefore measured in that condition. The compressive strength in the wet condition varied from 0.7 MPa to 3.6 MPa and the mean strength was 1.9 MPa. The compressive strength in the wet condition was lower than that in the dry condition and the mean ratio of wet to dry conditions was 0.67. The modulus of elasticity in the wet condition varied from 40 MPa to 240 MPa and the average value was 150 MPa. The modulus of elasticity in the wet condition was lower than that in the dry condition and the mean ratio of wet to dry conditions was 0.66. The results showed a great advantage for the destruction of urinary calculi in the wet condition.

In our other experimental reports, it was demonstrated that the detonation of a few mg of explosives produced a shock wave with a peak pressure of approximate 10 MPa in water [3] and expanded gas bubbles of 20 mL to 30 mL [4].

From the above-mentioned results, it has been shown that the power of even a small dose of explosive exceeds the limit of the strength of urinary calculi and MEL is therefore a satisfactory means of destruction for urinary calculi.

Conclusion

We studied the correlation between the chemical components and the mechanical properties of urinary calculi in order to find the explosive dose suitable for their destruction. All calculi could be classified into two groups: a high-strength calculus group and a low-strength calculus group, and most calculi belonged to the latter. The strength of urinary calculi in the wet condition was lower than that in the dry condition, and the mean ratio of wet to dry conditions was 0.67 for compressive strength and 0.66 for modulus of elasticity.

References

[1] Watanabe, H. and Oinuma, S., "Studies on the Application of Microexplosion to Medicine and Biology. Development of Special Explosive for the Experiments," *Japanese Journal of Urology,* Vol. 68, 1977, pp. 243–248.
[2] Watanabe, H., Uchida, M., Nakagawa, Y., and Kitamura, K., "Development and Application of Confined Blasting for Bladder and Kidney Stones," Urol.int. Vol. 42, 1987, pp. 3–29.
[3] Kondoh, K., "Studies on the Application of Microexplosion to Medicine and Biology. The Pressure Profile of Blast Wave in Buffer Liquid by Detonation of a Lead Azide Charging Chamber," *Japanese Journal of Urology,* Vol. 77, 1986, pp. 1716–1725.
[4] Watanabe, K., "Studies on the Application of Microexplosion to Medicine and Biology. Injury to the Dog Bladder by Microexplosion," *Japanese Journal of Urology,* Vol. 74, 1983, pp. 299–310.

Hiroki Watanabe,[1] *Yuji Nakagawa,*[1] *and Mutsumi Uchida*[1]

Tests to Evaluate the Mechanical Properties of the Ureter

REFERENCE: Watanabe, H., Nakagawa, Y., and Uchida, M., **"Tests to Evaluate the Mechanical Properties of the Ureter,"** *Biomaterials' Mechanical Properties, ASTM STP 1173,* H. E. Kambic and A. T. Yokobori, Jr., Eds., American Society for Testing and Materials, Philadelphia, 1994, pp. 275–282.

ABSTRACT: In 1975, we started a research project for the development of microexplosion lithotripsy. In this project, we investigated the mechanical properties of the urinary tract organs to clarify factors to prevent complications from the method. Tension and expansion tests were performed on the middle portion of the normal ureter taken from fresh cadavers in 1983.

A tension test was performed on eleven ureters in the longitudinal direction and seven in the transverse direction using a universal tensile tester. Tensile strength and maximum tensile stress in the transverse direction of the ureter were weaker than those in the longitudinal direction. Accordingly, it was presumed that ureteral injury first occurred in the transverse direction. The maximum tensile stress of the ureter was higher than that of the bladder, which was previously reported in another paper.

Expansive tests were performed on ten ureters. At the leakage point, the tensile strength and elongation ratio of the external diameter were approximately equal to the tensile strength and elongation ratio measured by tension test in the transverse direction.

It could be concluded from the results that microexplosion lithotripsy could be applicable even in the ureter under certain conditions.

KEYWORDS: ureter, mechanical property, tension test, stress, tension, elongation, expansion, yield point, leak point, tissue damage

The ureter is a tubiform organ that transports urine from the kidney to the urinary bladder. It is 24 to 30 cm in length and approximately 5 mm in diameter.

The wall of the ureter is composed of transitional cell epithelium under which lies loose connective and elastic tissue. External to these are a mixture of spiral and longitudinal smooth muscle fibers. The outermost adventitial coat is composed of fibrous connective tissue.

In pathology, the ureter is important because stones may gather in it. Small urinary calculi generated in the kidney occasionally fall into the ureter. When this obstructs the ureteral space, hydronephrosis occurs causing colicky pain and resulting in the disturbance of the renal function.

For the removal of these ureteral calculi, the only conventional technique was open surgery. In recent years, however, endoscopic lithotripsy has advanced dramatically and has replaced open surgery. Percutaneous nephroureterolithotomy is a method of extracting calculi. An endoscope is inserted into the kidney from the back by way of a channel. We were the first in the world to perform the method successfully in a single stage, in 1981 [1]. We also developed the original "pin-hammer lithotriptor" to crush calculi inside the ureter using the energy from a microexplosion, in 1985 [2].

---

[1] Department of Urology, Kyoto Prefectural University of Medicine, Kyoto, Japan, 602.

To complete these endoscopic techniques safely, the mechanical properties of the ureter had to be elucidated. For this purpose, we performed tension and expansive tests on the human ureter. The results of the tests were reported in Japanese [3] but we revised and summarized the mechanical test methods.

Tension Test

The middle portion of a normal ureter was taken from a fresh cadaver and was immersed in cold physiologic saline solution for 24 h to eliminate the effects of rigor mortis.

For the tension test, a special "I"-shaped cutter was newly devised. The test piece was molded in the I shape by chiseling with the cutter. The width of the test piece (w_0) was set to 5 mm. The width of the end portion, which was gripped in a holder, was a little wider than that of the test portion (Fig. 1). Test pieces were taken from both the longitudinal and transverse axes of the ureter.

A special holder for the test piece was also newly devised. On the surface of the portions gripping the test piece, small metal spikes were created to prevent slipping. The test piece was fixed between the two surfaces (Fig. 2).

The holder, to which the piece was fixed, was attached to a universal tester (TOM-200D, Shinko Co.). The depth (t_0) and the length (l_0) of the test portion of the piece were measured by a micro-caliper.

The cross-sectional area of the piece (S) was calculated from the depth (t_0) multiplied by the width (w_0) of the piece, which was presumed to be constant throughout the test, as given by the following values

$$t_0 = 1 \text{ mm} \qquad w_0 = 5 \text{ mm}$$

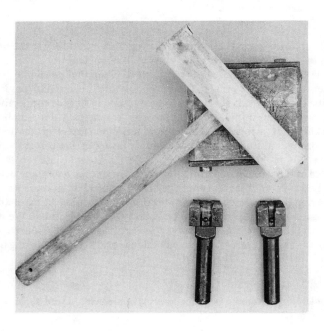

FIG. 1—*Special I-shaped cutter.*

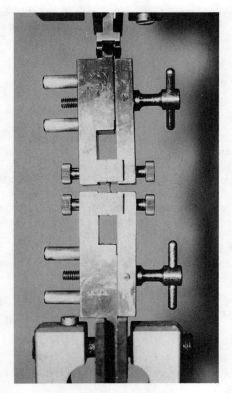

FIG. 2—*Special holder for the test piece.*

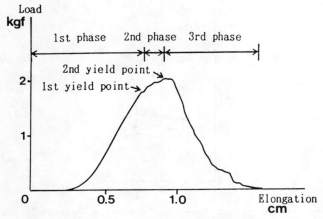

FIG. 3—*Stress-strain curve of the human ureter.*

The tension (T), strain (σ), and elongation ratio (ε) of the piece were also calculated as follows

$$T = F/w_0 \text{ (kgf/cm)}$$

$$\sigma = F/S \text{ (MPa)}$$

$$\varepsilon = \Delta l/l_0$$

where F is the stretching force, Δl is the elongation, and l_0 is the initial length.

The test piece was stretched at a constant loading speed of 5 mm/min. A stress-strain curve or load-deflection curve with three phases was obtained (Fig. 3). In Phase 1, the stress increased in proportion to the elongation, without apparent tissue damage to the test piece. In Phase 2, the degree of increase diminished and some wavering was observed in the curve. In this period, partial tissue rupture was occasionally noticed on the piece macroscopically. In Phase 3, the stress decreased suddenly, with advanced tissue rupture, and finally the piece separated into two portions. We defined the border between Phases 1 and 2 as the first yield point and that between Phases 2 and 3 as the second yield point.

The tension of eleven specimens of the ureter taken in the longitudinal direction was 2.0 ±

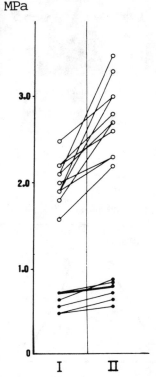

FIG. 4—*Strain of the human ureter.* ○: *Longitudinal direction.* ●: *Transverse direction. I: First yield point. II. Second yield point.*

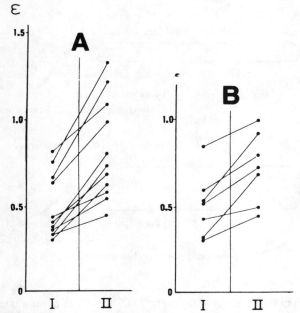

FIG. 5—*Elongation ratio of the human ureter. A: Longitudinal direction. B: Transverse direction. I. First yield point. II. Second yield point.*

0.21 kgf/cm at the first yield point and 2.8 ± 0.40 kgf/cm at the second yield point. The tension of seven specimens of the ureter taken in the transverse direction was 0.62 ± 0.10 kgf/cm at the first yield point and 0.75 ± 0.11 kgf/cm at the second yield point.

The strain of eleven specimens in the longitudinal direction was 1.96 ± 0.21 MPa at the first yield point and 2.75 ± 0.39 MPa at the second yield point. The strain of seven specimens in the transverse direction was 0.61 ± 0.10 MPa at the first yield point and 0.74 ± 0.11 MPa at the second yield point (Fig. 4).

The elongation ratio of eleven specimens of the ureter taken in the longitudinal direction was 0.49 ± 0.18 at the first yield point and 0.83 ± 0.27 at the second yield point. This means that the ureter stretched to 49% at the first yield point and to 83% at the second yield point. The elongation ratio of seven specimens of the ureter taken in the transverse direction was 0.50 ± 0.17 at the first yield point and 0.73 ± 0.19 at the second yield point (Fig. 5).

Expansive Test

For the expansive test, one side of the extirpated ureter was ligated. An 18G elastic needle was inserted into the other side of the ureter and then also ligated. The length of the ureter (L_0) was measured between the two ligations and the initial diameter (D_0) of the ureter was measured at the center of the ureter (Fig. 6).

A syringe was fixed to the universal tester and physiologic saline solution was injected into the ureter through the needle at a constant speed of 1.25 mL/min. The volume-pressure curve inside the ureter was obtained from the injected volume and the compressive force. After a time leakage of the injected saline solution from the ureteral wall was observed and the internal pressure ceased to increase. We named this the "leak point" (Fig. 7).

1) Initial condition

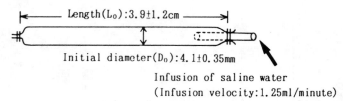

2) Leak point

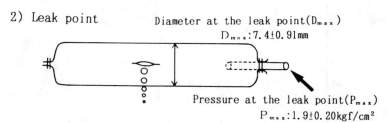

FIG. 6—*Expansive test of the human ureter.*

The increase ratio of the diameter of the ureter (ΔD) at the leak point was calculated by the following formula

$$\Delta D = \frac{D_{max} - D_0}{D_0}$$

where ΔD is the increased ratio of diameter, and D_0 is the initial diameter.

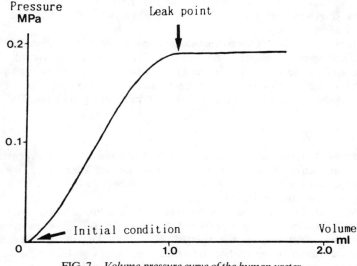

FIG. 7—*Volume-pressure curve of the human ureter.*

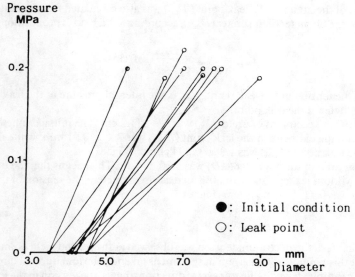

FIG. 8—*Correlation between the diameter and the internal pressure.* •: *Initial condition.* ○: *Leak point.*

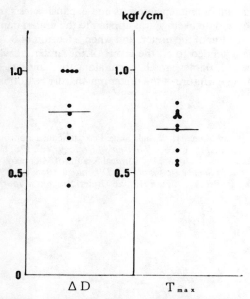

FIG. 9—*ΔD and T_{max} of the human ureter. ΔD: Increase ratio of diameter. T_{max}: Tension at leak point.*

The tension of the ureter at the leak point (T_{max}) was also calculated from the internal pressure (P_{max}) and the diameter of the ureter (D_{max}), according to La Place's proposition, as follows

$$T_{max} = P_{max} \times \frac{D_{max}}{2} \, (kgf/cm)$$

where T_{max} is the tension at the leak point, P_{max} is the internal pressure at the leak point, and D_{max} is the diameter at the leak point.

The length of ten specimens of ureter (L_0) was 3.9 ± 1.2 cm. The initial diameter (D_0) was 4.1 ± 0.35 mm, the diameter at the leak point (D_{max}) was 7.4 ± 0.91 mm, while the internal pressure at the leak point (P_{max}) was 1.9 ± 0.20 kgf/cm^2 (Fig. 8).

The increase ratio of the diameter (ΔD) was 0.80 ± 0.19. This means that the ureter could be expanded without leakage up to an 80% increase in diameter. The tension of the ureter at the leak point was 0.71 ± 0.10 kgf/cm (Fig. 9).

Discussion

In the tension test, the maximum tension was observed at the second yield point. The average tension at this point was 2.8 kgf/cm in specimens taken in the longitudinal direction, and 0.75 kgf/cm in samples taken in the transverse direction; that is, the tension in the longitudinal direction was four times stronger than that in the transverse direction. Furthermore, in the expansive test, the average tension of the ureter at the leak point was 0.71 kgf/cm, showing a very good coincidence with that in the transverse direction in the tension test.

Also, a good correlation was observed between the elongation ratio (ε) of the ureter in the tension test and the increase ratio (ΔD) of diameter in the expansive test.

Conclusion

From these experiments including tension tests and expansive tests, it was estimated that when a tension of 0.62 kgf/cm on average was applied to the ureter, damage started to occur along the longitudinal direction of the ureter, and when a tension of 0.75 kgf/cm on average was applied, the damage extended to all the layers of the ureter, at which point a leakage occurred. However, since little damage might occur along the transverse direction under tension of this extent, a complete rupture of the ureter may hardly be noticed.

References

[1] Saitoh, M., Watanabe, H., and Ohe, H., "Single Stage Percutaneous Nephroureterolithotomy Using a Special Ultrasonically Guided Pyeloscope," *Journal of Urology,* Vol. 128, 1982, pp. 591–592.
[2] Watanabe, H., Kondoh, K., and Uchida, M., "Clinical Results of Microexplosion Lithotripsy," *Proceedings of XXe Congrès de la Société Internationale D'Urologie* 1985, pp. 260–262.
[3] Nakagawa, Y., "Mechanical Property of the Human Ureter," *Japanese Journal of Urology,* Vol. 80, 1989, pp. 1481–1488.

Masahito Saitoh,[1] Katsumi Ohnishi,[1] Tadahisa Matsuda,[1] Hiroki Watanabe,[1] A. Toshimitsu Yokobori,[2] Takeo Yokobori,[2] and Fumiya Oki[3]

Mechanical Properties and Modeling of the Stress-Strain Behavior of the Urinary Bladder *In Vivo*

REFERENCE: Saitoh, M., Ohnishi, K., Matsuda, T., Watanabe, H., Yokobori, A. T., Yokobori, T., and Oki, F., **"Mechanical Properties and Modeling of the Stress-Strain Behavior of the Urinary Bladder *In Vivo*,"** *Biomaterials' Mechanical Properties, ASTM STP 1173*, H. E. Kambic and A. T. Yokobori, Jr., Eds., American Society for Testing and Materials, Philadelphia, 1994, pp. 283–289.

ABSTRACT: A stretch test *in vivo* for living materials was newly developed and applied to the dog bladder. The stress-strain curve of the normal living bladder was a downward convex and rose very slowly. The curve showed hysteresis and speed-dependence. These results proved that the mechanical property of the urinary bladder was essentially viscoelastic.

A computer analysis, based on the viscoelastic simulation model proposed by Glantz, was performed to evaluate the mechanical property of the bladder. Both proportional and exponential stiffness elevated in the extirpated bladder. In the denervated bladder, changes of the constants were not significant immediately after cutting the pelvic nerves; however, the proportional stiffness elevated remarkably two weeks after cutting. Compared with these abnormal bladders, the elastic constants of the normal living bladder were very low. The viscoelastic properties of the bladder and its low elastic constants seemed to account for the normal bladder function as a reservoir for urine.

KEYWORDS: stretch test, urinary bladder, viscoelasticity

The urinary bladder is a balloon-like organ that accumulates urine. The pressure inside of the bladder is extremely low and does not elevate when the urinary volume increases. This strange phenomenon has been discussed for many years, but still has not been satisfactorily explained.

A stretch test *in vivo* for living materials was newly developed, and analysis of the stress-strain curve for a normal living bladder provided a good explanation of this phenomenon.

Materials and Methods

A canine urinary bladder was explored under general anesthesia. A silk thread was inserted into the bladder puncturing it at two points 1 cm apart and both ends of thread were fixed to

[1] Associate professor, assistant, assistant, and professor and chairman, respectively, Department of Urology, Kyoto Prefectural University of Medicine, Kawaramachi-Hirokoji, Kyoto 602, Japan.

[2] Associate professor and Professor Emeritus, respectively, Department of Mechanical Engineering II, Tohoku University, Aramaki, Aoba-ku, Sendai 980, Japan.

[3] Assistant professor, Department of Physics, Kyoto Prefectural University of Medicine, Taishogun, Kyoto 602, Japan.

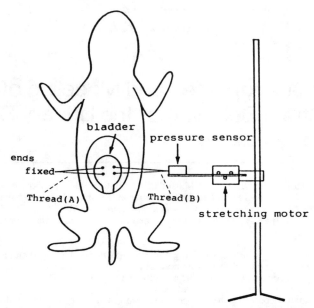

FIG. 1—*The experimental model of the stretch test in vivo. Thread (A) was inserted into the bladder puncturing it at two points 1 cm apart and both ends of thread were fixed to the operating table. Thread (B) was inserted in the same way and both ends were connected to a pressure transducer. The part of the bladder wall enclosed within the four puncture points of the two threads was stretched uniaxially at a constant velocity of* c = 5.0 cm/min.

the operating table. A second thread was inserted in the same way and both ends were connected to a pressure transducer. The distance between the two threads was approximately 2 or 3 cm and this was regarded as the initial length. The part of the bladder wall enclosed within the four puncture points of the two threads was considered to be the bladder strip for the purpose of the stretch test. The enclosed bladder wall was stretched uniaxially at a constant velocity of $c = 5.0$ cm/min (Fig. 1). The bladder was then contracted to its original length at the same velocity. The stress-strain curve obtained by this stretch test was recorded on a polygraph. The stretching velocity dependence of the bladder wall was studied by obtaining the stress-strain curve at different stretching velocities.

An industrial use pressure transducer (Orientec T1-1000-240, Japan) was equipped with a polygraph and monitored the stretch force. The bladder was empty when the stretch test was performed.

The simulation model for smooth muscle proposed by Glantz [1] was applied to analyze the mechanical property of the bladder. Theoretical analyses of the stress-strain curve based on Glantz's model were made by physical and computer analysis.

Glantz's model consists of two nonlinear elements and one damping element (Fig. 2). The following formula representing the stress-strain curve of the model was proposed

$$\psi = -\beta(\psi + \alpha)^2/\gamma + \beta(\psi + \alpha)C + \alpha^2\beta e^{\beta c t}/\gamma$$

where ψ is force, α and β are elastic constants, and γ is viscous constant.

According to their properties, α was designated as a proportional stiffness and β as an exponential stiffness. A computer analysis based on Glantz' viscoelastic simulation model was car-

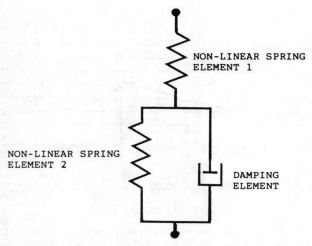

FIG. 2—*A mechanical model of the smooth muscle proposed by Glantz.*

ried out to evaluate changes of the curve under various conditions. Three constants for the dog bladder (α, β, γ) were calculated by the Runge-Kutta-Merson method from the most probable fitting between the actual stress-strain curve and the theoretical curve of Glantz's model. The software used for the Runge-Kutta-Merson method was a library program from Tohoku University.

Three constants (α, β, γ) were obtained for the normal bladder, the extirpated bladder, the bladder immediately after denervation, and the bladder two weeks after denervation.

Denervation was carried out by surgery. The complete nervous system for the bladder including the hypogastric and pelvic nerves was cut. All the tests were performed *in vivo* except for the test on the extirpated bladder. The bladder removed from the dog (extirpated bladder) was put into a saline solution at 37° centigrade temperature for 12 h and the stretch test was carried out in the saline using the same technique as for the normal bladder *in vivo*.

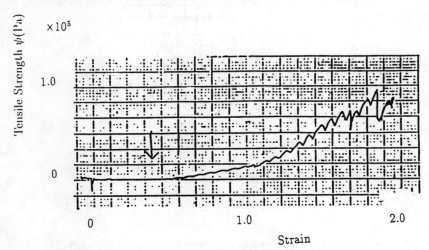

FIG. 3—*The stress-strain curve of the normal living bladder.*

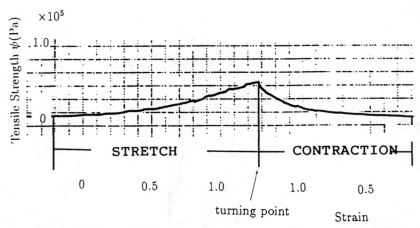

FIG. 4—*The hysteresis curve obtained by the stress-contraction test for the bladder.*

The Stress-Strain Curve

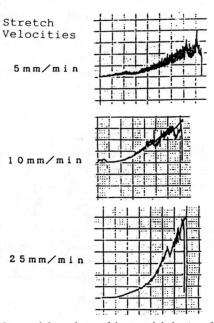

FIG. 5—*The speed dependence of the stretch behavior of the bladder.*

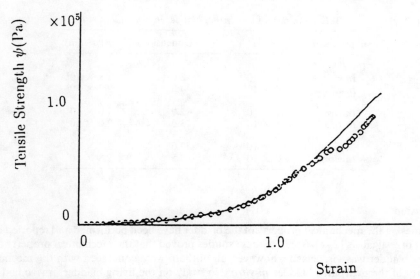

FIG. 6—*Theoretical stress-strain curve matches the experimental curve well. Solid line shows the theoretical one and the open circles line shows the experimental one.*

Results

Analysis of the Stress-Strain Curve

The stress-strain curve for the normal living bladder was a downward convex and rose very slowly (Fig. 3). The hysteresis loop of the stress-strain curve of the bladder was obtained by a stress-contraction test (Fig. 4). The stretching velocity dependence of the bladder wall (Fig. 5) was also recognized in the study of the stress-strain curve at different stretching velocities. These results proved that the mechanical property of the urinary bladder was viscoelastic.

The stress-strain curve for the denervated bladder and the extirpated bladder showed rapid elevation of the stretch force.

Simulation of the Bladder Wall by the Mechanical Model Proposed by Glantz

The theoretical stress-strain curve of Glantz's model obtained by computer calculation showed both a hysteresis loop and a speed dependence. The experimental and theoretical curves matched each other well (Fig. 6). These facts proved that the mechanical property of the bladder wall was well simulated by the mechanical model.

Evaluation of the Mechanical Properties of the Bladder

Three constants of the living dog bladder (α, β, γ) in different conditions such as normal bladder, extirpated bladder, the bladder after denervation, and the bladder two weeks after denervation were obtained by matching the experimental stress-strain curve with the theoretical one (Tables 1 and 2).

TABLE 1—α, β, γ of the normal bladder in vivo and in vitro.

Experiment	α(Pa)	β(No Dimension)	γ(Pa·min)
1			
In vivo	2.1×10^3	2.6	1.8×10^5
In vitro	5.0×10^3	4.0	2.2×10^5
2			
In vivo	1.7×10^3	2.0	1.0×10^5
In vitro	4.5×10^3	3.0	2.0×10^5
3			
In vivo	2.5×10^3	2.0	2.2×10^5
In vitro	7.0×10^3	3.5	2.8×10^5

Discussion

Studies on the mechanical property of the bladder have been performed and reported on by several investigators [2–4]. Some of these studies proved that the mechanical property of the urinary bladder was viscoelastic; however, all of them were concerned with the mechanical property of the extirpated bladder *in vitro*. No study on the living bladder *in vivo* had been done because a stretch test for living materials was not available. We succeeded in achieving such a stretch test *in vivo*. Our study demonstrated that the mechanical property of the living urinary bladder was different from that of the extirpated bladder. The stress-strain curve for the normal living bladder was a downward convex and rose very slowly. On the other hand, the curve for the extirpated bladder rose rapidly. The curve for the denervated bladder also showed a quickly elevated downward curve in a study two weeks after denervation. However, elevation was slower in the study performed immediately after denervation.

These facts were analyzed by computer calculation of the stress-strain curve. The three constants (α, β, γ) obtained by computer analysis showed the mechanical property of the bladder under different conditions well. The proportional stiffness α changed remarkably when the bladder was denervated or extirpated. The exponential stiffness β also changed when the bladder condition was changed, but the changes were not notable. The viscous constant γ seemed to be stable under the different bladder conditions. These results suggested that the spring components of the mechanical property of the bladder changed by denervation or extirpation, and that the dashpot component of the bladder did not change.

TABLE 2—α, β, γ of the denervated bladder in vivo.

Experiment	α(Pa)	β(No Dimension)	γ(Pa·min)
1			
Normal Bladder	2.2×10^3	2.5	2.5×10^5
Immediately After Denervation	2.0×10^3	4.0	2.5×10^5
2 Weeks After Denervation	5.5×10^3	2.7	2.0×10^5
2			
Normal Bladder	2.0×10^3	3.0	1.0×10^5
Immediately After Denervation	1.5×10^3	2.2	3.5×10^5
2 Weeks After Denervation	10.0×10^3	3.6	2.0×10^5
3			
Normal Bladder	2.0×10^3	2.3	2.0×10^5
Immediately After Denervation	3.0×10^3	2.0	8.0×10^5
2 Weeks After Denervation	8.5×10^3	2.8	2.5×10^5

Compared with these abnormal bladders, the elastic constants in the normal living bladder were very low. The viscoelastic properties of the bladder, and its low elastic constant, seemed to account for the normal bladder function as a reservoir for urine.

Conclusion

A stretch test *in vivo* for living materials was newly developed and successfully applied to the living urinary bladder. The stress-strain curve of the bladder was well simulated by the mechanical model proposed by Glantz. It was proved that the mechanical property of the bladder was essentially viscoelastic. The normal living bladder showed very low proportional stiffness, which must account for the normal bladder function as a reservoir for urine.

References

[*1*] Glantz, S. A., "A Constitutive Equation for the Passive Properties of Muscle," *Journal of Biomechanics,* Vol. 7, 1974, pp. 137–145.
[*2*] Alexander, R. S., "Mechanical Properties of Urinary Bladder," *American Journal of Physiology,* Vol. 220, 1971, pp. 1413–1421.
[*3*] Coolsaet, B. L. R. A., van Duyl, W. A., van Mastrigt, R., and Schouten, J. W., "Viscoelastic Properties of Bladder Wall Strips," *Investigative Urology,* Vol. 12, 1975, pp. 3551–3356.
[*4*] Susset, J. G. and Regnier, C. H., "Viscoelastic Properties of Bladder Strips, Standardization of a Technique," *Investigative Urology,* Vol. 18, 1981, pp. 445–450.

Future Directions

Helen E. Kambic[1]

Changing Strategies for Biomaterials and Biotechnology

REFERENCE: Kambic, H. E., "**Changing Strategies for Biomaterials and Biotechnology,**" *Biomaterials' Mechanical Properties, ASTM STP 1173,* H. E. Kambic and A. T. Yokobori, Jr., Eds., American Society for Testing and Materials, Philadelphia, 1994, pp. 293–301.

ABSTRACT: The basis for the design and fabrication of new substitutes for tissue regeneration and organ replacement resides in biomaterials science and in the emerging field of tissue engineering. Three design approaches employ materials that perform as inert, biometric or biodegradable interfaces with body fluids or tissues. Biomaterials can provide the substrate integrated with tissue engineered molecules, cells, extracellular matrix, or recombinant protein. The question remains as to how we begin to address the issue of quality, safety, and efficacy issues in experimental testing of these materials when used in medical applications. As federal government funding of research has decreased, industrial support of academic research and development has grown. As the complexity of the interactions between materials and biological tissues grows, biomaterials-based emerging technologies will prosper through an overall changing approach to basic and applied biomaterials research. How to meet these needs through industry and academia remain unresolved. Our priorities must include a major emphasis on quality and strict adherence to quality assurance issues in testing and analysis.

KEYWORDS: biomaterials, degradable polymers, ceramics, new directions, emerging technologies

Biomaterials used in medical devices are expected to perform a large variety of functions ranging from solid supports to pulsatile materials and biodegradable scaffolds. The rapid development of medical device technologies has been involved in composites and coatings, some with living cells, not just singular components, as was prominent in the past. Now scientists attempting to establish a chemical and physical basis for fabricating new substitutes for tissue and organ replacement have turned to the emerging field of tissue engineering. The basis for this all new technology remains the science of biomaterials.

The field of biomaterials does not exist alone but within the realm of biomedical engineering and this technology remains a multidisciplinary endeavor. This science based on chemistry, physics, and cellular and molecular biology feeds engineering efforts to make products for the benefit of man [1].

How to test and predict the performance of these products is one goal of ASTM Committee F–4. The purpose of this report is to illustrate some of the challenges and complexities of biomaterials testing in cardiovascular areas (vascular grafts, heart valves, interventional procedures) and in orthopaedic and dental applications. New analytical tools and strategies for analyzing biomaterials interactions must be employed to expand our understanding of both the cellular reactions and biomaterial response mechanisms involved.

---

[1] Project scientist, Department of Biomedical Engineering, The Cleveland Clinic, Cleveland, OH 44195.

The transition from experimental research to clinical acceptance depends on laboratory programs—good design, adequate testing, and quality control/assurances. Utmost in importance are good manufacturing and laboratory procedures.

Challenges and Existing Problems

In general, implanted metallic, ceramic/polymeric materials degrade in the body releasing constituent ions or components that, in time, may lead to an adverse response [2]. These reactions in the body elicit activation of inflammatory cells and with the subsequent release of cytokines, enhance fibroblast proliferation and collagen production. The formation of a fibrous capsule around the implant compromises the functional success of the implant. Minimizing such reactions could influence the durability and functional life span of implanted devices for clinical use [3].

The main obstacles in the use of nonbiological materials in cardiovascular implants are surface induced thrombus and embolism [4].

To understand these problems, three design approaches that are complementary yet quite different will be illustrated. One employs materials that are expected to perform as permanent inert interfaces with body fluids or tissue. The other, newer approaches apply bulk or surface modifications or incorporate cell linings or cellular components (extracellular matrix, hybrid devices, recombinant gene technology), or a combination thereof, that render biomimetic or biodegradable materials (Table 1).

Permanent Fixed Devices Vascular Grafts

Available synthetic materials for large blood vessel replacement (greater than 6 mm internal diameter [I.D.]) are composed of Dacron® or Teflon®, which bring about problems of compliance mismatch and thrombogenicity [5]. At the present time there are no clinically acceptable small diameter (less than 4 mm I.D.) synthetic grafts. One problem lies at the anastomosis where failure is due to anastomotic pseudointimal hyperplasia. Two general methods used for the development of small diameter vascular grafts include the concepts of (1) providing an inert material that will be ignored by the cellular systems of the body or, (2) producing a bioreactive material that will interact with specific cellular systems of the body [6].

The challenge at the anastomosis is the problem of how mechanical events occurring locally send signals to cells to increase their proliferative and synthetic activities with the release of PDGF (platelet derived growth factor), EGF (epidermal growth factor), and TGF-β (transforming growth factor-β).

In the clinical setting, myointimal hyperplasia occurs specifically at the distal anastomosis; the lesions more commonly associated with synthetic grafts rather than vein grafts manifest themselves relatively early (mean 16 to 24 months) in the postoperative period [10].

From a mechanical standpoint, compliance mismatch between the native vessel and synthetic graft has long been indicated as a cause of failure for small diameter prosthesis [11,12]. This hypothesis still remains unproven due to difficulties in isolating and in comparing two

TABLE 1—*Approaches to biomaterial design.*

Inert	Bioreactive Biomimetic	Biodegradable

important variables, namely, compliance and the graft surface characteristics in a given experimental model [13].

Heart Valves

Biomaterial associated calcification is the leading cause of failure and limits the functional lifetime of experimental blood pumps and polymeric heart valves [14]. To understand the mechanical determinants, a re-evaluation of implant geometry, controlled drug release, matrix incorporation, systemic therapy, and cuspal loading have been suggested to prevent bioprosthetic (chemically treated tissue) heart valve calcification. The assessment of heart valves with respect to clinical relevance necessitates the simulation of circulatory conditions and the applications of various measurement techniques [15].

These include velocity profiles, pressure drop measurements, energy loss, regurgitant volumes, fatigue testing, and washout. Protocols such as these evaluate potential hemolysis of the blood and predict contour of the cusps and durability of the valve design under cyclic loading conditions.

Mechanical durability remains a critical issue with the use of any prosthetic heart valve. The anti-coagulant therapy required to reduce the thromboembolic complication of mechanical valve prosthesis may result in hemorrhage.

To check the durability of valves, the materials and implant designs are tested in *in vitro* accelerated life cycle testers and testing specifications and with newly developed three-dimensional imaging techniques [16–17]. The correlation of *in vitro* valve durability data with the data from recovered *in vivo* implants has been inadequate [18]. More et al. [18] suggest dynamic loading as the predictive criteria for developing future valve designs. Their model describes wear in terms of applied dynamic load and design parameters such as contact geometry and material properties. As *in vitro* venous valve test system to measure venous hemodynamics influenced by muscle pumping activity, respiration, and filling pressure of the right heart has been developed by Lee et al. [19]. This hydraulic mock circuit mimics natural venous flow.

Coronary Interventional Procedures

Cardiovascular interventional procedures such as coronary stent implantation, directional atherectomy, aortic valvuloplasty, and the use of intra-aortic balloon pumps or circulatory support devices introduce not only the device but a myriad of guiding catheters, arterial sheaths, percutaneous energy transmission systems, skin buttons, and inflow grafts. Despite intensive anticoagulant and fibrinolytic therapy, the hazards associated with the use of these devices include a potential greater risk of arterial injury at the access site [20].

One aggressive approach for the treatment of stenosed atherosclerotic vessels has been the use of intravascular stents combined with interventional noninvasive angiographic techniques [21]. In a previous publication from our group, the titanium nickel alloy 5-mm-diameter intravascular stent was investigated as an adjunct for the treatment of symptomatic arterial dissection, early occlusion, and late restenosis resulting from percutaneous transluminal angioplasty (PTA) [22]. Our results evaluating stenotic arterial segments treated with angioplasty alone or with angioplasty plus intravascular stenting in atherosclerotic rabbits showed no significant difference in either the histopathologic changes or restenosis rates. The stent may not prevent diffuse atherosclerotic vascular disease.

In a recent study completed by Strauss et al. [23], in reviewing the European experience with stents placed in native vessels and bypass grafts, indicates a high incidence of late adverse clinical events in patients with stents. The thrombosis with the Wallstent limits its use.

The benefits for stenting for correcting the lumen of obstructed vessels must be balanced by the consequences of thrombosis. Escorcia et al. [24] point to the factors influencing thrombosis as the material of the stent, percentage of area covered by the device, lack of coating with anticoagulants, lack of aggressive systemic anticoagulation, and hemodynamics that may affect the blood flow. Stainless steel and tantalum are the materials in current use for stents; however, little has been reported on the mechanical properties, the amount of stent material [25–26], and the surface charge of the material used in these applications.

Escorcia et al. [24] have concluded that stenting in its current form to prevent coronary stenosis is (1) not justified, and (2) the stent remains an experimental device accepted as a "bail out" procedure when acute occlusion or dissection occur after routine percutaneous transluminal coronary angioplasty.

Metal Implants

Current problems in orthopaedics and dentistry involve the implant tissue interface. Corrosion susceptibility, the generation of wear debris, material fatigue, crack propagation, and the incompatibility of metals and alloys with the fluids and tissue of the body remain as major problems. The corrosion resistance of titanium and its alloys Ti-6Al-4V and Ti-2Ni had been studied for their uses, as both industrial and implant materials [27]. Their high resistance to corrosion was due to the stability and self repair capacity of the passivating film on the titanium alloy.

Recent studies by Healy et al. [28] have shown that during implantation, metal alloys, in particular, titanium, release corrosion products into the surrounding tissue and fluids even though it is covered by a thermodynamically stable oxide film [29]. Healy [28] has suggested changes in the mechanism that govern dissolution of the oxide and oxide surface chemistry; changes in kinetics, the oxide stoichiometry, composition, and thickness have been associated with release of titanium corrosion products *in vitro*. Such results imply that the chemical characteristics of dissolution products lead to a preferential accumulation of titanium species near the implant in the absence of wear related phenomena. The identification of these dissolution products in tissue located near titanium implants has yet to be determined.

An alternate approach to this problem has been the development of monolayer films on titanium. The monolayer surface coatings, onto bulk materials with defined chemical end group anchored by a siloxane network, have been used in regulating cell adhesion responses [30]. Such modified surfaces may alter our perception of mammalian cell adherence, bacterial adherence infection, and implant loosening and removal.

Ceramics

Ceramics have proven to be an ideal material for bone replacement characterized by their hardness. They were the choice for joint prosthesis development. Certain compositions of glasses, ceramics, and glass ceramics bond to bone and some bioactive ceramics will bond to soft tissue as well as bone [31]. The concept of bioactive ceramics was introduced by Hench [32] based on the hypothesis that the biocompatibility of an implant would be optimal if it promoted the formation of normal tissue at its surface and in addition establish a contiguous interface capable of supporting the loads that normally occur at the implant site.

The bioactive ceramics that bind to bone directly are divided into two groups: surface active ceramics (which include Bioglass®, Caravital® and Apatite-Wollastonite® containing glass ceramics [A-W, GC]) and the bioresorbable ceramics that include the tricalcium phosphate (α-TCP and β-TCP) and some forms of hydroxyapatite [33].

The significance of ceramic biochemistry remains controversial. Further characterization of the physical, chemical, electrical, and biological properties would provide an appraisal of their biocompatibility [34].

Certain compositions of silicate-based glasses and glass ceramic implants share common constituents such as CaO or P_2O_5 in their material. The bonding of bone has been associated with the formation of hydroxyapatite layer on the surface of the implant [35].

Many attempts have been made to design drug anticoagulant delivery systems capable of releasing drugs or hormones in a sustained manner without toxic effects over a prolonged period of time. One such system has been the aluminum-calcium-phosphorous-oxide (ALCAP) ceramics developed to replace traumatized bone [36].

Ceramic vehicles could be used to provide long-term release of drugs and, coupled with tissue engineering, serve as the receptacle for cell replicating systems. Bajpai [37] suggests that such methods would permit the implantation of an artificial organ without the threat of rejection because the ceramic would act as a mechanical barrier to the hostile elements of the bodily defense system.

Biodegradable Elastomers

Synthetic polymers in medical devices have a long history for the structural support and controlled drug delivery functions. The most widely used elastomers for cardiovascular applications have been the polyurethanes. The environmental stress cracking of polyether urethane pacing leads has demonstrated that surface degradation can compromise biocompatibility [38,39]. Ultra high molecular weight polyethylene (UHMWPE) for orthopaedic use has shown repeated wear and deterioration. Polypropylene in orthotic and prosthetic devices also degrades with time and usage.

The susceptibility of polyether urethanes to degradation *in vivo* by biological enzyme induction and hydrolysis compromises their mechanical properties and surface characteristics.

The design of biodegradable elastomers from a polyurethane structure has been suggested by Dahiyat et al. [40]. The search for the diisocyanate that will break down into a nontoxic diamine continues. The combination of a labile phospho ester chain extender and the abundant variations of the soft segment will provide the desired biodegradation and mechanical properties.

Synthetic biodegradable polyesters, in particular the homopolymers of lactic and glycolic acids, have been used for controlled release of drugs and biologicals [41].

Kobayashi et al. [42] have proposed that biodegradable materials would offer wider applications if they could be shaped *in situ* and adhere to living tissues. They have synthesized biodegradable ester urethane prepolymers which can be cured from the liquid to solid state upon contact in living tissue. Further characterization of the curing and biodegradability of these polymers is ongoing. This approach offers a new look into the development of surgical adhesives. A general review of the physico-mechanical properties of degradable polymers used for medical applications is well summarized in a recent review by Engelberg and Kohn [43].

Revolving Quality Issues

Quality is clearly one of the "hottest" topics in the business world today [44,45]. Health care organizations, once focused on applying new scientific and technological advances to heal the sick and cure disease, are now tackling the issues of escalating health care costs with increasing patient expectations and needs [46]. The current situation invites industry to make the appropriate changes. The quality crusade has reached every sector of American business including

TABLE 2—*Factors influencing patient care and profitability.*

- Managed Care Contracts
- Technology Changes
- Increasing Costs
- Access to State of the Art Equipment

medical services [*45*]. The factors that influence patient care and profitability are given in Table 2. The guidelines for the transition from research to clinical acceptance are outlined in Tables 3 and 4. How do we begin to address the issue of quality in experimental testing for materials and medical devices?

Support

Industry and academia play complementary roles in research and development. As the industrial support of academic research and development grows, the federal government funding has decreased over the decade [*44*]. Industry views such university-based consortia as a means of supporting basic research and product development and for accessing emerging technologies as means to stay competitive [*47*]. Without such associations, the university usually cannot advance a product to market and ensure commercialization; however, the university brings the innovative talent and creative thinking for future projects. Many disciplines are contributing questions and answers to the growing complexity of the interactions between materials and biologic tissues and are gradually changing the overall approach to biomaterials research [*48*].

Von Recum [*48*] states that these interactions will be defined on a molecular level and that biomaterials can be custom tailored for any time requirement and functional purpose; therefore, an essential requirement for this to happen is a multidisciplinary research approach through an academic environment.

The government has established new guidelines to include Medical Device Tracking under the Safe Medical Devices Act of 1990.

Hospitals are to submit reports to the FDA and to the implant device manufacturers of deaths, serious illnesses, and serious injuries related to medical devices.

Although the broadly worded legislation needs clarification by the FDA, serious illness or serious injury means an event that (1) is life threatening; (2) results in permanent impairment of a body function or permanent damage to the body structure; or (3) necessitates timely medical or surgical intervention to preclude such permanent impairment or damage.

All such reports on medical devices and compliance with this policy should be coordinated with the Quality Management office at their respective institutions. Although no specific

TABLE 3—*Experimental research → clinical acceptance.*

Programs:	• Good Design
	• Adequate Testing
	• Quality Control/Assurance

TABLE 4—*Device development.*

Predict Properties

Control Manufacture

Characterization

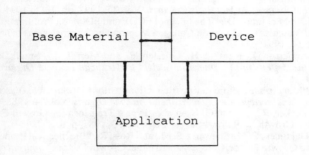

method of tracking has been outlined, the manufacturers would be required to trace, identify, and report to the FDA the patient's name and location within three working days.

The ruling applies to permanent implants (breast, penile, heart valves) and life-sustaining devices (defibrillators). A total of 35 devices made by more than 370 manufacturers are affected by the new rules.

New Direction for Research

Guidelines for Industry

Four basic phenomena are affecting research universities and the academic profile: the changing nature of research, the changing ethnic and gender mix among college students, the costs of doing research, and the pressures on universities to do more for industry, society, and the economy [49].

Based on the National Academy of Sciences Government Industry Roundtable in December 1991 in Washington, DC, research opportunities will go the direction of forming multi-disciplinary teams and more cooperative relationships within research institutions; growth in research funding will depend on the public perception of social value and political interests.

Summary

The science of biomaterials is changing and newer and more compatible medical devices and substitutes for tissue and organ replacement will develop based on the emerging field of tissue engineering.

Biomaterials-based emerging technologies will prosper through an overall changing approach to basic and applied biomaterials research. How to meet these needs through industry and academia remains unresolved. Industry must remain competitive to survive and universities must adjust to a multidisciplinary route to tackle the problems with biomaterials design and function. The priorities must be defined with major emphasis on quality and strict adherence to quality assurance issues in testing and analysis.

References

[1] Spector, M., "Biomaterials: Taming the Beast," *Journal of Biomedical Materials Research*, Vol. 26, No. 1, 1992, pp. 1–5.

[2] Black, J., "Does Corrosion Matter?" *Journal of Bone and Joint Surgery*, Vol. 70B, 1988, pp. 517–520.

[3] Christenson, L., Wahlberg, L., and Aebischer, P., "Mast Cells and Tissue Reaction to Interperitoneally Implanted Polymer Capsules," *Journal of Biomedical Materials Research*, Vol. 25, 1991, pp. 119–1131.

[4] Chandy, T. and Sharma, C. P., "Effects of Lipoproteins on Protein/Platelet Interaction on Polymers," *Journal of Biomedical Materials Research*, Vol. 25, 1991, pp. 1085–1094.

[5] Torrente, J. M. and Feldman, D., "The Effect of ECDF and PDGF on Proliferation and Interaction of Co-Cultured Vascular Cell Lines on Collagen Membranes," *Transactions of the Society for Biomaterials*, Vol. 14, 1991, p. 75.

[6] Connally, R., Anderson, J., Kambic, H., Griesler, H., and Merrill, E., "Small Diameter Vascular Prosthesis," *Transactions of the American Society for Artificial Internal Organs*, Vol. 34, No. 4, 1988, pp. 1043–1046.

[7] Griesler, H., "Macrophage Biomaterial Interactions with Bioresorbable Vascular Prosthesis," *Transactions of the American Society of Artificial Internal Organs*, Vol. 34, 1988, pp. 1051–1057.

[8] Mores, H. L., Tucker, R. F., Leof, G. B., et al., "Type β Transforming Growth Factor is a Growth Stimulator and a Growth Inhibitor," *Cancer Cells*, Vol. 3, 1985, p. 65.

[9] DiCorleto, P., Gajducek, C. M., Schwartz, S. M., and Ross, R., "Biochemical Properties of the Endothelium Derived Growth Factor: Comparison to Other Growth Factors," *Journal of Cell Physiology*, Vol. 114, 1983, p. 339.

[10] Painter, T. A., "Myointimal Hyperplasia: Pathogenesis and Implications. I. In Vitro Characteristics," *Artificial Organs*, Vol. 15, No. 1, 1991, pp. 42–55.

[11] Abbott, W. M. and Cambria, R. P., "Control of Physical Characteristics Elasticity and Compliance of Vascular Grafts" in: *Biological and Synthetic Vascular Prosthesis*, J. C. Stanley, et al., Eds., Grune & Stratton, New York, 1982, pp. 189–220.

[12] Clowes, A. W., Gronen, A. M., Hanson, S. R., and Reedy, M. A. "Mechanisms of Arterial Graft Failure," *American Journal of Pathology*, Vol. 118, No. 1, 1985, p. 43.

[13] Uchida, N., Kambic, H., and Emoto, H., et al., "Compliance Effects on Small Diameter Polyurethane Graft Patency," *Journal of Biomedical Materials Research*, Vol. 27, 1993, pp. 1269–1279.

[14] Schoen, E., Harasaki, H., Kin, K. M., Anderson, H. C., and Levy, R. J., "Biomaterial Associated Calcification: Pathology, Mechanisms and Strategies for Prevention," *Journal of Biomedical Materials Research*, Vol. 22A1, 1988, pp. 11–36.

[15] Reul, H. and Ghista, D. N., "The Design, Development, in vitro Testing and Performance of an Optimal Aortic Valve Prosthesis," in *Biomechanics of Medical Devices*, D. N. Ghista, Ed., Marcel Dekker, New York and Basel, 1980.

[16] "FDA Replacement Heart Valves—Guidance for Data to be Submitted to the Food and Drug Administration in Support of Applications for Premarket Approval," October 24, 1986.

[17] ISO Draft International Standard ISO/DIS 5840 ISO/TC150 cardiovascular implants—cardiac valve prostheses, submitted Feb. 11, 1988.

[18] More, R. B. and Silver, M. D., "Pyrolytic Carbon Prosthetic Heart Valve Occluder Wear: In Vivo vs. In Vitro Results for Bjork-Shiley Prosthesis," *Journal of Applied Biomaterials*, Vol. 1, 1990, pp. 267–278.

[19] Lee, D., Abolfathi, A., DeLoria, G., et al., "In Vitro Testing of Venous Valves," *Transactions of the American Society of Artificial Internal Organs*, Vol. 37, 1991, pp. M266–268.

[20] Muller, D. W., Shamir, K. J., Ellis, S. G., and Topol, E. J., "Peripheral Vascular Complications After Conventional and Complex Percutaneous Coronary Interventional Procedures," *American Journal of Cardiology*, Vol. 69, 1991, pp. 63–68.

[21] Sigwart, U., Puel, J., Mirkovitch, V., Joffre, F., Kappenberger, L., "Intravascular Stents to Prevent Occlusion and Restenosis After Transluminal Angioplasty," *New England Journal of Medicine*, Vol. 316, 1987, pp. 701–706.

[22] Sutton, C., Tominaga, R., Harasaki, H., et al., "Vascular Stenting in Normal and Atherosclerotic Rabbits," *Circulation*, Vol. 81, No. 2, 1990, pp. 667–683.

[23] Strauss, B., Serruys, P., Bertrans, M., et al., "Quantitative Angiographic Follow Up of the Coronary Wallstent in Native Vessels and Bypass Grafts (European Experience—March 1986 to March 1990)," *American Journal of Cardiology*, Vol. 69, 1992, pp. 475–481.

[24] Escorcia, E., and Hollman, J., "Current Status of Stents," *American Journal of Cardiology*, Vol. 69, 1992, pp. 687–689.

[25] Tominaga, R., Harasaki, H., Emoto, H., et al., "Effects of Stent Design and Serum Cholesterol Level on the Restenosis Rate," *Circulation,* Vol. 82, No. II, 1990, p. 656.

[26] Kambic, H., Tominaga, R., Emoto, H., et al., "Restenosis of Two Intravascular Stent Designs," *Transactions of the Society for Biomaterials,* Vol. 13, 1989, p. 281.

[27] *Corrosion and Degradation of Implant Materials, ASTM STP 684,* B. C. Syrett and A. Acharya, Eds., American Society for Testing and Materials, Philadelphia, p. 347.

[28] Healy, K. E. and Ducheyne, P., "The Mechanisms of Passive Dissolution of Titanium in a Model Physiological Environment," *Journal of Biomedical Materials Research,* Vol. 26, 1992, pp. 319–338.

[29] Ducheyne, P., Willems, G., Martens, M., and Helsen, J., "In Vivo Metal Release from Porous Titanium Fiber Material," *Journal of Biomedical Materials Research,* Vol. 18, 1984, pp. 293–308.

[30] Sukenik, C., Balachander, N., Culp, L., Lewandowska, C., and Merrit, K., "Modulation of Cell Adhesion by Modification of Titanium Surfaces with Covalently Attached Self-Assembled Monolayers," *Journal of Biomedical Materials Research,* Vol. 24, 1990.

[31] Hench, L., "Bioactive Ceramics," *Annals of the New York Academy of Science,* P. Ducheyne and J. Lemons, Eds., Vol. 523, 1988, pp. 54–71.

[32] Ducheyne, P., "Introduction to Bioceramics: Material Characterization Versus In Vivo Behavior," *Annals of the New York Academy of Science,* P. Ducheyne and J. Lemons, Eds., Vol. 523, 1988, pp. 1–3.

[33] Katani, S., Fujita, Y., Kitsugi, T., Nakamura, T., Yamamuro, T., Ohtsuki, C., and Kokuko, T., "Band Bonding Mechanism of β-Tricalcium Phosphate," *Journal of Biomedical Materials Research,* Vol. 25, 1991, pp. 1303–1315.

[34] "Significance of Porosity and Physical Chemistry of Calcium Phosphate Ceramics," in *Orthopaedic Uses in Bioceramics: Material Characteristics Versus In Vivo Behavior, Annals of the New York Academy of Science,* P. Ducheyne and J. Lemons, Eds., 1988, pp. 278–282.

[35] Li, R., Clark, A. L., and Hench, L., "An Investigation of Bioactive Glass Powders by Sol-Gel Processing," *Journal of Applied Biomaterials,* Vol. 2, 1991, pp. 231–239.

[36] Bajpai, P. K., Wyatt, D. F., Gelles, N. M., Stull, P. A., and Groves, G. A., "Use of Calcium Aluminate and Phosphorus Pentoxide Ceramics as a Bone Substitute," *Clinical Research,* Vol. 4, 1976, p. 524A.

[37] Bajpai, P. K. and Benghuzzi, H. A., "Ceramic Systems for Long Term Delivery of Chemicals and Biologicals," *Journal of Biomedical Materials Research,* Vol. 22, 1988, pp. 1245–1266.

[38] Stokes, K. and Chem, B., "Environmental Stress Cracking in Implanted Poly Ether Urethanes," in *Polyurethanes in Biomedical Engineering,* H. Planek, G. Egbers, and I. Syres, Eds., Elsevier Science Publishers, B. V. Amsterdam, 1984, pp. 243–255.

[39] Smith, K., Williams, D. F., and Oliver, C., "The Biodegradation of Polyether Urethanes," *Journal of Biomedical Materials Research,* Vol. 21, 1987, pp. 1149–1166.

[40] Dahiyat, B., Shi, F., Zhao, Z., and Leong, K., "Design of Degradable Elastomers for Medical Applications," *Proceedings of the American Chemical Society, Division of Polymeric Materials: Science and Engineering,* Vol. 66, 1992, pp. 87–88.

[41] Linhardt, R. J., in *Biodegradable Polymers for the Controlled Release of Drugs,* M. Rosoff, Ed., VCH Publishers, New York, 1989, pp. 53–95.

[42] Kobayashi, H., Hyon, S., and Ikada, Y., "Water Curable and Biodegradable Prepolymers," *Journal of Biomedical Materials Research,* Vol. 25, 1991, pp. 1481–1494.

[43] Engelberg, L. and Kohn, J., "Physicomechanical Properties of Degradable Polymers Used in Medical Applications. A Comparative Study,"*Biomaterials,* Vol. 12, 1991, pp. 292–304.

[44] Benton, W. C., "Statistical Process Control and the Taguchi Method: A Comparative Evaluation," *International Journal of Production Research,* Vol. 29, 1991, pp. 1761–1770.

[45] Williams, T. E., Benton, W. C., Jr., Fanning, W., Hankins, T. D., Kahas, G. S., "Quantitative Quality Descriptors for an Open Heart Program,"*Quality Progress,* Vol. 25, No. 4, 1992, pp. 29–32

[46] Anderson, C., "Curing What Ails U.S. Health Care," *Quality Progress,* Vol. 25, No. 4, 1992, pp. 35–38.

[47] Thayer, A. M., "Corporate Execs Weigh Evolving University/Industry R & D Alliances," *Chemical and Engineering News,* Vol. 70, 1992, p. 12.

[48] von Recum, A. F., "The Academic Environment of Biomaterials Science and Engineering," *Journal of Applied Biomaterials,* Vol. 3, 1992, pp. 63–71.

[49] Lepkowski, W., "University Research: Heyday of Science Seen as Over,"*Chemical and Engineering News,* Vol. 69, No. 49, 1991, p. 41.

Author Index

Subject Index

A

Absorbable composites, 256
Accelerated life testing, 9, 43
Adhesion, tissue, 65
Adhesive films and plastics
  hard tissue mechanical problems, 87
  overview, 1–5
  resins, 87
Alumina, in hip replacements, 111
Analysis of variance (ANOVA) experiment,
  96, 105-108(tables)
Anastomosis strength, 65
Anastomotic healing, 53
ANOVA. *See* Analysis of variance
  experiment.

B

Beads, 96
Biocompatibility, biomaterials *in vitro,* 167
Biological safety, 167
Biomaterials
  applications, 212
  cell-to-materials interaction, 167
  emerging technologies, 293
  flexure test specimens, 212
  in oro-maxillo-facial applications, 167
  in vitro, 167
  interactions, 293
  metallic, 148
  pericardial testing, 19
Biomechanics, dynamic properties of bone,
  127
Biomedical engineering applications, 77
Biomedical polymers
  applications, 77
  in mechanical heart valves, 44
Biomer blends, 245
Bioprostheses, 19
Bladder, urinary, mechanical properties,
  283, 288(tables)
Blood compatability
  cardiovascular implant materials, 9
Bonding agents, 87

Bone, dynamic properties, 127
Bones, fracture healing, 142

C

Calcium chloride blends, polyurethane, 245
Calculi, urinary, 267
Callotasis, 142
Callus, mechanical properties, 142
Cardiovascular materials
  implants, 9
  overview, 1–2
  prostheses, design, 9
Cell-to-material interaction, 167
Ceramic/metal modular head/taper
  systems, 111
Ceramics, 293
Chemical components, urinary calculi, 267
Cholesterol-lipid solution, 9
Coatings, porous, tensile strength, 96
Cobalt-chrome, 156
Collagen, 19
Compact bone, dynamic properties, 127
Complex modulus, 225
Composite biomaterials
  absorbable composites, 256
  fiber reinforced polymer, 193
  overview, 3–4
  polymers, mechanical properties, 212
  polymethyl methacrylate, 225
  resins, 87
Corrosion, 148, 156
Creep rupture modeling, 77
Crevice corrosion, 156
Crosslinking, 19

D

Damage, biomaterials—overview, 1–5
Deformation cyclic loading, biomaterials
  blood compatability, 9
Degradable polymers, 293
Delrin, 43, 45(table), 77
Dental adhesives, 87
Dental composites, resin, 87